Acclaim for Jerry Avorn's

POWERFUL MEDICINES

"Expressive [and] well-documented. . . . Dr. Jerry Avorn brings convincing data and sharp analysis to *Powerful Medicines*, his timely, challenging appraisal of health policy." —*The Boston Globe*

"This is an authoritative, stunningly comprehensive, and beautifully written work about a subject that ought to interest every American. At last: a smart Harvard doctor who knows drugs, understands FDA and regulatory policy, and has a sense of humor. Unbelievable!"
  —Donald Kennedy, Ph.D., Editor in chief, *Science;* President Emeritus, Stanford University; Former Commissioner of the FDA

"Deepens a reader's understanding of the complex cost-benefit analysis involved with prescription drugs." —*New York Post*

"*Powerful Medicines* is a must-read for anyone interested in the use, abuse, and economics of prescription drugs. The issues it addresses are central to the ongoing debate about how to reduce the cost and improve the quality of health care in America." —Senator Edward M. Kennedy

"Provides insight into one of the central medical debates of our time: how to ensure that prescription drugs are affordable, effective and safe."
  —*American Scientist*

"Passionate and well-informed. . . . [Avorn] goes beyond articulating the problems and makes many creative suggestions about how we can do better." —*Annals of Internal Medicine*

"In *Powerful Medicines,* Dr. Avorn brilliantly demonstrates the corrosive effects of commercial influence over medical research, education, and clinical care. This impressive book demonstrates the adverse effects such privatization can have on the health care system and ultimately on patients." —Bernard Lown, M.D., Winner of the Nobel Peace Prize, Professor Emeritus, Harvard School of Public Health

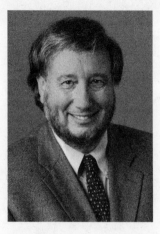

JERRY AVORN, M.D.

POWERFUL MEDICINES

Jerry Avorn, M.D., is a professor of medicine at Harvard Medical School and chief of the Division of Pharmacoepidemiology and Pharmacoeconomics at Brigham and Women's Hospital in Boston. An internist, geriatrician, and drug researcher, he is the author of more than two hundred papers in the medical literature on medication use and its outcomes, and one of the most frequently cited researchers in the field of social science and medicine.

POWERFUL MEDICINES

POWERFUL MEDICINES

The Benefits, Risks, and Costs of Prescription Drugs

JERRY AVORN, M.D.

Revised and Updated

VINTAGE BOOKS
A Division of Random House, Inc.
New York

FIRST VINTAGE BOOKS EDITION, AUGUST 2005

The Library of Congress has cataloged the Knopf edition as follows:
Avorn, Jerry.
Powerful medicines : the benefits, risks,
and costs of prescription drugs / Jerry Avorn.—1st ed.
p.   cm.
Includes bibliographical references.
1. Drugs—Prescribing—United States. 2. Pharmaceutical industry—
United States—Costs. 3. Drugs—Side effects—United States.
4. Prescription pricing—United States. I. Title.
HD9666.5.A94 2004
338.4'3615'0973—dc22   2003066119

Vintage ISBN 1-4000-3078-1

Author photograph: Jeffrey Thiebauth

www.vintagebooks.com

Printed in the United States of America
10 9 8 7 6 5 4 3 2 1

For Karen, Nate,
Andrew, and Muz

CONTENTS

INTRODUCTION TO THE UPDATED VINTAGE BOOKS EDITION ix

PROLOGUE: DIFFERENT STROKES 3

PART ONE: BENEFITS

1: THE PREGNANT MARE'S LESSON 23

2: LEAVING THE DARK AGES BEHIND, MOSTLY 39

PART TWO: RISKS

3: THE FAT IS IN THE FIRE 71

4: TOO SWEET TO BE TRUE 85

5: COLD COMFORT 96

6: GETTING RISKS RIGHT 102

7: THE MOST VULNERABLE PATIENTS 126

8: ENTER DOCTOR FAUSTUS 139

9: IMPERFECT MEASURES 149

CONTENTS

10: WHOSE RISK IS IT, ANYWAY?   160

11: A BALANCING ACT   172

PART THREE: COSTS

12: LIVE CHEAP OR DIE   189

13: FILLING THE PIPELINE   198

14: WHAT THE TRAFFIC WILL BEAR   217

15: NAVIGATING THE THIRD DIMENSION   235

PART FOUR: INFORMATION

16: SIGNALS, NOISE, AND THE BIG VOID   269

17: INFORMATIONAL KUDZU   292

18: DEVISING AN ANTIDOTE   313

19: THE EMPEROR'S FASHION CRITICS   339

20: SAME LANGUAGE, DIFFERENT ACCENTS   348

PART FIVE: POLICY

21: PULLING THE FACTS TOGETHER   359

22: TURNING KNOWLEDGE INTO ACTION   388

23: MARKETS AND MEDICINES   401

EPILOGUE: THE TRIPLE-EDGED SWORD   417

NOTES   421

INDEX   437

INTRODUCTION TO THE
UPDATED VINTAGE BOOKS EDITION

The Longest Year in Prescription
Drug History

Through a striking set of coincidences, the original hardcover edition of *Powerful Medicines* appeared at the same time as a string of dramatic drug-related events that instantly brought its subject matter to the center of public awareness and debate. Throughout 2004, the media and medical journals spotlighted revelations and questions about medication risks, benefits, and costs that illustrated most of the issues raised in the book. I have revised the text in light of these developments and will continue to update its website, www.powerfulmedicines.org, to cover new issues, insights, and references as they emerge in this fast-moving field.

In the spring, clinical trials yielded the disturbing news that popular SSRI antidepressants (such as Prozac, Paxil, and Zoloft) could actually *increase* suicidal thoughts and attempts in adolescents and children. When the drugs were first introduced in the late 1980s, there had been anecdotal reports of such problems, but they were based on the clinical impressions of a few psychiatrists who were caring for severely ill people, or the observations of patients treated in routine practice, in whom a host of confounding factors could have explained away the findings (Chapter 6). As a result, it had been hard to tell whether the problem was being caused by the medications themselves or by the depression they were designed to treat. Not so for the new clinical trial data that came to light in 2004. All the study patients had the same psychiatric condition and were being systematically studied in randomized clinical trials of the effect of these drugs in young people. In these new studies, the subjects randomly allocated to take the drug were *more* likely to develop suicidal thoughts than those given a dummy pill, a difference that could not be blamed on doctors' drug preferences or patients' underlying illnesses. Other controlled trials found that suicide risk also rose in young subjects given the SSRIs for problems such as obsessive-compulsive disorder and anxiety—conditions not normally associated with high rates of self-destructive behavior.

What explained this influx of new clinical trial data for a drug class that had been on the market for well over a decade? Like many medications, the newer antidepressants were widely used in children and adolescents but had never been well studied in age groups at either end of the life cycle—another by-product of the nation's quick-as-possible drug approval process (Chapter 7). The companies were not willing to conduct new pediatric studies without an economic incentive. They received an offer from Congress that promised a very lucrative result: if a company tested one of its drugs in young people, the government would extend its patent by six months—a windfall for products whose annual sales approximated $1 billion or more. It wasn't necessary for the new studies to show that the drug actually *worked* in young people; conducting the trial alone was enough to win the valuable patent extension. The new findings about increased suicide risk in teenagers taking SSRIs emerged accidentally from a series of clinical trials that wasn't even done to study side effects.

The pediatric antidepressant revelations raised new questions about how drugs could remain on the U.S. market for up to fifteen years and suddenly turn out to have severe and potentially lethal risks—a theme that recurred several times in *Powerful Medicines'* first year on the shelves. Those of us who study drug side effects had long been aware that the U.S. drug safety surveillance system was not working well (Chapter 21), and that the FDA was having great difficulty in dealing with hazards that were discovered in products it had approved. The antidepressant crisis and those that followed brought these defects to national prominence.

The problem turned out to have multiple layers, each more worrisome than the last. By law, drug companies must inform the FDA about adverse effects that arise during their clinical trials. But in this case, the agency had failed to aggregate, analyze, and inform the public about the very reports it had in its own files. At first, its efforts were hampered by an astonishing flaw in the data. In many of their antidepressant studies, the companies hadn't used a uniform method to record suicidal thoughts, gestures, or attempts. (The manufacturers may not have anticipated an *increase* in suicidal symptoms, but you'd expect them to track these problems systematically anyway, to look for a reduction.)

A researcher familiar with the FDA's investigation told me about some of the problems caused by the chaotic systems used to record adverse events. To describe medicated patients who reported intolerable feelings like "wanting to jump out of my skin," some companies used the term "activation" in reporting the results to the FDA—a benign-sounding term that could have positive connotations. One young study subject became agitated during a school exam and stabbed himself in the neck with a pencil; the episode was reported to the FDA as an "accidental injury" rather than as an attempt at self-harm.

Lacking a consistent measure of the problem, the FDA eventually resorted to a cumbersome next-best plan: it asked the manufacturers to perform a word search through all the free text collected in their clinical trial reports to look for terms that might describe suicidal thoughts or gestures. This flailing produced some surprising results. For example, in responding to a computerized search for the letters "g-a-s," which might have been used if subjects had employed car exhaust fumes or ovens to try to kill themselves, the computer would instead expel a host of stomach complaints, from "gastric upset" to "excessive gas." This combination of sloppiness and subterfuge in drug company accounts was similar to the flawed reporting we had seen earlier with drugs like the diabetes treatment Rezulin (Chapter 4) that delayed the FDA's ability to address its dangers for years.

In defending themselves, the antidepressant makers said they were not obliged to warn doctors and patients of these findings, because in no single study did the increase in suicide risk rise to the level of statistical significance. This numerical shortfall was neither surprising nor relevant. Clinical trials are designed to measure whether the study drug is better than placebo, which should be an easily measured outcome. But the number of patients studied in these trials is rarely large enough to pass conventional statistical tests in assessing rare side effects such as suicide. Each company could fall back on that excuse as long as it looked only at its own studies, and the FDA did not call them on it.

Another attribute of our industry-dominated drug evaluation process further obscured the truth. It turns out that the results of clinical trials (including the discovery of unexpected side effects) are considered to be the property of the drug companies that conduct or pay for those trials, and are not available to the public. The FDA usually goes along with this unseemly triumph of corporate prerogative over public health. Yet even if the increased rate of side effects wasn't made public by any one company (and who would want to be the first to raise the issue in such a lucrative market?), the same dangers were cropping up in studies submitted by several manufacturers. The agency was painfully slow in putting the big picture together on behalf of the millions of kids and teenagers who were prescribed these drugs.

Even if no single company had access to adverse effects rates in its competitors' products, the FDA had access to all the data. But in the ongoing disarray of its Office of Drug Safety (Chapter 21), the agency was slow to aggregate all the trial findings in order to examine the link between SSRIs and suicide more systematically. When it eventually did so, the evidence of increased risk turned out to be compelling. Yet even as that insight emerged within the agency, its bureaucrats managed to commit an even worse misstep.

This aspect of the antidepressant crisis of 2004 opened a window on what became known as the "culture of denial" within the FDA itself. One of its drug safety researchers, Dr. Andy Mosholder, combined the data from all the adolescent SSRI trials and analyzed them together. He found that young subjects who were randomly assigned to take drugs such as Paxil or Zoloft were twice as likely to make suicidal gestures or have suicidal thoughts as the subjects given placebo—a difference that, with the larger numbers of subjects involved, did have statistical significance. Before this analysis was released, the British government had previously warned that these drugs were simply too unsafe to be used in children or teenagers— an embarrassing development for the American regulatory authorities as well as for the companies that made the drugs. In early 2004, the FDA convened a meeting of an advisory panel of scientists to determine U.S. policy in light of the British warning. But Dr. Mosholder's supervisors did not allow him to report his full findings to the advisory panel. They argued that the results were still inconclusive, and that the analysis would have to be redone from scratch by outside researchers at Columbia University. Dr. Mosholder's report was suppressed, but a year later the Columbia team came to virtually the same conclusion.

Taken together, by late 2004 these data finally became compelling enough for the FDA to place a "black box" warning on the official labeling of antidepressants. The new language pointed out—after tens of millions of patients had been prescribed the drugs—that they could raise the risk of suicide in young people. The wording was weaker than the outright prohibition the British had employed, but even the milder U.S. warning soon came under assault by the industry and by psychiatrists. Within weeks, the FDA backed away from its cautionary language and quietly omitted the phrase stating that the drugs could cause self-harm.

More insight into the nation's capacity to identify the risks from this class of drugs came from an unexpected quarter. Working independently, New York Attorney General Eliot Spitzer found that the FDA's dossier on antidepressant risks in young people was incomplete, because at least one company had suppressed the results of some of the clinical trials it had conducted and never submitted them to the agency. Spitzer charged that GlaxoSmith-Kline publicized the results of studies that favored its antidepressant, Paxil, while burying the results of others that showed the drug didn't work very well. Now the risk-assessment situation took on a new level of complexity that was particularly worrisome for those of us—prescribers, researchers, policy makers—who try to evaluate drug benefits and risks. How can we synthesize what is known about a drug's effectiveness and safety to help patients and doctors make informed choices, if data are selectively suppressed? The British medical journal *Lancet* expressed the problem astutely:

> Published data suggest a favourable risk-benefit profile for some SSRIs; however, addition of unpublished data indicates that risks could outweigh benefits of these drugs (except [Prozac]) to treat depression in children and young people. Clinical guideline development and clinical decisions about treatment are largely dependent on an evidence base published in peer-reviewed journals. . . . Drug sponsors who withhold trial data (or do not make full trial reports available) undermine the guideline programme, which can ultimately lead to recommendations that are ineffective, cause harm, or both.

Defenders of the use of SSRI antidepressants in children and teenagers quickly pointed out that doubling the likelihood of suicidal thoughts or attempts might be a reasonable price to pay for all the clinical good these drugs could do for young patients. This trade-off of potentially lethal side effects in a few unlucky patients in exchange for a therapeutic benefit for many is just the kind of Faustian bargain we doctors are forced to make every time we write a prescription. To put the question precisely, if crassly: How many additional suicide attempts would we accept in a drug that lifted the terrible burden of depression from much larger numbers of young people? We have formal ways to compare such sour apples and sweet oranges (Chapters 8–11), although they're not entirely satisfying. But in the end, most of the trials didn't even allow us to consider a trade-off of greater suicide risk in some patients versus the resolution of depression for many of them. Amazingly, the new clinical trials in young people did not produce any evidence of benefit for most of the SSRIs studied. Only Prozac produced a modest improvement; Paxil and Zoloft did not, although that result was not widely disseminated. That is the most upsetting—and least widely known—aspect of the adolescent antidepressant debacle.

In the wake of the antidepressant revelations, legislators and researchers called for a mandatory registry of all clinical trials in order to prevent selective disclosure of favorable studies. The pharmaceutical industry responded that its participation in such a registry should be voluntary, which of course would severely compromise its effectiveness. There was less discussion of a far more important underlying issue: as long as the nation continues to allow most clinical research on drugs to be conducted by and for the companies that manufacture these products, who stand to gain or lose literally billions of dollars over their results, we are not going to get all the answers we need to our questions about drug efficacy and safety . . . or feel secure that the right questions are even being asked.

PAINFUL REVELATIONS

Barely a month after *Powerful Medicines* was published, an even larger storm erupted over the safety of the painkiller Vioxx. Concerns about its cousins, the other Cox-2 inhibitors Celebrex and Bextra, quickly followed. The story mushroomed into the greatest prescription drug crisis in generations and raised further worries about what we know about drug risks and what we should do about them. Equally disconcerting were two subthemes: what we *don't* know and why we don't know it. My group's research findings drew me deep into this controversy.

At least since 2000, researchers have been aware of evidence that Merck's Vioxx, widely used for arthritis and pain, might also increase the risk of heart attack. In that year, a randomized clinical trial known as VIGOR found that patients given Vioxx experienced four times as many heart attacks as patients given naproxen (sold over the counter as Aleve and other brands). Merck contended that this was because naproxen *prevented* heart attacks, not because their drug caused them. In 2001 and 2002, additional articles in medical journals raised further concerns about a possible Vioxx–heart disease risk. Yet Merck did not conduct another clinical trial specifically designed to address this problem, and the FDA did not demand that the company do so. (Documents later showed that Merck had designed and was ready to implement a clinical trial known as VALOR to test the Vioxx–heart attack question, but senior company executives canceled the plan just before the study was to have started.) Dr. Jeff Drazen, editor in chief of the *New England Journal of Medicine,* later observed that this insouciance was tantamount to smelling smoke coming from your kitchen as you leave for work, not checking on it, and then calling a neighbor from work later in the day to see if your house is on fire.

Several groups, including my own research team at Harvard, became interested in the problem early on. In 2002, my colleague Dr. Dan Solomon and I published a paper showing that naproxen might have a very mild heart-protective effect, but nowhere near large enough to explain the higher number of heart attacks in patients given Vioxx in the VIGOR study. We next wanted to use the methods detailed in *Powerful Medicines* (Chapters 6 and 21) to conduct our own observational study to find out whether patients taking Vioxx in routine practice were having more heart attacks than expected. Despite the importance of this kind of research, the

National Institutes of Health and the FDA provide very little funding to support it, so we applied for an unrestricted research grant from Merck to conduct the project. In approving the grant, Merck signed off on our proposed research design and assigned Dr. Carolyn Cannuscio of their research staff, who had just completed her doctoral work in epidemiology at Harvard, to act as a liaison with us for the duration of the study. Led by Dr. Solomon, our group studied thousands of patients with heart attacks and tracked what medications they had been taking. The study confirmed that patients taking Vioxx had higher heart attack rates than comparable patients taking other, similar drugs (Chapter 13).

On learning of our findings, Merck asked us to publish the results in a way that would soften their impact; we refused. The study was already in page proofs at the nation's premier cardiology journal, *Circulation,* when we got another call from the company. We were informed that if we didn't change our description of the results, Dr. Cannuscio's name would have to be removed from the paper, apparently to distance the company from the findings. We pointed out that they couldn't force us to remove her name, because she had been a collaborator on the project. But unlike university-based drug researchers, scientists in industry are often required to accept restrictions on what they can publish about their work. It appeared that Dr. Cannuscio had agreed to such a constraint in her contract with Merck: days before the journal went to press, Carolyn called Dan and told him she was being obliged to have her name removed from the paper.

With the request now coming from her, we had no choice but to comply. We removed her name but added an acknowledgment thanking an unnamed epidemiologist who participated actively in all aspects of the project. But the change came so late in the process that the web-based edition of the paper had already been disseminated with Carolyn's name on it. An alert *Wall Street Journal* reporter picked up the discrepancy in authorship between the two versions of the publication, did some research, and published this article on the front page of the paper's business section:

MERCK TAKES AUTHOR'S NAME OFF VIOXX STUDY

In the sedate world of medical journals, this could be called The Case of the Vanishing Author. Stepping into thorny ethical territory, drug titan Merck & Co. ordered the name of one of its epidemiologists purged from the list of authors on a research paper—after the study produced an unflattering portrait of a blockbuster drug Merck happens to make.

Once the study was published, Merck issued a statement assailing its design and its findings and criticized the very methodology it had previously approved.

The most damning evidence on Vioxx eventually came from the company itself, in a clinical trial it was conducting—not to get to the bottom of the heart attack question but to justify the additional use of its drug for the treatment of colon polyps. The study did not include the kind of patients who could have best clarified the heart attack risk issue; in fact, it excluded anyone with evidence of active coronary heart disease. Despite this, when the study's safety monitoring board performed a periodic check of clinical outcomes, it found that patients assigned to take Vioxx rather than placebo were having twice as many heart attacks and strokes as the control group. Merck could no longer deny the connection and halted the study. On September 30, 2004, the company withdrew Vioxx from the market worldwide.

The story did not end there, of course. Other clinical trials, likewise not designed to study heart disease, also began to show unexpected increases in cardiovascular events in patients taking other Cox-2 drugs. Celebrex was incriminated in studies designed to determine whether the drug could prevent cancer, and Bextra in a trial of patients undergoing heart surgery. Hundreds of thousands of anxious patients asked their doctors: What exactly are the risks of these drugs? In exchange for what added benefit? And how do we know? The nation again marveled that despite five years of use by tens of millions of patients, and public and private expenditures of tens of billions of dollars, there was still not enough firm information to answer these questions. Benefit-risk trade-off questions again swirled about: How much additional pain relief or stomach protection is worth what increase in the risk of heart attack, stroke, or death? What is the best way to come up with these numbers, and what should then be done with them? By whom? Had I written *Powerful Medicines* as a student textbook, I couldn't have invented a better set of midterm exams. The problem was that these were not exercises: they were population-wide crises that affected millions of patients and produced, we now believe, thousands of preventable hospitalizations and many avoidable deaths.

As with the antidepressant-suicide question, there was an ironic twist to the "How much extra benefit is worth the risk?" paradox. For the vast majority of patients, none of the Cox-2 drugs had ever been shown to provide more pain relief than older products like aspirin or ibuprofen (Motrin). Despite this, the media had been encouraged to hype these products as "super aspirins," implying (as the manufacturers were not permitted to do directly) that they were stronger analgesics. They weren't, and some very intensive marketing was needed to persuade people to use pills that cost about $3 each instead of older ones that cost pennies. It worked; use of these drugs extended far beyond people at increased risk for gastrointestinal side effects. Studies from our group and others showed that thanks to over-the-top marketing to doctors and patients alike, most users of Vioxx and Celebrex didn't have any of the conditions that would have justified the need for (and additional cost of) that extra gastrointestinal protection.

Detailed evidence of the risk of Vioxx had appeared in the medical literature since 2000, but when Merck finally withdrew the drug from the market in 2004, the company's CEO said that he and his colleagues were shocked when they first saw the polyp trial data documenting the problem. (On appearing with him on a television program as he uttered these words of astonishment, my mind flashed to the scene in *Casablanca* in which Inspector Renault exclaims that he is *"Shocked! Shocked!"* to learn that gambling was going on in Rick's café . . . just as the croupier hands him his winnings.) Perhaps annual sales of $3 billion would make it hard for any company to choose to study a hazard that could (and did) take such a profitable blockbuster off the market. In the wake of the withdrawal, several clinical trial experts calculated the size and expense of a study that could have been done as early as 2000 to clarify the problem; the price tag of that research would have been a fraction of the nearly $100 million Merck spent alone on direct-to-consumer ads for Vioxx each year.

It was alarming to see how small a role three important facts played in the debate. First was the observation that for most patients Vioxx, Celebrex, and Bextra were no more effective than older drugs like ibuprofen (sold as Motrin, Advil, and several other brand names). Second, the only supposed advantage the newer drugs had—a reduction in the risk of stomach bleeding—was of minor importance for most of the patients who took these drugs, because they were at exceedingly low risk of this complication in the first place. This advantage was so unimpressive for Celebrex and Bextra that the FDA did not even allow their manufacturers to mention it in their advertising. There was even evidence that the modest stomach-protective effect of Vioxx might have been reduced or eliminated if patients were taking low-dose aspirin, which many of them needed to protect their hearts. Finally, it is likely that taking a gastrointestinal drug like Zantac or Prilosec along with any of the older drugs would probably have achieved the same pain relief and stomach protection for most patients, at a much lower cost. Those GI drugs could also be combined with the humble aspirin, which has the well-proven property of preventing rather than causing heart attacks. The aspirin makers just didn't have as big an ad budget.

Instead of weighing these issues, the debate centered on what would be an acceptable level of heart attack and stroke risk to trade off for the supposed advantages of the Cox-2 drugs. The frenzy reached its peak in a three-day FDA advisory committee meeting in February 2005, which reviewed the evidence that all three of the drugs in this class raised the risk of heart attack or stroke. The committee's surprising recommendation: allow Merck to bring Vioxx back onto the market, since its risks were shared by Celebrex and Bextra. An analysis of the committee's voting pattern showed that ten of the thirty-two panel members had financial ties to the companies that made the drugs being evaluated. Those with such ties were ten times more likely to vote in the drugs' favor than were members without such ties. Had they recused themselves from the vote, the group would have voted against allowing Vioxx or Bextra to be sold.

The story of Vioxx and its sister drugs will no doubt continue for years, as one of the more dramatic developments in the evolution of U.S. drug policy. It will also serve as a compelling illustration of how relevant pharmacoepidemiology can be in informing drug decisions, both at the bedside and in Washington. Spin-off developments will also continue for the foreseeable future. My work on completing this introduction has just been interrupted by an unannounced early-morning home visit from several FBI agents who want to interview me about possible criminal activities by Merck in its development and marketing of Vioxx. Watch www. powerfulmedicines.org for updates.

THE FDA UNDER FIRE

The antidepressant and Cox-2 crises also provided two new case studies for several of the issues raised in the original hardcover edition of *Powerful Medicines* concerning when we need to conduct randomized clinical trials and when we should use observational studies of routine practice to define medication risks (Chapter 6); the drug companies' occasional practice of suppressing data that cast their drugs in a poor light (Chapters 3 through 5) while actively publicizing those with favorable findings (Chapter 17); and the FDA's inability to perform adequate safety surveillance for widely used drugs (Chapter 21). This last problem received wide public attention in 2004 and 2005 and was blamed on several possible causes. First was the inherent difficulty of making these risk-benefit trade-offs, even in the best of circumstances. But the problem was compounded by the agency's internal disarray, especially the atrophy of its Office of Drug Safety.

These issues became front-page stories in the fall of 2004 when Dr. David Graham, an FDA drug safety researcher, took the agency's internal crisis public. In widely televised testimony, he warned a congressional hearing and a stunned nation that the FDA was incapable of protecting the nation from preventable drug safety crises. At a dramatic Senate Finance Committee hearing, Dr. Graham warned that the culture within the FDA had changed from protecting the public health to protecting the interests of the pharmaceutical manufacturers. Since 1992 these companies have been paying much of the agency's operating budget, and they have become some of the largest donors to campaign funds and the lobbying firms that increasingly shape governmental programs (Chapter 16). Graham reported that the agency's system for monitoring drug side effects was badly broken, and that he and others in its Office of Drug Safety were frequently criticized by superiors for bringing up disturbing findings about the adverse effects of drugs the FDA had approved. Readers of the hardcover edition of *Powerful Medicines* found ample evidence of the agency's difficulties in assessing the safety of marketed drugs; the events of 2004 brought this embarrassing reality to the attention of a much wider audience.

PAYING THE PIPELINE

The antidepressant and Cox-2 debacles provided vivid examples of risk-benefit assessment in chaos. But what about that third element in the equation that *Powerful Medicines* addressed—costs? The year provided ample case studies of that dimension as well. The first cost-related crisis was the unexpected disappearance of half the nation's flu shot supply in the autumn of 2004. The vaccine was being manufactured in England by an American company, Chiron, in a plant where the FDA had previously found quality control problems. Yet the agency was caught unawares when British inspectors found these problems to be so severe that they shut down production because the vaccine would be contaminated. Another problem of regulatory ineptitude, true, but what does this have to do with economics?

Half the nation's flu vaccine supply suddenly vanished because of the same overreliance on marketplace economics that taints other aspects of U.S. drug policy (Chapter 23). For years, companies had been leaving the vaccine field for more profitable areas, such as drugs for allergy and heartburn. No intervention was necessary, we were told by the free marketeers: if vaccines are so unprofitable that companies stop making them, their price will go up because of scarcity, and other manufacturers will naturally rush in to fill the gap.

It didn't happen that way. By mid-2004, the nation had become dependent on only two corporations for its entire flu vaccine supply. When Chiron could no longer manufacture its product, the remaining vaccine supply had to be restricted so that there would be enough to cover the very sickest patients, primarily the elderly and the chronically ill. Even they faced long lines and hours of waiting for their shots—only to be told, in many cases, that a clinic's allotment had run out. President Bush proposed buying vaccine from Canada— the nation he frequently condemned as the source of risky counterfeit drugs that endangered all those Americans who couldn't afford to fill their prescriptions at U.S. prices. Late in the flu season alternative supplies were found, but the rescue arrived too late for many patients who had initially been forced to forego immunization. In an ironic turnaround, some states ended the flu season with sizable but unusable stashes of vaccine tailored to that year's virus. These would go to waste, because each winter requires a vaccine tailor-made to the genetics of that year's virus. Contrary to the promises of the free marketeers, the silent hand of the marketplace hadn't precisely regulated supply and demand; it had just given us the finger.

Other economic case studies also developed after the book's publication, often along predictable lines. When President Bush rushed the new Medicare prescription drug benefit through Congress within just a few days in December 2003, many in Washington knew that its projected cost of $400 billion over the coming decade was artificially low. It was less widely known then that the administration had calculated more realistic numbers, but suppressed their release to Congress until after the bill passed. By early 2005, the ten-year estimate had grown to more than $700 billion for the years that the benefit would actually cover. Some facts pushed aside during its hasty passage reasserted themselves, as facts sometimes do. The legislation had omitted some key provisions that could have encouraged more cost-effective drug use. Much of its unaffordable cost would be driven by the drug industry-written provision that Medicare could not negotiate with manufacturers for better prices. Serious economic and political questions began to arise about whether the program could survive in its original form.

BLUE MEDICINE VS. RED MEDICINE?

The public and many elected officials may have been surprised to learn about the unexpected dangers of antidepressants and the Cox-2 drugs, the disarray that both crises revealed about the FDA and the nation's drug safety surveillance system, and the emerging unaffordability of the much-vaunted Medicare prescription drug benefit. A reader of the original hardcover edition of *Powerful Medicines* would not have been. In 1848, the great German pathologist Rudolf Virchow wrote, "Medicine is a social science, and politics is nothing but medicine on a larger scale." He might have added that this insight applies equally to good medicine and bad medicine. If Virchow was right, then one of the more important medical events of the Longest Year took place on November 2, 2004, when conservatives assumed firmer control of the U.S. presidency, House of Representatives, Congress, and judiciary. The policy considerations in Part Five of *Powerful Medicines* will be played out in that context. Fortunately, that section contains a number of ideologically androgynous proposals whose implementation could proceed regardless of the political color wars that dominate current policy discourse. Creative change remains possible within states, specific health care systems, and individual practices.

Until recently, worries about pharmaceutical makers' influence on FDA decisions, or concern about the industry's role in crafting drug benefit policies, were often written off as the paranoid whinings of out-of-touch liberals. Yet the developments outlined above are beginning to change the thinking of people all along the political spectrum. Mounting public concern over governmental disarray in detecting and managing drug risks, coupled with the growing fiscal crises caused by uncontrollable drug expenditures in the private and public sectors, will probably drive reform regardless of the political complexion of Washington. Several states are establishing systems to import prescription drugs from Canada, as well as programs to inform doctors in a noncommercial way about prescribing affordable drugs. The FDA is expected to develop tougher new processes to improve the detection of adverse drug events and its capacity to warn about them. And as he left office, outgoing Secretary of Health and Human Services Tommy Thompson mused that he wished the new Medicare drug benefit had allowed him to press manufacturers for better pricing. In big enough doses, reality can sometimes prove stronger than ideology.

One final development merits mention in the very busy year since *Powerful Medicines* was first published. Someone once observed that changing a medical school curriculum is like trying to move a graveyard, but some progress is being made in this direction, with no exhumations required. Several years ago Dr. Arnold Gold, a senior neurologist at Columbia University, and his wife, Dr. Sandra Gold, created a small foundation to try to help medical schools refocus on the social and humanistic aspects of being a physician—values that sometimes get short shrift in modern curricula. They quietly established a national movement of "White Coat Ceremonies" in which faculty mentors present medical students with that symbol of the profession at the start of their careers, along with an eloquent restatement of the basic values of being a healer. Similar events help young doctors mark the critical transition from classroom work to their years of clinical training. These ceremonies are now conducted in most of the nation's medical schools, providing special moments in the development of young physicians all over the United States. The Drs. Gold were taken with the spirit and message of *Powerful Medicines* and have arranged for it to be distributed to medical students as part of their training. Several small charitable organizations are providing additional funding for this purpose, sometimes by "adopting" specific states or medical schools. It may be another decade before the systematic study of drug risks, benefits, and costs is covered fully in medical training programs, but thanks to the Golds and other kindred spirits working at the local level, progress has begun all over the country.

Jerry Avorn, M.D.
Boston, May 2005

POWERFUL MEDICINES

PROLOGUE: DIFFERENT STROKES

It is much easier to write upon a disease than upon a remedy. The former is in the hands of nature, and a faithful observer with an eye of tolerable judgement cannot fail to delineate a likeness. The latter will ever be subject to the whim, the inaccuracies, and the blunder of mankind.

—WILLIAM WITHERING (1741 – 1799),
the discoverer of digitalis

A SIN OF OMISSION

I had never seen Dr. Vasily so shaken. He had always seemed the very image of a wise, seasoned clinician. A primary-care doctor in the community who admitted his patients to a high-powered teaching hospital, he had gently borne decades of mild condescension from the faculty in his role as LMD, or local medical doctor. The hospital and its specialists relied on LMDs for a steady supply of admissions, but in teaching rounds they were often the butt of case presentations that centered on missed diagnoses or poorly made decisions. Typically, in these cautionary tales, some damage was done by the LMD to a patient PTA (prior to admission), the error then being set right by the hospital-based physicians. Yet we all knew that Dr. Vasily was special; he was always there for his patients, and while he had only published two articles in medical journals back in the early 1980s, he had a solid grasp of a surprisingly wide domain of practical medical knowledge, on topics ranging from kidney failure to depression to acne. Its breadth often dwarfed the narrower expertise of his more specialized colleagues.

This morning, his eyes were moist and he looked exhausted. Overnight he had admitted a patient who had collapsed at home, a seventy-four-year-old retired mailman who had been his patient for over twenty years. "The family called me around eleven to say that Stan was making a cup of tea in the kitchen and they heard a thud; they found him on the linoleum having a seizure. I met them in the ER around midnight; the interns had stabilized him and sent him off for a CAT scan. Turns out he flipped a large clot into his middle cerebral artery and knocked out a big piece of his right frontal lobe."

I told Dr. Vasily I'd never seen him so upset over a case before.

"The clot came from his heart," he explained. "He had been in and out of AF for years." AF is atrial fibrillation, a cardiac condition in which the atria—the smaller antechambers of the heart—quiver uselessly instead of contracting at just the right moments to pump blood into the muscular ventricles that adjoin them. AF is itself not a life-threatening condition most of the time. But when the atria don't contract normally, blood clots can form on their flaccid walls. Those clots can later break loose and be propelled into the circulation—including that of the brain. That is what happened to Stan; now he was lying in bed unconscious and breathing heavily, his mouth an open circle, his tongue dangling off to one side—a poor prognostic indicator the interns call a "positive Q sign."

"Last year I brought Stan in for pneumonia, and we almost lost him," my colleague recalled. "I had a run-in with one of the interns who demanded to know why I wasn't anticoagulating him." Using a drug to thin the blood in an AF patient prevents the clots from forming, reducing the chance that one of them will break off and float downstream into the brain. But the drugs that do this also increase the risk of bleeding, which can itself be fatal. "The little *putz* even copied a journal article and put it in Stan's record for me to see, showing how anticoagulants cut the incidence of stroke by two-thirds. Of course I knew that. I had just admitted another patient I *did* anticoagulate for her AF; she came in with a massive hemorrhage and died not long after. I didn't want to be responsible for that kind of thing again. Maybe I should have . . . I don't know. That intern is a resident now; he was in charge in the ER last night. He remembered. You should have seen the look he gave me."

Stan recovered only limited use of his left side and never regained the ability to speak normally, walk independently, or feed himself. He could utter only a few words, including the "Thank you" he croaked to Dr. Vasily as he was discharged to the chronic rehab facility that would be his home for the rest of his life.

A BAD CASE OF THE SNIFFLES

We assume that if you can get something over the counter for your cold it must be safe, and that there are people whose job is to monitor that pretty carefully. Millions use these products, and if any of them posed an important danger, we expect that someone would have done something about it. And what company in its right mind would want to market a pill for the common cold that could paralyze you?

Ethel Coryza, a twenty-three-year-old secretary living near Olympia, Washington, had a cold. Apart from some nasal congestion, she was in fine health: no medical problems, no prescribed medicines, no allergies. She felt great except for that damn stuffy nose. She went to a local supermarket and surveyed the rows of familiar over-the-counter cold remedies: Contac, Comtrex, Dimetapp, Coricidin. She picked one of them, took it, and went to work. Later that day, she developed a terrible headache while she was driving home, worse than any she'd had before. That evening her family noticed that she was behaving oddly and took her to the hospital. By this time her speech had become slurred and she was having trouble moving her right arm and leg. An emergency CAT scan showed a surprising finding: there was a bright, egg-shaped stain deep in her brain tissue on the left, the part that controls movement and sensation on the right side of the body. An intracerebral hemorrhage—a bleed into the brain—was causing her headache, unusual behavior, and partial paralysis.

To determine the cause of this strange lesion would require looking at the arteries supplying Ethel's brain. A large-bore needle was inserted into her groin, into the femoral artery, and upward. Through it, a delicate catheter was threaded upstream into her aorta, past the heart, and into her neck, entering the carotid artery. X-ray dye was injected through the catheter to fill the main blood vessels supplying that side of her head; additional pictures were taken. Instead of the uniform, clean, spaghetti-like image of healthy cerebral arteries, there were multiple constricted regions of vascular spasm on one side. This produced a characteristic appearance of "beading" in the main artery, like some kind of deadly necklace strangling her brain from the inside. A careful workup revealed none of the usual causes for this kind of vasculitis: she didn't have high blood pressure or any clotting disorder, no obscure autoimmune diseases, didn't abuse drugs. She was just a healthy young woman who had a cold.

Her doctors' attention turned to the over-the-counter remedy she had taken for the first time that morning. Its active ingredient was phenyl-propanolamine, or PPA—a tamer cousin of amphetamine, from which it differs chemically only minimally. Reports had appeared in medical journals over the years describing previously healthy people who had used over-the-counter PPA for nasal congestion or as a weight loss aid (its other common use) and developed sharp elevations in blood pressure, unbearable headaches, or—as in Ethel's case—the symptoms of a stroke.

Unknown to the public and to nearly all physicians, throughout the 1980s and 1990s a debate had been smoldering over whether these drugs were safe enough to be left on the market. As early as 1985, the U.S. Food and Drug Administration (FDA) had declined to classify PPA as safe. Congressional hearings were held in the Senate and in the House about PPA risks. But PPA-containing products continued to be sold widely, generally without any mention on their packaging of the risk of stroke. It wasn't until 2000 that the *New England Journal of Medicine* published a definitive epidemiologic study conducted at Yale University, showing convincingly that PPA, in doses routinely sold over the counter, did indeed increase the risk of intracerebral hemorrhage by three- to eighteenfold, particularly in women. A few months after that report appeared, the FDA declared the drugs to be unsafe and they were removed from the market.

The PPA in dozens of cold remedies was immediately replaced by an equally effective decongestant, pseudoephedrine (commonly marketed as Sudafed), which does not pose the same stroke risk. This was done with remarkable speed; the industry had known since the early 1980s that the FDA might ban PPA use, and plans for the substitution had been in place for years. The companies had resisted the reformulation for so long, most observers agree, because of concern that the switch could have a negative impact on revenues.

MULTIPLE SYSTEM FAILURE

There is no single explanation for what happened to Irma Washington. She admitted to being "no big fan of doctors," and even though she had been careful about taking all her children to the pediatrician whenever the Medicaid program would pay for checkups, she wasn't keen on seeking medical attention for herself. Her blood pressure had shot up when she was pregnant with her fourth child, Vaneesha, and she had to stay in the hospital for two weeks until she delivered. "High blood" ran in her family, but she figured she didn't need to do anything about it as long as she felt well. At age thirty-five, when Vaneesha was two, Irma had her blood pressure taken by a nurse at the pediatric clinic, who found that it was 190 over 105—a very high number for anyone, and particularly worrisome in a relatively young black woman. The nurse told Irma to cut down on salt and to go see a doctor. On the day she went back to the clinic, the doctors didn't get to see all the patients who were waiting, so she was given an appointment to come

back another time. But that morning her s⌐
wouldn't take him, so she had to stay home

When she was in her forties Ms. Wa⌐
again at a neighborhood health fair, an⌐
nurse-practitioner there insisted that Irn⌐
the community health center. Her pressure ⌐
immediately started on a thiazide diuretic, one o⌐
blood pressure drugs. Since Irma had kids under ⌐
Medicaid covered the cost of her prescription, which wa⌐
since the drug was generic. The clinic was busy that day and t⌐
have time to give Irma the lecture she had planned, to explai⌐
blood pressure would require lifelong medication to keep it under con⌐
order to prevent a heart attack or stroke or kidney damage.

Irma didn't think she really needed to take those pills, but the nurse
seemed honest and she liked coming back to the clinic every few months to
hear that the pressure was down to a "normal" number. It wasn't often that
someone told her she was succeeding at something.

One day Irma showed up at the clinic to find the door locked; a hand-
written sign told patients to go to the big municipal hospital center across
town. The neighborhood health center had closed because of budget cutbacks, but she could still get care at the hospital outpatient clinic. No one
knew what had happened to the nurse she knew, but Irma was given an
appointment for the following month with one of the clinic doctors.

Earlier that year, Irma had begun to notice some numbness and tingling
in her arm. She didn't tell her kids about it, but it was enough to make her
feel that maybe she should pay more attention to her "high blood." The
new doctor renewed her thiazide prescription and told her to return in three
months.

At the next appointment she had a different new doctor. This one didn't
seem old enough to have graduated from medical school (he had, three
months earlier), but he said the medicine she had been taking was out-
moded, and much newer drugs were available. (He had learned this the
preceding week, during a dinnertime talk, "Modern Concepts in Anti-
Hypertensive Therapy," at one of the nicer local restaurants. The food and
the knowledge were provided by a company that manufactured a calcium-
channel blocker, a different kind of blood pressure medication. The speaker
failed to mention that a national panel of experts on hypertension treatment didn't share the company's view. But unlike the company, the national
panel had no budget for dinner speakers.) Irma's new doctor stopped her
thiazide and started her on a calcium-channel blocker. Neither Irma nor
the young doctor knew it, but the switch meant that the cost to Medicaid
went from $55 to $600 a year.

...gton took her new pills fairly regularly. She didn't notice any ... she felt, except that her ankles got a little puffy. The doctor ... her heart and gave her another drug to treat that. On her third ... d he wouldn't be there next time because his rotation at that hos- ... ending, and he was going somewhere else to learn to be a derma- ... t. He gave her the name of the new doctor who would take his place. ... became an annual ritual, but Ms. Washington tried to make it to the ... patient clinic at least a few times each year, especially if her headaches ...re bad.

When Vaneesha turned eighteen, Ms. Washington got a letter from Medicaid. It explained that because her youngest child wasn't a minor anymore, Irma no longer qualified for coverage. The next time she went to get her blood pressure medicine, the pharmacist said the one–month bottle would cost her $52.85. She said she'd come back later with the money, but she couldn't, and she didn't. Irma was working two minimum-wage jobs, at a McDonald's by day and as a janitor by night, but neither provided health insurance. Someone at work said she should try going back to her old drug if it was cheaper, but she didn't see any point in taking something that was outmoded. She figured that as she got older her high blood might come down, and she was really trying to watch her salt.

Two weeks shy of her fifty-fifth birthday, Irma Washington went to the emergency room of the county hospital because she felt "like someone is splitting my head open with an ax." Her blood pressure on admission was 220 over 115, though it was impossible to tell whether this was a new problem (no one there had seen her before) or related to her developing stroke. Intravenous medications were given to manage her hypertensive crisis, and as she progressed into a coma she was transferred to the intensive care unit (ICU). Years of uncontrolled severe hypertension had taken their toll on her kidneys, and within a day she was in renal failure. Plans were made for emergency hemodialysis. A diligent medical student managed to find her old files in the record room. "She was seen here on and off for years for bad hypertension," he reported. "Looks like she was a big non-complier."

The rapid swings of her blood pressure in the first days of that admission were too much for her overburdened heart, and on day three she suffered a massive heart attack. As a result, not enough blood was being pumped to the mesenteric artery supplying her intestines, leading to "dead bowel syndrome." A surgical team was mobilized to remove the affected portions of her intestine; plans were being made to coordinate the abdominal surgery with her kidney dialysis when her heart stopped around noon on day four. The ICU team decided not to attempt resuscitation because of the brain damage that had already resulted from her stroke. Her brief hospitalization would end up costing over $12,000, though Medicaid would refuse the bill, as she was no longer enrolled. The hospital would have to cover those costs from its long-since-depleted Free Care fund.

The day Irma died, the resident in charge of the intensive care unit got a call from the ER. "What ever happened to that Washington woman we sent up a few days ago?" asked the intern who had admitted her. "Just want to get some follow-up."

"Flatlined just now," answered the ICU resident. "Turns out she was a longtime noncompliant hypertensive. Seen here a few times in the clinic. First her brain went, then the kidneys, then the heart, then the gut. Multiple system failure."

"Too bad," replied the ER intern. "I may need that bed. We're just working up another uncontrolled hypertensive down here with the worst headache of her life. Make sure housekeeping turns things around fast."

Multiple system failure, at several levels.

TEN MINUTES MORE

I first heard about "the Levine sign" during my internship. It was initially described by the eminent cardiologist Samuel Levine, who established one of the world's first coronary care units in the 1950s at the hospital where I now work, then called the Peter Bent Brigham Hospital. Dr. Levine had observed that if you ask a patient with chest pain to describe his symptoms and he raises his hand to his sternum and makes a fist to convey the crushing nature of his pain, the chances are good that he's having a heart attack rather than an obstructed gallbladder, indigestion, a bleeding ulcer, or any number of other possible diagnoses. Even with the advent of sophisticated blood tests and radionuclide scans, it is an observation that has withstood the test of time.

Tommy O'Rourke arrived in the emergency room of his local hospital gasping for air, his face ashen and contorted with pain. He hadn't been this scared in all his seventy-eight years of life. When the doctor on duty asked what was wrong, he responded with a positive Levine sign. Oxygen was administered, blood drawn, and an electrocardiogram taken. It showed extremely elevated S-T segments, indicating that a portion of heart muscle was being starved for oxygen because the artery supplying it with blood had shut down. His chest pain had first begun some four hours ago; Tommy had been taken by the ambulance driver to the nearest emergency room, even though his usual doctor worked at the larger teaching hospital ten minutes farther away. The policy was to get patients with chest pain to the closest facility so that doctors could administer an intravenous "clot-busting" drug to dissolve the obstruction, or to perform coronary angioplasty, in which the blockage is reamed out mechanically through a catheter inserted into the heart. Use of the clot-busting medications had become widespread during the 1990s. The drugs could be given in any facility where an intravenous line could be started, unlike the more difficult angioplasty procedure, which required more highly trained doctors and specialized facilities. It was assumed that both procedures worked equally well, and that the clot-busting drugs were as safe in elderly patients like Tommy as they were in the younger heart attack patients on whom most of the initial studies had been done.

As it turned out, both assumptions were flawed. The original clinical trials evaluating the thrombolytic drugs had enrolled inadequate numbers of elderly patients, even though most heart attacks occur in older people. The drugs had become widely used before it was clear that their risks in older patients were not quite the same as in the younger subjects studied in the trials. Specifically, the clot-busters were likelier to blow a hole in the cerebral arteries of older patients than younger ones. It took several more years before adequate head-to-head trials randomly assigned patients having heart attacks either to receive a thrombolytic drug or to undergo angioplasty. Most found that the patients randomized to angioplasty had significantly fewer deaths—and fewer strokes.

Both treatments had been in widespread use for many years; why did it take so long to do this obvious comparison? It was no one's responsibility to do so. The cardiologist who conducted one large trial that was eventually published in 2002 had tried for years to persuade the National Institutes of Health to fund it, but it had demurred, citing more pressing research priorities.

As a result, when Tommy had his heart attack, controversy continued in many communities over whether drugs or angioplasty was safer or more effective, and many doctors remained unaware of the connection between old age and the higher risk of stroke from thrombolytic drugs. Since the local community hospital didn't have the resources to perform angioplasty, Tommy was given the clot-dissolving drug instead. His heart attack turned out to be a modest-sized one, the kind that usually leads to fairly complete recovery. Not so for the stroke he had, which was devastating. Would his odds have been better if he had been driven the extra ten minutes to his usual medical center and treated there with angioplasty instead? Perhaps. Would he have had a stroke anyway? There is no way to tell, but the clinical trial statistics indicate that the likelihood of that complication would have been substantially lower.

Not all of Tommy's luck was bad. He had seven children, and six of them lived nearby. Once he was released from the rehabilitation facility three weeks later, unable to speak or walk, they each took turns having him live with them for two months out of the year, and providing him with the round-the-clock care he needed until his eventual death seventeen very long months later. "When it came," his daughter said, "it was truly a blessing."

NEWER IS BETTER

Paul was a bright young pharmacist who had worked for years at a teaching hospital in California. With another new baby at home, he couldn't make ends meet on an academic salary. "I'm going over to the Dark Side," he said jokingly when he called me to let me know he had accepted a job at a pharmaceutical company. The hours, as well as the salary, would be much better—though he'd miss the patient contact and intellectual stimulation of his old job.

Paul went to work for a multinational drug giant that had a strong market presence in psychoactive and dermatologic drugs, but was weaker in the lucrative cardiovascular field. His first assignment was to act as a sales representative for Posicor, the company's newly marketed blood pressure product. Like most drugs, it had taken many years and hundreds of millions of dollars to develop. "The product looks promising, but there are some questions about its pharmacokinetics," Paul told me. Pharmacokinetics describes the way a drug makes its way through the body: how it is absorbed, distributed through the tissues, broken down to inactive substances by the liver, and eventually excreted. New drugs are subjected to extensive testing of each of these component steps, but in the rush to market a new product, not every potential problem is evaluated exhaustively.

Meanwhile, in another part of town, the professional life of one primary-care physician, whom we'll call Dr. Brady, was changing for the worse. His group practice had been bought by a large managed care company, and the corporation had set up new productivity standards for physicians. To meet them, he had to get to the hospital by 6 a.m. to make rounds on his inpatients so he could be in the office by eight o'clock to see the first appointments of the day. Lunch was a quick take-in sandwich while he caught up on lab and X-ray results; the afternoons were reserved for walk-in patients with urgent problems and for rounds in the nursing home, where he cared for two wards of wheelchair-bound patients, most of them demented. He was back in the hospital by five o'clock if one of the inpatients had gone sour, and ended his day back at the office to confront stacks of administrative and billing paperwork. Evenings were for catching up with the family if he got home in time, and reading the three or four medical journals he subscribed to.

The time with the medical journals was the hardest to give up, and the easiest. The hardest, because keeping up with new developments was one of the best parts of his life as a doctor. Through it, he felt he was participating in the great chain of basic research, clinical trials, and practical application that had once made him feel that medicine was the finest calling there was. Reading the journals was also the easiest part of his day to cut back on, because he caught no flak if he missed a few issues of the *New England Journal of Medicine* or the *Journal of the American Medical Association*. But there was flak if he didn't round on his inpatients, or wasn't in the office when a patient's angina flared, or if he missed covering his staff's payroll one week.

This made it harder for Dr. Brady to keep track of medical progress, not to mention all the new drugs his patients saw advertised on television and came in asking for. Most of those products hadn't even been discovered when he was in medical school. Here, for once, he had some support. Each day, advisers would come to the office to update him on when to use the newest medications, giving him concise, easy-to-understand explanations of how each one worked and what its advantages were.

His waiting room was usually full of people in anguish, in pain, or both, who confronted him with questions he couldn't always answer, or demanded relief he couldn't always provide. They were mostly elderly and poor, and many hadn't finished high school. But these consultant-educators were young, bright, attractive, engaging, affable, well dressed. If he was tied up, they would wait for him, sometimes for hours, or come back when he had a few spare minutes. They'd take him out to lunch, or bring in his favorite dish from a local restaurant. Their teaching materials were simple, colorful, short, and punchy. They could even arrange for some of his poorer patients to get sample drugs for free, at least initially. Dr. Brady was confident that even though each of these people worked for a different pharmaceutical company, they were still giving him solid, useful information about the latest developments. And it was much quicker, not to mention more pleasant, than slogging through all those journals he didn't have time for now anyway.

And so Dr. Brady had a visit one day from Paul, the hospital-pharmacist-turned-sales-rep. He brought some Posicor mugs and pens for the doctor and his office staff, as well as stacks of notepaper and "Posicor"-labeled stick-on pads. One especially catchy teaching tool was a leaflet shaped like a cell phone; when you opened it, a microchip inside made a ringing sound and delivered a recorded message about the virtues of the new product.

"What do you think about these advances in blood pressure therapy, Dr. Brady?" Paul queried.

The doctor confessed that he didn't have much time to keep up with his reading lately, and asked Paul what he was referring to. Paul replied by asking him how he was managing his newly diagnosed hypertensive patients.

"With thiazides or beta-blockers," Dr. Brady replied, citing the two oldest and best-studied drugs for that condition.

"Well, those old workhorses have certainly been around for a long time," Paul responded with a smile. "But fewer and fewer doctors are actually starting new patients on them anymore." He rattled off a half-dozen company-funded studies documenting possible side effects of the older drugs. "Most of the specialists I've come across are using the newer products now, especially for their patients who are just beginning a lifetime of therapy." He described the excitement he was encountering now that these doctors were starting to use Posicor. The ten minutes of medical education were nearly up, and it was time for Paul to move in for the close.

"I'll tell you what," he said, seamlessly rising, turning, heading for the door, and reaching into his large sample case. "Why don't you take these samples and try Posicor out on the next ten new hypertensives you see. I'll leave you with some materials on its clinical trial results. . . . You'll find these charts the most interesting." He pointed to the centerfold in a four-page glossy handout, replete with bold headlines, pictures of smiling patients, and a few graphs. "I'll come back in a month, and you can let me know how it's working. The doctors in our Scientific Affairs Department are particularly interested in reports from cutting-edge practitioners like yourself. And here's a laser pointer for you, for the next time you give a talk. And an extra one for that bright son of yours—Timmy, isn't it? Just don't let him shine it in anyone's eyes! We got a deal?"

"Sure," said Dr. Brady, holding out his hands for the samples and trinkets.

The next day, Sally Lentman came in for her annual physical. A thin woman in her early sixties, she began her visit by tremulously handing the doctor a wrinkled sheet of paper filled with numbers. "They have a new nurse at the plant now," Sally explained, "and she does these blood pressure checks whenever you want. I remember you said last time you were worried that my pressure was getting a little high, so I had her test it a few times." Dr. Brady looked over his own notes from Sally's last appointment several weeks earlier. He had written: "BP 160/92 this visit; rising over last year. If still up next time, will start Rx." The numbers on Sally's crumpled sheet, in a neat feminine hand, each with its own date, were similar: 165/95, 172/90, 168/96, 177/97. That day's reading in the office was 180/95. Dr. Brady made Sally his first Posicor patient, adding it to her list of medications. Since she was already having a hard time paying for them all, she was delighted to get the free samples.

After a few days on the drug, Sally complained to her husband that her muscles ached and that she felt dizzy every time she stood up. He worried that the problem might be her blood pressure, so he made sure she had taken all of that day's Posicor and her other heart medicines, and sent her to bed early. Around 3 a.m., he heard her making gurgling noises and couldn't wake her. In panic, he called 911; when the EMTs arrived her pulse was 40 and her blood pressure barely measurable. The doctors at the hospital were eventually able to get her pulse and pressure back up with a mix of adrenaline-like drugs, but in combination with the acute kidney failure she had developed, the prolonged low pressure had taken a toll. Sally had what we call a watershed infarct: the parts of her brain at the far end of their arterial supply had perished first with the pressure drop. Brain cells deprived of circulation long enough generally don't come back to life when their blood supply is restored. The resulting stroke rendered her unconscious and able to make only the most rudimentary twitches in response to what neurologists euphemistically call "deep stimulation." She remained in that state for three weeks, when the family reluctantly agreed to turn off her mechanical ventilator and other life-support systems.

There hadn't been much in the initial Posicor package insert warning about the potential for death if it was combined with several other commonly used drugs. Dr. Brady was sure of that, since he checked right after he had gotten the call from Sally's husband. The doctor hadn't actually read the package insert that Paul had given him that day with the free samples—*no one does,* he reminded himself. Like all of them, it went on for page after page in tiny print. But now Dr. Brady went back like a man possessed and reread the original FDA-approved information to see if there was some warning he had missed about potentially fatal drug-drug interactions with the other medications Sally was taking. *It just wasn't there.*

In the coming months, it would become much clearer that the drug could occasionally drop a patient's pulse to a dangerously low rate, and if taken together with several commonly used cardiovascular drugs it could prevent patients' livers from metabolizing them normally, causing the other medications to build up to toxic levels. Critics would later point to evidence of the potential problem that had been available before the drug was approved, and suggested that this had been a disaster waiting to happen. After it was in use for just a year, the manufacturer agreed to take Posicor off the market, citing unanticipated pharmacokinetic interactions. Some time later, Paul left the company. A number of suits are pending against the drug maker.

GONE FISHING

Ben Snow had always loved the climate in Vancouver, British Columbia. Resting on the rugged coast of Canada's westernmost province, Vancouver is stroked the year round by moderating breezes off the Pacific, producing weather that is surprisingly mild for a city so far north. Medical care for Mr. Snow and his wife, Molly, was covered by the province's health insurance program; he got to pick his doctor, and the government paid the bills. Those weren't high, but they were frequent: Ben had elevated cholesterol and blood pressure, and "some ticker problem" whose name he could never pronounce. The province paid for his medicines as well, as it did for all citizens over sixty-five. Each morning, he dutifully took the pills he had been on for years: his cholesterol-lowering pill, two different pills for high blood pressure, a drug to control his irregular heartbeat, and a single baby aspirin, "though I don't see why, I'm no damn baby anymore."

When he turned seventy, Ben and his wife took half their life savings and bought a cabin in the woods an hour outside Vancouver, near a stream with wonderful trout fishing. The house became a gathering place for his sons and grandchildren too; Ben taught them how to cast their lines into just the right spot halfway across the river, next to a little waterfall. In the summer of his seventy-fourth year Ben had a heart attack and had to spend two weeks in intensive care. But he pulled through fine, his doctor added a new drug to his list of medicines, and in September he was back at the cabin, "pretty much as good as ever." A bout of shortness of breath that winter led to a new diagnosis of congestive heart failure and another new drug, which got him back to his old baseline. By the time the Snows were in their eighties, their grandkids were bringing their own children to visit the cabin. Ben liked to say that the day he showed his five-year-old great-granddaughter how to cast her line into the trout stream "was the happiest moment of my whole life."

The winter that he turned eighty-seven, there were no trips to the cabin because Ben came down with a bad case of bronchitis, which quickly turned into bacterial pneumonia. It took several courses of antibiotics and a long stint in intensive care to put him right, but he was over it by the spring, and felt well enough for the annual ritual of planting his vegetable garden. The family trips resumed. The grandchildren bought property on an adjacent lot and a small family compound of modest cabins took shape.

One Saturday night in September, when Ben was ninety-two, the Snows drove from the cabin into town to buy some maple syrup for a pancake breakfast they planned for the whole family the next morning. On their way back, their car was struck by a drunk driver doing eighty-five miles per hour. They were both killed instantly.

ETHEL CORYZA of the stuffy nose, Tommy O'Rourke with the heart attack, and Sally Lentman, whose doctor started her on the new blood pressure medication, all had strokes that were likely caused by the drugs they took. But it's even more important to realize that Stan, the mailman with atrial fibrillation, and Irma Washington, who had so much trouble navigating the health care system, suffered their strokes because they *didn't* get the drugs that could have prevented them. In the end, regardless of the path each patient took to get there, their dismal neurological fates were similar— about the same tragic outcome as if each had been struck in the head with a tire iron during a mugging. While the cause of the brain damage inflicted in a mugging is fairly straightforward, thinking about causation and preventability in these patients is more complicated, and much more interesting.

What is old Ben Snow doing in this list of patients? He is there because he *didn't* have a stroke, and he's the most common case study of all. Most of the time people take their medications without incident and benefit from them—often enormously. For thousands of days, Ben Snow woke up each morning, took his pills, lived his life, and went to bed without having a stroke. Each of Mr. Snow's "nonstroke" days was made possible at least in part by the drugs he took. Most of them were produced by years of painstaking research in the public and private sectors, tested rigorously in large, costly clinical trials often conducted by their manufacturers, prescribed for him by doctors who made just the right decisions over and over for decades. And while it is obvious on what days Ms. Coryza and Mr. O'Rourke and Ms. Lentman had their strokes, it's much harder to think clearly about the many days on which Mr. Snow *didn't* have his. In the end, he was done in by someone else's use of another drug, alcohol, that causes more chemically induced disease and death each year than all medications put together. (Add in the illness and death caused by a different drug, tobacco, and the combined risks from all prescription medications wouldn't even fit on the same scale.)

How much of Mr. Snow's blissful stroke-free old age can we credit to the medicines he took? Might clean living, smart chromosomes, and good luck have gotten him intact to age ninety-two without benefit of any prescriptions, or any medical care at all? It's impossible to know for sure. But we do know from studies of tens of thousands of people just like him that using drugs properly to manage high blood pressure, cholesterol, and cardiac disease sharply reduces the risk of stroke, heart attack, and other devastating outcomes. As a doctor, would I want to have all patients' odds improved in that way? You bet. At the risk of what side effects? That question is a bit tougher. And how much should society pay for the benefits that these powerful medicines provide? That's a separate $200 billion question—the amount Americans spend each year on drugs.

Benefits, risks, and costs don't exist inside a given drug molecule; they become real only when that molecule is inserted into the life of an individual patient, as he or she interacts with clinicians and moves through the health care system. To use a computer analogy we will return to later, prescription drugs are like the high-tech hardware of medical care, whereas the information, systems, and relationships that shape their use are the software that makes it all work beautifully—or crash. Both components must be understood in order to grasp the impact that medications have on health and illness, and to optimize those outcomes. While our main focus will be on prescription drugs, it is sometimes arbitrary whether a given medicine falls under this socially defined rubric, and a few of our examples of benefit and risk will be found on the other side of this dividing line.

TAKING DRUGS CAN hurt you; not taking drugs can hurt you. Tens of millions of people are alive today who would be dead without their medicines, and tens of millions more have far less life-crushing disability because of prescriptions their doctors have written. Some others—though mercifully a much smaller number—become disabled or die when a drug's risk-benefit balance goes horribly wrong. Each year sees the introduction of new discoveries that hold enormous clinical promise if used well, and each year the nation's pharmaceutical bill is considerably larger. The price of our drug appetite now takes an ever larger bite out of already strained health care budgets. It has grown at an unsustainable annual rate of 15 to 19 percent over the last few years, making prescription drugs the fastest-rising component of all health care expenditures.

The central idea of *Powerful Medicines* is that every drug is a triangle with three faces, representing the healing it can bring, the hazards it can inflict, and the economic impact of each. All of us—doctors, patients, regulators, taxpayers, insurers, policy makers—must learn to balance these three dimensions better if we are to get the maximum benefit from this most common and powerful of all health care interventions. Following the model of medical education, we will explore these relationships through case studies, often situations in which that balance was upset. At times our approach will resemble a teaching and quality-control exercise employed in many hospitals, the weekly "morbidity and mortality" conferences often referred to by interns as M&Ms. Each of those sessions focuses on one or more patients who did poorly when they shouldn't have, retracing the facts and decisions occurring at each step throughout a given episode of care. It's an uncomfortable process, but enormously useful for learning how to do things better.

Some of our examples will explore problematic decisions made by regulators, pharmaceutical companies, or physicians. This is not because people at the FDA or drug companies or practitioners are normally bad at what they do, any more than the lesson to be drawn from M&M rounds is that interns and residents are normally inept. Rather, as we are learning from the emerging field of medical errors research, it is often *the system* that shapes decisions for good or for ill—the incentives that drive behavior, the culture of expectations about information or standards of practice, the regulations that do or don't exist and how thoughtfully they're enforced. Just as morbidity-and-mortality rounds are not designed to make individuals feel bad (though that is sometimes an unavoidable result), the main goal here will be to learn how we can do a better job on these fronts in the future. All of us have much to learn.

As a physician, I instinctively focus on the causes and amelioration of people's illnesses rather than dwelling on wellness. As an epidemiologist, I find it helps to think about medical problems and achievements in terms of the *populations* that comprise those patients. And as a health policy researcher, I obsess over why parts of the health care system fail and how we can fix them. Despite the enormous good they do, medications provide a fascinating lens through which we can focus on the improvements needed in each of these domains.

This is not a "Just Say No to Drugs" book. Medications are one of the finest achievements in all of science, and when used appropriately the good they do far outweighs their harm. But just what *is* appropriate use? How can we know when good outweighs harm? And what is a reasonable cost to pay for this balance? With the ante rising annually on each of these fronts, we need a better grip on how to maximize the potentially awesome good of medicines, contain their often preventable harm, and manage their increasingly burdensome expense.

Most doctors make sound prescribing decisions much of the time, and most drugs are both effective and reasonably safe. The Mr. Snows are far more common than the other cases presented above. But if the revolution in therapeutics through which we are living is to reach its full potential, we have to understand what lies behind the stories of the other patients as well, so that there can be even more "uninteresting" cases like Ben Snow in the coming years.

THE BOOK IS DIVIDED into five parts: "Benefits," "Risks," "Costs," "Information," and "Policy." In the section on benefits, we will explore the surprisingly fragile nature of a seemingly simple determination: whether or not a drug works. In the section on risks, we will visit the various settings in which a drug's adverse effects are assessed, from the bedside to the courtroom to research centers such as the one I head at Harvard. Our goal will be to figure out whether the connections between tragic medical outcomes and the use of particular drugs are causal or casual, to use an old epidemiological pun. The third section will tackle the increasingly burdensome cost of medications, and how we pay for them—one of the most pressing current policy debates. The fourth section, on information, will investigate the flow of good data, factoids, and hype that shapes the prescriptions a doctor writes. The journal papers that are published, the ones that don't get written, educational programs for physicians ranging from rigorous university-run courses to lavish company-sponsored gourmet infomercials—all compete to influence the clinical decisions my colleagues and I make. The final section, on policy, will consider how the U.S. health care system could—indeed, must—bring each of these dimensions into harmony so we can deliver this most important medical intervention intelligently, equitably, and affordably.

Much of what follows is based on my experiences as a physician and researcher. It is written from a personal perspective, and will draw heavily on the studies I have done with many talented colleagues over the years. This is not at all because my group's work is the most important source of information in these areas—far from it. Rather, it is because this is the perspective from which I can offer "the story behind the story" of our investigations and other adventures. The personal voice usually has to be edited out before a clinical note is written in a patient's medical record, a paper is published in a journal, testimony is delivered before Congress, or an expert report is submitted to the courts. But this perspective can yield important insights that would otherwise go unreported.

In the long-standing tradition of medical education, we will make frequent use of case studies, one of the most effective ways to render complex issues both accessible and engaging. The patients and doctors described, including those above, are based on individuals I have cared for or known about, or cases reported in clinical journals, or composites of these; all names and identifying characteristics have been changed to protect privacy and confidentiality. For conciseness, I will generally refer to prescribers as physicians, although I recognize that nurse-practitioners and pharmacists in many states also prescribe drugs, often with great acumen. I request the indulgence of these colleagues for this wording.

Extensive notes at the end of the book can be used to relate this material to the medical literature and other sources for further exploration, or can be ignored. The notes also include references to related websites, so that any reader with an internet connection can delve more deeply into many of the areas we will touch on. Updates and addenda will be periodically posted to the book's website, www.powerfulmedicines.org, along with automatic links to papers cited and other relevant internet sites. The goal of all that follows will be to relate the issues we discuss to improving the health of individuals. That is the highest purpose of all powerful medicines, however far some of the protagonists we will meet may stray from this central goal.

PART ONE: BENEFITS

1: THE PREGNANT MARE'S LESSON

In a former British colony, most healers believed the conventional wisdom that a distillation of fluids extracted from the urine of horses, if dried to a powder and fed to aging women, could act as a general tonic, preserve youth, and ward off a variety of diseases. The preparation became enormously popular throughout the culture, and was used widely by older women in all strata of society. Many years later modern scientific studies revealed that long-term ingestion of the horse-urine extract was useless for most of its intended purposes, and that it caused tumors, blood clots, heart disease, and perhaps brain damage.

The former colony is the United States; the time is now; the drug is the family of hormone replacement products that include Prempro and Premarin (manufactured from pregnant mares' urine, hence its name). For decades, estrogen replacement in postmenopausal women was widely believed to have "cardio-protective" properties; other papers in respected medical journals reported that the drugs could treat depression and incontinence, as well as prevent Alzheimer's disease. The first large, well-conducted, controlled clinical trial of this treatment in women was not published until 1998; it found that estrogen replacement actually increased the rate of heart attacks in the patients studied. Another clinical trial published in 2002 presented further evidence that these products increased the risk of heart disease, stroke, and cancer. Further reports a year later found that rather than preventing Alzheimer's disease, the drugs appeared to double the risk of becoming senile. The studies resulted in a reduction, but not an end, to the long-term use of these products.

For decades, these were among the most widely prescribed drugs in the nation. How did we get such an important question so wrong for so long?

Despite the deer-in-the-headlights astonishment with which the nation greeted the 2002 report that hormone replacement caused more harm than good, signs of trouble had been emerging for several years. The estrogen debacle was a case study waiting to be written, and its story can tell us much, both good and bad, about how the health care system evaluates and deploys medications. The fabric of modern medical care is woven of the belief by doctors and patients that the prescription drugs we use have been exhaustively studied and shown to work. The spectacular downfall of estrogen replacement therapy drew attention to the question of just how we determine that a drug actually "works," and why the system broke down in this very high profile case. For years, I've studied how we know what we know about drug benefits and risks, an inquiry I think of as "pharmaco-epistemology." The hormone replacement story is a perfect cautionary tale in this domain; it has much to teach us about how fragile our knowledge base can be concerning a drug's ultimate effects.

The word "estrogen" itself comes from the Latin *oestrus* and the Greek *oistros,* which mean "gadfly" and, by extension, "frenzy." The roots were chosen by early physiologists to depict the sexual arousal the hormones can cause in animals. They are also related to the semantic lineage of the word "ire," which in turn derives from the Old English words for "haste" and "zeal" as well as from the Greek *heiros,* or "holy." I can think of no better linguistic pedigree for a once-sacred clinical concept that was promoted in haste and defended with zeal, and whose demise precipitated both frenzy and anger. Most important for the present context, the estrogen story has become a gadfly that is provoking a reconsideration of just how we know what we know about a drug's effectiveness.

The shared delusion about long-term hormone replacement therapy started innocently enough. For centuries, women of a certain age (and their spouses) knew that the end of regular menstruation was often accompanied by the onset of uncomfortable hot flashes, insomnia, and a drying of the internal surface of the vagina. As the new science of physiology developed in the 1900s, these changes were understood to result from a falloff in estrogen production by aging ovaries. If a reduction in natural estrogen was the cause of these problems, then maybe restoring a woman's estrogen to premenopausal levels might ameliorate them. By mid-century it was possible to create a pharmaceutical product that would enable women to replenish their own flagging hormone by ingesting it in pill form. Pregnancy sharply increases the production of estrogens, and they are copiously secreted in the urine. Someone figured out that horses could be used as mass-production hormone factories for this purpose, and pregnant mare's urine provided Premarin with both its ingredients and its brand name.

By the 1970s, with the support of Ayerst (now Wyeth), the manufacturer of Premarin, Madison Avenue magic redefined the normal age-related reduction in estrogen levels into a new syndrome, "ovarian failure." This novel disease concept was featured prominently in medical journal advertisements for Premarin, which was presented as its logical treatment. And so a normal age-related change took its place alongside kidney failure, congestive heart failure, and liver failure as a newly discovered illness in need of treatment. (I don't intend to belittle the discomfort associated with the hot flashes, vaginal dryness, and other symptoms that accompany menopause, or to suggest that they should not be treated for short periods simply because they are normal. What is at issue is lifelong "replacement therapy.")

Things began to go astray when the temporary management of menopausal symptoms became transformed into a belief that ovarian failure was itself a treatable risk factor for other dread conditions, just as elevated cholesterol or blood pressure was. If that were true, then lifelong drug management would be necessary to tame this risk and prevent a host of horrible clinical outcomes. The concept was fed by public fascination with the idea of a pharmacological fountain of youth for women. The Dupont company had already introduced the motto "Better Living Through Chemistry" to promote its line of household products; a few years later my own generation would co-opt that phrase more ironically in defense of psychedelics. In the same spirit, the 1966 best-seller *Feminine Forever* popularized the notion that a woman's aging (and quite explicitly, her loss of sexual appeal) was now preventable, thanks to pharmaceutical research. Its author, Dr. Robert Wilson, was a gynecologist who took on the curing of menopause as a personal crusade, to save the millions of women who "suffered sweeping metabolic disturbances that literally put them in mortal danger." His views were a twisted precursor of the argument that anatomy isn't destiny; but he seemed to warn that without proper medical attention, physiology could become tragedy:

> Though the physical suffering from menopausal effects can be truly dreadful, what impressed me most tragically is the destruction of personality. Some women, when they realize that they are no longer women, subside into a stupor of indifference. . . . I rest my case on the simple contention that castration is a bad thing and that every woman has the right—indeed, the duty—to counteract the chemical castration that befalls her during her middle years.

A new magic bullet could replace, molecule for molecule, the female hormones that failing ovaries could no longer secrete. *Feminine Forever* brought this message to women and their doctors all over the country, supplemented by well-placed articles in women's magazines and news releases describing this bold, modern treatment. The company could not legally advertise the drug for long-term use, since it had not presented clinical data to the FDA demonstrating the promised benefits. But it could support numerous educational programs put on by hospitals, medical schools, and medical communications companies, with the understanding that they would promote lifetime-use messages. Premarin's manufacturer heavily but quietly subsidized the distribution of Dr. Wilson's book as well as these prolific "public information" campaigns. Authors friendly to Wyeth and the gospel of estrogen wrote articles that appeared by the dozens in medical journals and women's magazines from the 1970s to the late 1990s. (We will return to the role of pharmaceutical companies in shaping beliefs about drugs in a later chapter.)

Prolonged use of pharmaceutical estrogen came to be known as hormone replacement therapy, or HRT; the very name gave legitimacy to the treatment by connoting the restoration of a vital bodily ingredient that went pathologically missing at menopause. The logic was appealing, but appealing logic alone has resulted in some of the very worst drug treatments in human history. After all, the second-century texts of Galen helped keep medicine in the Dark Ages for centuries with their supremely logical but completely incorrect theories of how derangement of the four humors caused most human disease.

HOW WE WENT WRONG

Some of the apparent evidence favoring HRT came from measurements of surrogate outcomes—laboratory markers used as stand-ins for real clinical events. It takes years of study to show that a treatment eventually lowers the rate of heart attack or stroke, but one can demonstrate changes in patients' blood tests in just a few weeks or months, using far fewer subjects at a fraction of the cost of a full-scale, long-term clinical study. Here is how the logic of the surrogate outcome worked. It was known that patients with high levels of the "bad" cholesterol LDL and low levels of the "good" cholesterol HDL were more likely to suffer from heart disease and stroke. Estrogens were shown to lower LDL and raise HDL in the blood, so it seemed reasonable that they would eventually reduce the risk of cardiovascular disease. Hormone therapy was also found to produce apparently beneficial short-term effects on several other more arcane measures of vascular function.

The logic of estrogen replacement was bolstered even more compellingly by voluminous epidemiological evidence, only some of it correct. The argument began with the observation that until late middle age, women have dramatically lower rates of heart disease and cardiac death than men. But once menopause occurs, a woman's risk of cardiovascular disease begins to catch up to that in men of the same age. Next came a series of observations that were even more seductive. Several papers reported that postmenopausal women who took estrogen had less heart disease than women of the same age who did not. Replacing the estrogen a woman could no longer make for herself didn't just prevent hot flashes and keep the vaginal tissue supple; it also seemed to maintain the heart and its arteries as healthy as those of younger women.

Additional observational studies seemed to uncover other connections as well. Long-term estrogen users were reported to have less incontinence, Alzheimer's disease, and depression than women of the same age who remained bereft of estrogen replacement. Here as well there were plausible biological mechanisms to explain the observed associations. In many older women, incontinence results from the thinning and shrinkage of vaginal tissue that occur when natural estrogen levels drop; adding pharmaceutical estrogen, either in pill form or as a cream applied directly to the affected areas, perhaps reversed these changes. The explanations for Alzheimer's disease and depression were more tenuous, since we still have little understanding of the basic causes underlying these conditions. Nonetheless, the papers reporting reduced rates of each illness usually included fascinating sections proposing possible mechanisms of such effects, related to the presumed effects of estrogen on derangements in brain chemistry.

There was still the problem of cancer. In the 1970s, it became clear that estrogen replacement increased a woman's risk of developing cancer of the endometrium, the lining of the uterus. Bathing this tissue in extra estrogen for so long provided hormonal stimulation far beyond what those cells expected in their retirement years, and led to a higher rate of malignancy. HRT advocates responded that this problem could be handled with regular endometrial biopsies; at the first sign that cells were becoming cancerous, they could be removed. Or the drug regimen could be altered to a more natural format by combining the estrogen with another female hormone, progestin, to mimic the normal premenopausal cycle more closely. The addition of progestin would help protect the uterus from estrogen overdrive and help it to catch its cellular breath, preventing it from becoming overstimulated and then cancerous.

Alternatively, a few zealots (all men, as far as I can tell) even argued that given the obvious benefits of long-term estrogen replacement, the simplest way to prevent endometrial cancer would be just to cut out that pesky uterus. After all, once it had finished its purpose of childbearing it was a useless organ whose only final act could be malignant transformation. The

United States already had the world's highest rates of hysterectomy, often performed for indications now considered questionable, such as heavy periods or abdominal pain of unclear origin. But cooler heads prevailed, and for a woman who kept her uterus the estrogen-progestin combination worked well to eliminate the excess risk of uterine cancer; the most widely used product was Wyeth-Ayerst's Prempro. Women who had already undergone hysterectomy could take the straight stuff, marketed primarily by Wyeth as Premarin.

The use of Premarin and related products soared—not just for management of symptoms related to menopause itself, but also for all those other age-defying preventive purposes as well. It was conventional wisdom during my early years of practice that enlightened physicians put their older female patients on estrogen replacement for life as soon as they reached menopause. Besides the apparent protective effects of HRT on the heart, estrogen replacement also caused a reduction in bone-thinning osteoporosis, reducing the risk of fractures that can be so devastating in older women. Yes, there was also an increase in the frequency of breast cancer, but elaborate calculations based on the expected reduction in heart disease and fractures showed that those benefits would far outweigh the breast cancer, blood clots, and other problems the drugs were known to cause.

The Food and Drug Administration allowed Wyeth to advertise its products only for the management of menopausal symptoms such as hot flashes and insomnia, as well as for preventing age-related loss of bone mass—the only outcomes for which the company had submitted clinical outcome data. But beyond their text the Premarin ads conveyed a more comprehensive vision of feminine youthfulness. The words may have stuck to the letter of the law, but the larger message was carried in color photos of robust middle-aged women, their hair barely flecked with gray, romping zestily along a beach with a large dog or virile-looking husband. This notion was reinforced by virtually unanimous assertions of the benefits of HRT that could be found in nearly all textbooks. Hundreds of continuing education programs for doctors, many of them supported by Wyeth, were offered at professional society meetings of gynecologists or primary-care physicians. The groups that arranged these sessions were permitted to bring in experts of their choosing who could, in turn, say whatever they wished about the drug; this was beyond the pale of the direct company promotion that the FDA controlled.

THE BIRTH OF DOUBT

In the early 1990s, some voices of skepticism began to be noticed. Granted, numerous studies seemed to show that estrogen users had lower rates of several diseases when compared to age-matched nonusers. But nearly all these insights had come from epidemiologic analyses. Such studies follow users of a specific drug as well as nonusers and track their fates, adjusting the results for differences such as age and preexisting illnesses. In the studies of HRT use and heart disease, numerous adjustments were also made for cardiac risk factors such as smoking, diabetes, high blood pressure, and even family history.

But purists argued that the findings came solely from *observational* studies of people who did or didn't happen to be taking the drug. That's not the kind of evidence the FDA requires: a clinical trial in which patients are put on Treatment A or Treatment B and then followed forward in time. With HRT so widespread, some began to ask whether such an experimental study should be conducted to demonstrate convincingly the preventive effects everyone expected. To accomplish this, instead of simply observing rates of disease in users and nonusers, researchers would have to randomly assign women to take estrogen or a dummy pill, and follow them for years; neither the women nor their doctors would be told who was getting which treatment.

At first, opposition to this idea was deafening. Hadn't numerous observational studies from a wide variety of settings already shown that estrogen users suffered less heart disease than nonusers? Those analyses had included enormous numbers of people, and were done by some of the best epidemiological researchers. It might even be unethical to conduct a clinical trial in which some women are randomly assigned to receive a dummy pill instead of estrogen over so many years. The people randomized to the placebo group would be denied a treatment that was commonly accepted as effective and even lifesaving.

But others pointed out that in the absence of a well-conducted placebo-controlled trial, it would indeed be ethical to do such a study, because we didn't *really* know that estrogen was effective for these purposes. Further, the treatment did have known side effects, including cancer. Some argued that the hard evidence against estrogen treatment was just as compelling as the evidence in favor of it, making such a study both scientifically useful and morally acceptable. Yet even those who agreed that the question was unresolved admitted that it could be impractical to mount this kind of trial: it might be too hard to recruit enough gynecologists and patients willing to let a flip of the coin decide whether or not they would use this standard and accepted treatment, given how many doctors and patients believed so firmly in its value.

Unnoticed by most of the combatants, the Food and Drug Administration continued to keep a clear head throughout the emerging debate. Although often criticized for its stodginess on this point, it steadfastly stuck to its polestar principle that a drug cannot be considered effective for a given purpose unless that effect has been demonstrated in well-conducted clinical trials in which patients are randomly assigned to a given treatment or to a placebo or comparison drug and followed forward in time. Premarin had been approved for marketing in the first place by showing in small, brief trials that it was better than placebo at reducing the severity of the immediate menopausal symptoms of hot flashes and vaginal dryness. (Later clinical studies also demonstrated its capacity to reduce bone loss.) The official product description approved by the FDA for Premarin and similar drugs never went beyond its use for these purposes, or indications, and no studies were ever presented to the FDA to back up the widespread presumption that the drug was good for women's hearts. For years, from the manufacturer's perspective none had to be; doctors were prescribing it to millions of women based on that belief anyway.

Despite these behind-the-scenes debates, the use of HRT continued on a massive scale throughout the 1990s. The absence of official FDA approval for the use of Premarin to prevent heart disease was readily dismissed with the following argument that a seasoned clinician might make: "There's plenty of epidemiological evidence in the medical literature that these drugs work for many different purposes. Once a drug is on the market, you can't expect a company to spend the millions of dollars needed to run new clinical trials to convince the FDA about every new use; it's just too costly. Estrogens are approved for the symptoms of menopause, the drugs are out there, and now it's up to the doctor to decide how to use them." The FDA doesn't object to such "off-label" use by physicians and makes no attempt to curtail it, admitting that many drugs have additional legitimate uses even if a manufacturer didn't go through the cumbersome effort of conducting new controlled clinical trials to prove each effect to the government's satisfaction. More and more observational studies were published, some supported by the drugs' manufacturers and some by the National Institutes of Health, showing that regular HRT users had lower rates of a wide variety of diseases compared to ex-users or nonusers.

In the end, it was probably the women's movement that ensured the question would be settled once and for all by a randomized trial. If the most widely used drug in the country were being taken by men, feminists asked, what are the chances that it would never have been evaluated by the same criteria used for every other drug? Studies of illnesses that primarily afflicted women were being shortchanged, women's health advocates contended. Many of the important multicenter heart disease trials mounted by the Veterans Administration, not surprisingly, had included vanishingly small numbers of women or none at all. Research on illness in women became a hot political issue at the National Institutes of Health.

The NIH was reluctant to touch this potential time bomb, and did not initially leap at the chance to supply funding. So researchers also approached Wyeth, arguing that after so many decades of sales, the manufacturer had an obligation to fund research on whether the promised heart disease benefit of its drugs was real. For its part, the company realized it could be commercially useful to prove its products' preventive effects once and for all, so as to gain FDA permission to promote this effect openly. Eventually, NIH also began its own studies under the umbrella of the new Women's Health Initiative, or WHI.

Many feminist health advocates applauded the new studies. Others pointed out trenchantly that once the patriarchal medical research establishment finally got around to spending millions of dollars to study drugs in women, the centerpiece of the effort was a trial that withheld one of their best-loved medications from half the subjects in the study. Still, against all odds thousands of subjects were recruited into several clinical trials in which they were randomly assigned to take either estrogen or a dummy pill for years.

THE RETURN OF SCIENCE

The first study to yield results was a Wyeth-funded trial that focused on estrogen use in women with preexisting cardiac disease. It had the wonderful acronym HERS, for Heart and Estrogen-progestin Replacement Study. Amazement followed publication of its findings in the *Journal of the American Medical Association* in 1998. The study that never needed to be done, that had withheld life-giving hormonal therapy from thousands of women in an obsessive exercise of pseudoscientific misogyny, found that subjects given estrogens had significantly *more* heart attacks in the first year of the study than did comparable women given placebo. The hormone group also had higher rates of blood clots and gallbladder disease.

The HERS findings created understandable anxiety for the investigators running the ongoing NIH Women's Health Initiative study. The paradigm had now flipped. A trial that hadn't seemed worth doing, because everyone knew that estrogens protected the heart, might itself be putting women in harm's way—not in the placebo group, but in the estrogen group. Was it safe for the women receiving estrogen to continue in this new trial? Was it ethical? Over sixteen thousand women across the nation were by now enrolled in WHI. HERS had restricted enrollment to women with preexisting heart disease; might estrogens have quite different effects in the healthier women now in the WHI study? And if WHI were terminated, it would foreclose the possibility of ever mounting another randomized trial to learn whether estrogens could prevent Alzheimer's disease, or depression, or anything else. But could doctors continue to administer a treatment to thousands of women even after they knew it might not reduce risk, and might even increase it? In hearing about the dilemma the researchers faced, my thoughts naturally turned to the Deep South.

Historians have Waterloo; moralists (as we'll see again in a later chapter) have Sodom and Gomorrah; jurists have Nuremberg. All were once low-profile places that became eponyms for turning points in human affairs. Medical ethicists have Tuskegee, Alabama. One of the most notorious case studies in the morality of medical research was the lengthy experiment that took place in that quiet city from the 1950s to the 1970s. Doctors observed poor young black men with syphilis for years to learn about the course of the disease in its untreated state—even though penicillin had been widely available since the 1940s and was known to be an effective remedy for this debilitating illness. Word of the study eventually leaked out in the 1970s and touched off a public uproar; the experiment was hastily stopped and the subjects were belatedly offered the same treatment that syphilis patients outside the study had been receiving routinely for years. Decades later, President Clinton invited some of the experiment's survivors to the White House to witness his formal apology on behalf of the nation.

The design of the Tuskegee experiment was so loathsome that its legacy became a touchstone for medical researchers all over the world. If a question of potential harm to patients arose in the design or conduct of a clinical trial, someone might underscore an objection by warning, "We don't want another Tuskegee." Now, the ghost of that project hovered over a modern study that was its mirror image: administering sex hormones used by mostly well-to-do aging white women to preserve their feminine physiology. Echoes of the Tuskegee aftermath must have drifted through the investigators' minds: *Doctor, do you mean to say that you kept these people in the study even after it was known what the risks were, just to see what would happen to them?*

We've now come upon our first example of the struggle to balance the benefits and risks of a drug. It is a dilemma with which we physicians wrestle (or should) every time we write a prescription; it is one that patients take on, consciously or unconsciously, every time they fill or don't fill that prescription. The conflict is at its starkest in designing a drug trial, but it emerges routinely in clinical practice as well. Once the HERS results were known, what was the right course of action for the doctors running the NIH's Women's Health Initiative? They could abort their study, or continue as if HERS had never happened, or do something in between. What would be the most ethical way to treat the women enrolled? Equally important, for the benefit of women in general, now and in the future, which course would yield the most useful medical information about the benefits and risks of these drugs? Were these two perspectives compatible?

A middle course carried the day. Stopping the new trial early would cut off all possibility of learning about the effects of HRT in patients *without* preexisting heart disease—knowledge that could be vitally important over the coming decades. Much more could still be learned about how best to protect women's health, proponents argued, if the trial were allowed to continue—including answers to questions about the hoped-for benefits of estrogen for Alzheimer's disease, depression, incontinence, and other conditions of aging. But if the new trial confirmed the HERS findings, imagine the anger that might be felt (and acted upon) by the women assigned to take estrogen and suffered heart attacks. Would Tuskegee-like questions be hurled at the study leaders and at the federal agencies that funded the trial, with recriminations and litigation continuing for years to come?

The issue here balances on a sharp concept with a gentle name: *equipoise.* This is the state of knowledge necessary for the ethical and scientifically appropriate conduct of any clinical trial in humans. If I were forced to replace this with a less elegant term, it might be "confusion." Equipoise exists if a well-informed researcher truly cannot know whether an experimental treatment is better than, equivalent to, or worse than another potential treatment for a given patient. After much anguished debate, the WHI trialists in 1998 decided that they were still in a state of equipoise over whether estrogen protected the heart in women without cardiac disease, or had no effect, or in fact damaged it. But however comfortable the investigators were, the women in the WHI study would have to be informed of the latest findings so they could decide for themselves whether to continue as experimental subjects. A mailing went out to the thousands of participants, reporting the HERS findings so they could make informed choices about their participation in the trial.

Other disturbing blemishes soon began to appear on estrogen's previously creamy complexion. In 2001, the American Heart Association rewrote its guidelines on prevention and stated that estrogen should *not* be assumed to have any protective effect on the heart. The same year, another study produced worrisome data suggesting that estrogens could also increase the risk of stroke. Most large clinical trials convene a data safety monitoring board to periodically review interim findings, to make sure that patients in one treatment group are not doing substantially worse than those in the other. In May 2002 the WHI safety monitoring board reviewed the outcomes to that point and found that in this trial too, the women assigned to the hormone replacement group were developing heart disease at a higher rate than those in the placebo group. The same was happening for breast cancer, strokes, blood clots, and gallbladder disease. On the other side of the ledger were a much smaller benefit in the risk of colon cancer, and the expected reduction in hip fractures—although there were several safer drugs on the market for this purpose that did not have estrogen's downsides. In July 2002, thirty years to the month after the first revelations about the Tuskegee experiment became public, the WHI leadership announced that it would be unethical to allow their trial to continue.

Even after the trial was halted, researchers continued to pore over the voluminous data that had already been collected. An analysis of mental functioning had been another key part of WHI from the start, to determine whether HRT did indeed delay the onset of senility or prevent it altogether, as the observational studies had suggested. Quite the opposite was found. Cognitive function was not better in the women randomized to estrogen, and even seemed to be worse, with the treated patients appearing twice as likely to develop the symptoms of Alzheimer's disease. A study in Britain that followed over a million women confirmed that estrogen users had a risk of breast cancer that was 66 percent higher than that of nonusers. In a particularly chilling calculation, its authors determined that HRT use in women aged fifty to sixty-four had produced 20,000 *more* cases of breast cancer than would have been seen in the United Kingdom without HRT. A drug taken by tens of millions of women to preserve their health and youth turned out to be worthless for that purpose and instead caused heart disease, cancer, stroke, blood clots, and perhaps even brain damage.

AN INTELLECTUAL AUTOPSY

How could this have happened? How did clinical practice lurch forward for so long and so far in the absence of solid evidence about what these products did? These are not obscure side effects caused by an arcane drug; cardiovascular disease is the single most important cause of disability and death in the industrialized world, and HRT products were among the most widely prescribed drugs in America for years. During all that time, why did it take so long to determine whether they actually worked the way they were supposed to?

It wasn't anyone's job to make that determination. As we saw, the National Institutes of Health had initially avoided the question for years. This probably had less to do with gender bias than with the NIH's strong preference for funding basic science studies and its relative lack of interest in more mundane applied research questions about the effects of existing medications. For its part, Wyeth had received permission from the FDA to market its products for the temporary management of the symptoms of menopause. For decades, the company was content to have doctors prescribe it to women for other purposes even though the FDA had never approved such use; the company found it easier and safer to ride (as well as drive) the tide of prevailing medical and public opinion. The company's belated support of the HERS study in the 1990s was an attempt to assemble the evidence that the FDA required before it would allow advertising to promote the drugs' cardio-protective property. No one at the company expected the results that emerged; if they had, they are unlikely to have sponsored the study.

Where was the FDA during all those years? It does not usually insist that a company study aspects of a drug not related to its official labeled use, and the FDA doesn't have a budget to conduct clinical trials of its own. Until very recently the agency didn't see its role as monitoring *how* drugs are used in practice; rather, it stuck closely to its authority to simply say yes or no to the initial entry of a given product onto the market. What doctors and patients did with it after that decision, the FDA believed, was none of its business. That attitude has recently begun to change, but the old ways were firmly in place for all of HRT's halcyon years. It also allowed Wyeth to adopt a *Who, me?* approach to how doctors prescribed its drugs. As long as the company didn't directly promote estrogen's preventive powers through printed advertisements or sales calls to doctors, the prevailing law held it blameless for what other people did with its product.

The only real hero to emerge from this complicated story is the randomized controlled trial. On the guilty side is its country cousin the observational study, which the estrogen debacle indicted as a codefendant or at least as an unintentional coconspirator. An observational study is just what its name implies: the passive evaluation of outcomes in large numbers of people who did or didn't end up taking a certain drug. The rationale is that over time, given enough numbers, one can eventually sort out the role of the drug in causing those outcomes.

In performing such research (and I do), we can adjust for differences such as age or race and deploy an impressive array of epidemiologic methods to try and correct for other differences in underlying clinical factors between users and nonusers. If all this works extremely well, the hope is that we can retrofit these observational data to nearly simulate a real clinical trial, in which the groups of drug takers and nontakers are virtually identical because people were randomly assigned to one treatment or the other. We will see in later chapters that observational research can be a valid and even indispensable way to study drug side effects and to answer questions that the randomized trial design cannot hope to address. However, it's dangerous to use observation-only studies to measure the *effectiveness* of a given treatment, as the HRT example has taught us. The problem is this: patients who end up taking a certain drug can differ in important and unmeasured ways from those who do not, even if they appear to be otherwise similar.

As we look back at it, the estrogen story has some of the attributes of a Greek tragedy. It all began with the protagonist's inherent flaw: in this case, the inability to distinguish *association* (the fact that two events often occur together) from *causality* (the conclusion that one event causes the other). Then there's hubris. Pride leads the protagonist to attempt feats that are beyond him, setting the stage for his flaw to bring about the inevitable downfall. Hubris is a common occupational hazard among scientists. Archimedes famously boasted that if he had a lever long enough and a place to put the fulcrum, he could move the world. Many of us who do epidemiologic research are sometimes blinded by a similar bold belief: if we have a large enough sample of subjects (some of the databases we use contain millions of people), enough information on possible confounding factors, enough statistical savvy, and a big enough computer, we think we can replicate the experimental precision of a randomized trial. According to this view, one can simply observe patterns of drug use and outcomes in free-living populations, and then apply complex epidemiological techniques to square away all the differences between those who took a given medication and those who did not. This is supposed to render the users and nonusers perfectly comparable, so that any differences in their medical fates must have been caused by the drug that the users took. (An elaborate set of computer programs was recently developed to facilitate such manipulation of large-scale observational data. It employs hundreds of complex differential equations to predict the course of disease and the impact of specific treatments in vast populations; its developer named it "Archimedes.") However well this approach works in studying the occurrence of side effects, it is much feebler when we try to use it to measure a drug's effectiveness, at least with our current state of knowledge and skill.

It is becoming clearer how all those observational studies of estrogen and heart disease led to conclusions that were so wrong. In some studies, HRT use was assessed using patients' own self-reports on a questionnaire that was updated only every year or two. (These surveys were not originally designed for research in drug epidemiology.) Human memory is fallible, especially in recalling events so remote. Worse, the method caused estrogen users who developed heart disease and then stopped HRT to be erroneously depicted on the next survey as nonusers, obscuring the effect. Such self-report questionnaires also tended to reduce important risk factors such as hypertension and diabetes to simple YES/NO responses, even though the severity of these conditions can be enormously important in predicting the risk of heart attack.

Even more important, it's now clear that women who chose to take estrogen and stay on it for years were quite different from women their age who didn't, even if they had the same blood pressure, rates of diabetes, or cholesterol levels. The estrogen users (whom we should really call the estrogen choosers) had better access to medical care and tended to be more highly educated, wealthier, and more prevention-oriented than their otherwise identical non-estrogen-choosing sisters. These differences may have contributed to the apparently lower rates of heart disease and death seen in estrogen users in the observational studies, even after adjusting for a whole host of other cardiac risk factors.

In hindsight, another clue might have come from a curious observation made years earlier in some of the first large-scale studies of medications to prevent heart disease. In those trials, patients were randomly assigned to take either an active drug or an identical-appearing placebo for several years, without knowing which group they were in. At the study's end, participants who failed to take their experimental pills as directed ended up having more heart disease events than those who took their pills faithfully. That wasn't surprising, except for one fact: the lower rate of heart disease among good versus bad compliers *also occurred in the placebo group.* What was going on here?

The patients who were conscientious about taking their dummy pills every day were also probably conscientious about taking all their other medications, trying to quit smoking, watching their weight, and all those Good Things that our grandmothers and primary-care physicians keep telling us to do. By contrast, the sloppy compliers to the study drug (even if it was placebo) were probably also being less careful about all those other health-related behaviors too.

For a long time, this arcane story about improved outcomes in people who comply well with placebo served primarily as an intriguing anecdote to lob into an otherwise dull lecture on clinical trial design. But in light of the estrogen study findings, the lesson took on more importance. In the ill-fated epidemiological studies, regular ongoing estrogen use over several years was probably a *marker* for other behaviors that actually do prevent heart disease. The women who quit taking estrogen after only a few months landed in the "non–current user" category in those observational studies. They may also have been inconstant users of their blood pressure medication, their cholesterol-lowering medication, and their treadmills. Even the studies that attempted to control for heart disease risk factors apparently missed such subtle but clearly important differences. This is known in epidemiology as "residual confounding," the methodological equivalent of dressing elegantly for a formal dinner party and leaving your zipper wide open.

The tens of thousands of extra breast cancers, pulmonary emboli, strokes, and other drug-related side effects that were caused by the use of estrogens in millions of women didn't have to happen. Together, they amount to one of the largest epidemics of drug-induced illness in modern times. This raises disturbing questions that will be addressed throughout the book. How do we know whether a drug actually works as intended? How are its adverse events monitored and addressed? What benefits justify what risks? What should companies be required to prove about the effectiveness and hazards of their products? How does our massive regulatory apparatus decide which drug effects will be studied, and by whom? How do we physicians make prescribing decisions, and from where do we get our information? Who if anyone is responsible for looking out for how well or carelessly drugs are being prescribed?

In the 1970s and 1980s, hormone replacement therapy was the poster child for the brave new world that modern pharmacology was making possible. By the start of the present century, it had become a symbol for the excesses and lapses that can mark the darker side of prescription drug use in America. If HRT is an example of how things can go wrong in determining whether a drug works or not, it can also teach us a great deal about the tools we can use to get these vital questions right.

Before leaving the story of estrogens and heart disease, a small amendment to the historical record is necessary. It's not quite accurate to imply that no large-scale trials of estrogen's effect on the heart were published before 1998. In fact, a well-designed clinical study was conducted as far back as the 1950s. It sought to determine whether patients assigned to take long-term estrogen would have fewer heart attacks than those randomized to placebo. That study clearly demonstrated that estrogens conferred no protection on the heart, but did cause side effects that made the approach too dangerous to use clinically. Its conclusive findings put an end to the use of estrogens for this purpose in the patient group in which they were tested—men.

2: LEAVING THE DARK AGES
BEHIND, MOSTLY

> When it came to the plague, sufferers were treated by
> various measures designed to draw poison or infection
> from the body: by bleeding, purging with laxatives or
> enemas, lancing or cauterizing the buboes, or applica-
> tion of hot plasters. . . . Medicines ranged from pills of
> powdered stag's horn or myrrh and saffron, to potions
> of potable gold. Compounds of rare spices and pow-
> dered pearls or emeralds were prescribed, possibly on
> the theory, not unknown to modern medicine, that a
> patient's sense of therapeutic value is in proportion to
> the expense.
>
> —BARBARA TUCHMAN,
> *A Distant Mirror*

How quaint. How . . . *medieval.* The estrogen debacle was unsettling because we take it for granted that prescription medications
will work as expected, just as we assume that when we turn on the
tap to get a drink there won't be any sewage in the water, when we accelerate
to eighty on the interstate we won't find a five-foot pothole around the next
bend, and when we make a bank deposit the money will still be there when
we go to withdraw it. Thanks to the daily intrusion of big government into
our lives, these safeguards usually work with reassuring precision—so well
that we have come to accept them as natural. But there is nothing natural or
automatic about what lies behind them.

Water purification, highway construction, the supervision of financial markets, and the regulation of drugs are all complicated, unnatural, active processes. They don't happen spontaneously; each requires a vast infrastructure of continuous public- and private-sector interaction to function. When this works well, it is testimony to the complexity of these processes, not to their simplicity. It's only when a rent occurs in this delicate fabric— an outbreak of waterborne infection, a collapsed overpass, a failed bank, a drug that kills—that the public gets a fleeting glimpse of the awesome machinery that is usually at work preventing such disasters. The aberrant event is condemned, analyzed, corrected, and then forgotten, until the next one. But the delicate mechanisms that prevented thousands of other similar events from occurring continue to hum along on background in the hard drive of society—silently, invisibly, and usually effectively.

In this chapter, we will look at what lies behind the assumption that the prescription drugs prescribed and taken in such large volumes in the United States actually work better than powdered stag's horn or rare spices—an assumption that is usually correct. Surprisingly, our ability to be sure about this most basic attribute of medicines is both recent and fragile. The hormone replacement example reminds us how easily this process can go wrong. It goes right more often, and how that happens is even more interesting.

IT WAS ONLY fairly recently—the second half of the twentieth century—that rigorous evaluation of drug therapies became routine. What passed for pharmacology during all of human history before that was summed up well by a physician in the late nineteenth century: "I firmly believe that if the whole *materia medica* [all available drugs] could be sunk to the bottom of the sea, it would be all the better for mankind, and all the worse for the fishes." This judgment was not made by some Victorian-era Ralph Nader but by the dean of Harvard Medical School, Oliver Wendell Holmes, father of the Supreme Court justice.

Holmes' insight accurately reflected the quality of the drugs of his day: most were potions of uncertain composition and unproven effectiveness. They were sold by individual practitioners, hucksters, or small companies, unencumbered by any requirement that the products had to work, had to contain what they claimed to contain, or were nontoxic. Only a few of the compounds used in medicine at the beginning of the twentieth century did anything useful: morphine and its derivatives (extracted from poppies) to relieve pain, digitalis leaf (from the foxglove plant) for an ailing heart, aspirin (from willow bark) for fever and inflammation, and a handful of others. It's been estimated that during this time, the average patient consulting the average physician had only about a fifty-fifty chance of benefiting from the encounter. Voltaire's insight still prevailed: a prescription was something prescribed by the doctor while waiting for nature to cure the illness.

Things are dramatically different today. As we saw in the Prologue, judicious use of anticoagulants in patients with atrial fibrillation can reduce the risk of stroke by two thirds. For patients with osteoporosis who are at high risk of breaking a hip, medications to strengthen the bones can cut the chance of that devastating outcome by half. Antipsychotic medications have helped to empty the nation's state mental hospitals, and enable many schizophrenics to lead lives that are at least functional, and sometimes almost normal. Putting a heart attack patient on a drug of the beta-blocker class will markedly lower the chance of death in the following year. Prescribing an ACE-inhibitor medication to a diabetic will slow the development of the kidney failure that is so common in these patients; the same drugs will also lower the death rate in patients with congestive heart failure. Antibiotics have transformed infections that were once universally fatal into brief hospitalizations or, increasingly, conditions that can be managed at home.

The litany is a long one, and we can only touch on its highlights here. Our successes have been greatest in diseases of the heart and blood vessels. Using medications to lower blood pressure reduces the risk of stroke by 35–40 percent, and of heart attack by about 25–30 percent. In patients with cardiac disease, drugs that lower cholesterol also reduce the risk of heart attack by 20–30 percent and of stroke (in patients under seventy) by about 17 percent. The humble aspirin, in doses so low as to be once thought homeopathic, can cut the rate of heart attack by a third in susceptible patients, and of stroke by 16 percent. So great are the cardiovascular benefits of medications, and so ample is the evidence of their effectiveness, that two British doctors recently proposed with complete seriousness that a standardized "polypill" combination containing many of these ingredients should be concocted and administered routinely to everyone over age fifty-five. Drawing on scores of previous studies, they calculated that doing so could reduce heart attacks, strokes, and cardiac deaths by an astonishing 80 percent or more. While their proposal was controversial, it gave testimony to the magnitude of benefit we have come to expect of medications, as well as the wealth of data available on which to base such recommendations.

How do we know all this, and how did we get there?

A COGNITIVE REVOLUTION

The idea that treatments have to be proven effective before they can be used is a remarkably new invention. Even today, prescription medications are one of the few medical interventions that have to meet this standard. In the operating room, new surgical procedures can be introduced without anyone having to prove that they are better than older operations, or even that they work at all. As late as 2002, a widely used orthopedic procedure, knee surgery performed through a fiberoptic endoscope, was found to be no better than a sham operation in relieving patients' joint pain. Psychotherapy has had a similarly bumpy history of unevaluated outcomes. Only recently with the advent of the newer antidepressants have psychiatrists and psychologists conducted respectable trials to pit their skills against the pills—with modest results for both sides. The medical device industry has traditionally faced lower hurdles than the drug industry in winning FDA approval. A manufacturer must show that the device isn't dangerous, which is a nice idea, but if it can be depicted as similar to other devices already approved for the same purpose, the company may not be required to demonstrate how well a new product actually works.

Elsewhere in medicine, laboratory and radiological tests do not have to meet any tough criteria of clinical usefulness. The recent fad of whole-body CAT scanning, shamelessly promoted to find Early Evidence of Bad Things Hidden Inside, has become a lucrative service provided to patients who have too much money to spend on medical care. These costly tests have themselves spread like rapidly metastatic tumors, in the absence of data that they do anything except increase the median income of radiologists. Even after decades of use of the respected mammogram, we are still trying to figure out which patients actually benefit from it. And in 1994 the nation took a great leap backward in freeing the makers of over-the-counter "supplements" from the bothersome constraints of both science and honesty in hawking their wares.

Prescription drugs thus occupy a special position in the pantheon of medical interventions. An idea that we take for granted so readily today—that a medication must be proven to work before it can be marketed—was a long time in coming. For most of the history of medicine, what physicians knew about medications was based more on received wisdom than on experimental data. For the hundreds of years that medical practice was dominated by the ancient teachings of Galen, an apprentice physician was not expected to understand data from experiments, but to memorize concepts and recipes based on arcane humoral relationships, regurgitating the same wrong ideas that had been passed down from physician to apprentice over the generations. This uncritical spirit underlay much of therapeutics until the beginning of the twentieth century, and vestiges of it survive today in some quarters.

Our modern approach to prescription drugs is the product of two historical streams that came together only recently. The first was the political evolution that gave governments the authority to decide what products could be sold as medicines and how they could be promoted. The second was the scientific evolution that accorded experimental data priority over received wisdom. Both trends reached their zeniths at the end of the twentieth century, and both are now under attack.

GIVING GOVERNMENT CLOUT

Responding to the travesties of a completely unfettered marketplace, the Progressive movement of the early 1900s called for the establishment of minimum standards to regulate the quality of foods and drugs that Americans consume. The Pure Food and Drug Act of 1906 marked the first official recognition that the wholesomeness of what people put into their bodies was too important to be left exclusively to the haphazard control of unregulated commerce. At this early stage, purity was the main concern; it would be several decades before the nation was ready to involve government in determining whether medications had any useful effects, or whether their inevitable risks were worth incurring to achieve that effectiveness.

A further requirement, that those ingredients be nonlethal, was not put into place until more than three decades later. In 1937, over a hundred patients died—many of them children—after taking a sulfanilamide product that had been manufactured with a toxic solvent. In the wake of this tragedy, named the Massengill Massacre after the company that produced the tainted drug, Congress strengthened the Pure Food and Drug Act to allow the federal government to require that drug products not be poisonous. But there was still no requirement that the drugs needed to work. That criterion was resisted for decades by manufacturers who successfully lobbied against the idea, depicting it as unbearably onerous government regulation of the free market. The notion was put forward again by Senator Estes Kefauver of Tennessee in the early 1960s. His bill was headed for certain legislative defeat in a Congress that was convinced government had no business intruding into commercial transactions among drug companies, physicians, and patients. Languishing on Capitol Hill, the Kefauver legislation was saved by another tragedy.

Thalidomide was being widely used overseas as a sedative and antinauseant, and was particularly popular among pregnant women. Its approval in the United States had been slowed by a diligent FDA medical officer named Dr. Frances Kelsey, who wasn't convinced that the manufacturer had adequately demonstrated its safety. The struggle was portrayed by many in the drug industry as another instance of a boneheaded, inept federal regulator unnecessarily delaying the availability of an important new product to the American public. Then reports began to appear in Europe of babies born with grotesque abnormalities of their arms and legs. Instead of normally formed limbs, the affected infants grew little malformed appendages that resembled flippers. Because this was such a rare aberration, it didn't take long to determine that the mothers had something in common: they had all taken thalidomide during the first trimester of their pregnancies, the period during which the basic architecture of the limbs is laid down in the developing fetus. Dr. Kelsey was transformed from an anonymous bumbling bureaucrat to a legendary public servant who saved untold numbers of American families from needless misery.

It suddenly seemed plausible that a government agency could protect the public health by evaluating drugs, and the Kefauver Act was passed by Congress in 1962 without a dissenting vote. This was a watershed in the nation's approach to medications, and an important development for the science of pharmacology as well. The new law completely changed the way doctors and patients thought about drugs. For the first time, the federal government, through the Food and Drug Administration, could require that a prescription medication had to be proven effective before it could be sold as a drug in the United States.

But what, exactly, does "effective" mean?

In 1962, armed with its new powers, the FDA faced a marketplace full of existing medicines that had never been shown to work, or were bizarre combinations of products whose use in tandem had little pharmacologic rationale. So great was the entrenchment of useless products in American medicine that it would take over twenty years to fully implement this new evidentiary requirement for drugs already in use. Like the oversized jet-fin appendages on the backs of late-1950s cars, many of those products had been seen as important modern developments in their day:

- Marax, a combination asthma medication whose original formulation included bronchodilators to open constricted airways, which made sense, along with barbiturates, potentially addictive respiratory depressants, which did not.
- Bellergal, a combination product containing doses of stimulants and sedatives in amounts too small to have any physiological effect, marketed primarily for treating hypochondriacal women.
- a combination of estrogen and tranquilizer, in case the Bellergal didn't work.
- antibiotic combinations containing streptomycin, often used to treat sore throats and colds. Such combinations fostered the development of bacterial resistance, and the unnecessary streptomycin occasionally caused permanent deafness.

• Pavabid, a preparation made from the by-products of morphine production, heavily promoted for its ability to open up blood vessels in the brain to restore mental functioning to senile patients. It has never been shown to work.

Powdered pearls were not on the list.

To clean up this swamp of useless and occasionally dangerous nostrums, the FDA launched DESI, the Drug Efficacy Study Implementation program, soon after passage of the Kefauver Act. Through DESI, the FDA commissioned studies of the several thousand products on the market that had no discernible evidence of usefulness. The task turned out to be more difficult and time-consuming than many had expected. Years after its inception, the DESI program was still trying to persuade scores of manufacturers to produce evidence that specific daffy products were better than a sugar pill for any purpose whatsoever. Many companies were understandably slow in responding to this challenge, putting the FDA in a bind: Should these evidence-free drugs be summarily removed from the market, or should the companies be given year after year to conduct the clinical trials needed to determine whether they worked or not? The procrastinators prevailed, and the FDA had to come up with a new categorization for such limbo drugs, to be listed in the small print of their promotional materials: *"The Food and Drug Administration has determined that this product is 'possibly effective.'"* The nonbureaucratic translation for "possibly effective": "There is not a shred of solid evidence on the entire planet Earth that this drug is of any use whatsoever for any purpose known to man or beast, but the manufacturer has successfully demanded additional years to study it, and we don't have the political clout to take it off the market until that unbearably lengthy foot-dragging process has run its course."

The DESI program finally finished its work more than two decades later in the mid-1980s, ending the painful adolescence of American drug therapy. Over two thousand pharmaceutical zits had been squeezed out or dried up by themselves. A small number of bad products managed to escape the process, like the PPA (phenylpropanolamine) cold remedies that caused Ethel Coryza's stroke. But for the most part, the new authority given to the FDA in 1962 meant that from that time on, pharmaceutical products had to be proven to work before they could be marketed. No more would the American public be subjected to groundless claims for totally useless products promoted for use in arthritis or senility or cancer or liver disease. Never again—until the mid-1990s.

The adoption of this requirement of efficacy, and the start of our slide back toward sloppier standards for some products, comprise one of the great intellectual and public policy adventures of modern times. It took a

struggle that lasted for generations to wrest our understanding of therapeutics from the dead grip of received wisdom and place it in the more
agile hands of experimental science. But why is it so difficult to distinguish
drugs that work from those that don't? It seems intuitive: Patients given
effective treatments will get better and patients given ineffective treatments
won't, right? And shouldn't we be able to predict which treatments will
work based on known principles of physiology and pharmacology? No on
both counts.

THE SCIENTIFIC EVOLUTION

The second transformation, the conceptual shift that gave priority to experimental science, proved even more difficult than the political one. As hard
as it was to develop a governmental infrastructure to regulate prescription
drugs, it took even longer to build the scientific infrastructure that would be
needed to guide those new powers.

The apparently simple task of determining whether a drug *really works*
turned out to be dauntingly complex. To begin with, many diseases have
trajectories that are hard to predict. A host of illnesses from ulcers to
influenza to depression often get better on their own whatever the patient
or doctor does. "My doctor gave me these pills, and my symptoms were
gone in a week!" A good thing—otherwise the problem would have taken
seven days to resolve.

Even treatments that work may be only partially effective. Or they may
work extremely well, but only for a particular variant of the disease. Think
of penicillin-type antibiotics, which have impressive powers to cure one
type of bacterial pneumonia but are less effective in pneumonias caused by
different kinds of bacteria, and useless in pneumonias caused by viruses.
Does penicillin "work" in treating pneumonia? Yes, maybe, and no,
depending upon what the infectious organism is. This was a particularly
challenging problem before we were able to distinguish one kind of microbe
from another: a century ago, we knew only that these patients had bad
lung infections with high fever and a sputum-producing cough, and often
died. As a result, even the most astute clinician observing which patients
improved on particular therapies would have had a hard time picking out
the ones that were truly effective. Similar confusions today bedevil our
attempts to discover drugs in oncology because of our inability to distinguish among the different causes of malignancy, referring to them all somewhat simplemindedly as "cancers." The same ignorance applies to our
medieval understanding of the different causes (and therefore treatments)
for the "depressions." Even for a given disease, we are learning that patients

with different genetic characteristics will respond differently to the same drug.

Another problem in determining whether a given drug works is the well-known placebo effect, from the Latin for "I will please." This is one of the commonest causes of symptomatic improvement in conditions in which the patient's subjective state plays a key role. The list of such diseases is long and includes angina, anxiety, arthritis, asthma, depression, dyspepsia, headache, insomnia, itching, menstrual symptoms, and diverse other kinds of pain. The placebo effect owes part of its impressive power to the human tendency to see causal relationships even where they don't exist, a phenomenon well known in cognitive psychology and in philosophy—recall the fallacy of *post hoc, ergo propter hoc:* "After this, therefore because of this." I gave the patient an herbal poultice on Monday, and by Friday he was better. It must have been the poultice.

Things become even more complicated when we realize that the placebo effect also has a real physiological dimension. As a military physician during World War II, Harvard anesthesiologist Henry Beecher cared for men who sustained horrific wounds that guaranteed them a respite from combat. He was struck with the soldiers' capacity to tolerate these severe injuries even before they received any painkiller. The observation led to Beecher's lifelong study of the body's ability to control the sensation of pain. Years later, neuroscientists discovered that the brain can synthesize its own endogenous versions of morphine, which were named endorphins. Some wondered whether these substances might be related to the capacity for self-analgesia that Beecher observed, or the relief so commonly reported by subjects who are given placebo pills in pain studies.

Naloxone is a drug that blocks the brain effects of opioids (the substances that include narcotics such as morphine, heroin, and cocaine) as well as the body's own endorphins. A pivotal paper published in the British journal *Lancet* in 1978 placed the once touchy-feely placebo effect firmly in the realm of hard-science neuropharmacology. The study started out as a typical pain experiment: volunteers were given an inert placebo and, as expected, a substantial proportion of them reported that it reduced their pain. But when these subjects were given the opioid blocker naloxone, it blocked the placebo benefit as well. This suggested that the placebo effect results in part from a person's capacity to secrete homemade narcotics within the brain itself.

More recent studies using sophisticated imaging techniques took this line of inquiry even further. In a study of pain sensation reported in *Science* in 2002, a Swedish team mapped areas of brain activity in volunteers who were given either an injection of a morphine-type drug, an injection of placebo, or no treatment at all. Those who responded to the placebo showed activation of the same brain area as those who received the narcotic medication, suggesting that morphine and placebo may exert their pain-relieving effect through a common neural pathway. To further research in this area, the National Institutes of Health recently initiated an interdisci-plinary grant program, "The Science of the Placebo." This expanding area of research has profound implications for how we study medications and how we decide whether or not they work.

If an inert substance can trigger specific neurochemical events that then produce clinical effects, it gives new meaning to the once-dismissive phrase "It's all in your head." And even without invoking neurochemistry, we know that the placebo effect is also accompanied by more old-fashioned psychological processes like expectation and conditioning. The more a medicine may be helped along by the patient's own capacity to experience relief, the more we need to measure whether a new drug is truly better than a sugar pill. If not, we could just prescribe the sugar pill. After all, it's an affordable product with an enviable safety record.

A POWERFUL TOOL EMERGES

In assessing drugs, the forces of confusion have a lot on their side: the unpredictable and self-limited nature of many diseases, the diversity of their underlying causes, the variability in how well any given treatment works, and the patient's tendency to experience benefit from inert sub-stances. Little wonder that for millennia, medicine was a random collection, of bogus remedies whose uselessness was exceeded only by the confidence that both healers and patients placed in them. People recovered from many illnesses no matter what was done for them, and the occasional treatments that actually worked didn't work all the time. In this prescientific environ-ment, we had no way to distinguish the few things that were effective from the majority that were not—a recipe for pharmacological chaos. What was missing was a systematic way to evaluate a given treatment—not to deter-mine whether it *makes sense,* since most ineffective treatments make sense in one system of thought or another, but whether it actually *works.* Consid-ering how obvious this approach is, it is astonishing what a small role it played in medicine's first several thousand years, and how vulnerable it is even today.

The first recorded clinical trial was an evaluation of the currently popu-lar Mediterranean diet. Its results weren't published in a medical journal, but in the Bible, in the first chapter of the Book of Daniel. After conquer-ing Jerusalem, the Babylonian king Nebuchadnezzar ordered the master of his eunuchs, Ashpenaz, to go find some nice smart Jewish boys and make them royal advisers. During their training they were to be nourished from the king's own stores of meat and wine. Among those chosen were Daniel and his three pals, who were redesignated Shadrach, Meshach, and Abednego so their old-country names wouldn't limit their career advancement. Daniel drew the line at another kind of assimilation: he refused to defile himself with the king's *traif* food during the three-year internship. The bureaucrat Ashpenaz worried that if he replaced the royally prescribed regimen with a less effective generic substitute, he could get into big trouble: "I fear that my Lord the King, who allotted food and drink to you, will notice that you look out of sorts, unlike the other youths of your age—and you will put my life in jeopardy with the king."

Daniel had been selected because he was "cunning in knowledge and understanding in science," so he proposed an experiment to the master of the eunuchs, whom we can consider the biblical equivalent of today's Food and Drug Administration:

> "Please test your servants for ten days, giving us legumes to eat and water to drink. Then compare our appearance with that of the youths who eat of the king's food, and do with [us] as you see fit." He agreed to this plan of theirs, and tested them for ten days. When the ten days were over, they looked better and healthier than all the youths who were eating of the king's food. So the guard kept on removing their [royal] food and the wine they were supposed to drink, and gave them legumes.

When the four were eventually presented to the king, they made a very good impression and were given tenure in the royal service. In the years that followed, perhaps because of Daniel's methodological savvy, the king "found them to be ten times better than all the magicians and exorcists throughout his realm." One suspects that they were subjected to ongoing harassment by the Babylonian food and beverage industries, but the Bible is silent on this point.

If I were asked to peer-review the experiment of Daniel et al., I'd quibble with some aspects of their study design: there may have been baseline differences between the subjects and the controls, they were not allocated to treatment groups randomly, the outcome measures ("looking out of sorts") were not precisely specified *a priori*, and there is no mention of obtaining informed consent from the subjects or approval of the project by an institutional review board. But these are small objections when we consider that it was the first clinical trial ever done.

Despite the power of this method, such commonsense evaluation was mostly disregarded over the next two thousand years of scientific thought. The cool gaze of science can feel threatening to an authority-based system of knowledge, and it's bad for business if you're a shaman or a purgative salesman. In part because of such opposition, medicine for the most part forgot about the experimental approach to therapeutics for nearly two millennia. Throughout that time, treatments continued to be based primarily on authoritative texts and expert opinion, both of which were usually wrong.

Another exclamation point in the punctuated evolution of therapeutic thinking didn't come until the Enlightenment. It resulted from the work of a Scottish naval physician named James Lind (1716–1794). Serving on the royal warship *Salisbury,* Lind regularly saw sailors getting sick and dying of scurvy, a very common illness among seamen of his time. We now know that the condition results from a dietary deficiency of vitamin C, but nothing was known of vitamins then, nor of the cause of the disease. Its victims bled into their gums and muscles, developed purplish skin lesions, and wasted away. Treatments abounded, but none had any impact on the course of the illness. I first learned about Lind's work during a medical meeting in Edinburgh. Our group was given a tour of the exquisite Georgian building housing that city's Royal College of Physicians and its remarkable library. The works of Vesalius, Lister, and Audubon were reverently displayed in sealed glass cases like saintly relics in a cathedral. A local member of our group pointed out one first edition with special pride: Lind's 1753 masterwork, *A Treatise on the Scurvy.* "The Scots invented the clinical trial, you know," he observed. (My Scottish friends often point out that some indispensable aspect of modern life was invented by a Scot, and often they're right.) Apart from Daniel's biblical health food experiment, the claim has something going for it. Stuck aboard a long sea cruise with 350 men who predictably began to suffer and die of scurvy, Lind devised one of the first systematic experiments in the history of medicine:

> On the 20th of May 1747, I took twelve patients in the scurvy on board the Salisbury at sea. Their cases were as similar as I could have them. They all in general had putrid gums, the spots and lassitude, with weakness of their knees . . . and had one diet common to all.

Lind's breakthrough was his decision to assign the twelve men arbitrarily to six different kinds of treatment: he put two each on a regimen of either cider, elixir vitriol, seawater, vinegar, oranges and lemons, or a purgative made of nutmeg, garlic, mustard seed, myrrh, barley water, and tamarind. (This last recipe turned out not to do much for the scurvy, but in a smaller dose it would probably make a great vinaigrette for an endive-and-watercress salad.) The old book in the glass case at the Royal College contained Lind's description of what he found:

They continued six days under this course. . . . The consequence was that the most sudden and visible good effects were perceived from the use of the oranges and lemons; one of those who had taken them being at the end of the six days fit for duty. . . . The other was the best recovered of any in his condition; and being now deemed pretty well, was appointed nurse to the rest of the sick.

The fruit, rich in vitamin C, cured the sailors' nutritional deficiency, even though it would take more than a century before anyone understood the biochemistry involved. Lind's discovery led the British admiralty to supply its ships with ample quantities of citrus fruits on each voyage, helping to bring an end to scurvy at sea and giving rise to the appellation "Limey" for Englishmen. (The lime also proved to be a fine complement to the plant-derived quinine extract the British began to prescribe in other parts of the empire to prevent and treat malaria; this nutraceutical was most enjoyably consumed as gin and tonic.)

Another legacy of Lind's discovery is a website the Royal College of Edinburgh launched in his honor, a modern monument to the clinical trial and the evidence-based medicine movement. It offers teaching materials for physicians, historians, and even schoolchildren about how treatments are evaluated, "to introduce people to the characteristics of fair tests, and to illustrate how these tests have evolved." In the 250th year after Lind's publication, the Royal College scheduled a commemorative James Lind Symposium to mark its anniversary: "From Scurvy to Clinical Guidelines: How Can Clinical Research Lead to Better Patient Care?"

TESTING THE CURE

It is hard to know which is more amazing: the power and simplicity of the experimental approach pioneered by Lind or its neglect over the next two hundred years. Even today, it is an ongoing struggle to separate the wheat of important medicinal breakthroughs from the chaff of ineffective treatments. To see how these issues play out in contemporary medicine, we can return to Barbara Tuchman's example of powdered staghorn for the treatment of plague, cited at the start of this chapter. Unlike its metaphorical namesake or the famous epidemic that precipitated the Hebrews' escape from Egypt, the real plague is a specific disease caused by the bacterium *Yersinia pestis*. As the Black Death, it laid waste to millions throughout Europe in the fourteenth and fifteenth centuries.

Updating Tuchman, we can explore the issue of drug efficacy by picturing a modern attempt to figure out which products on her list of treatments might actually work against the plague. Let's put a team of medieval alchemists in a time machine and drop them into the present. We can imagine that researchers at a contemporary university-based lab have been funded by the National Institutes of Health to explore a new compound they isolated from the antlers of stags, and that there is some biochemical evidence it might be effective against *Yersinia pestis* and could therefore be a valuable weapon in the treatment of plague. Conceptually, this is no more far-fetched than the idea of drugs extracted from African tree frogs, Pacific yew trees, or the venom of snakes, all of which have given rise to modern medications in wide use today. Consider yourself one of the alchemists who becomes CEO of a new biotech start-up we can call Stagogen, developed to commercialize the researchers' product. (This is not that big a stretch either; in the go-go days of the 1990s biotech feeding frenzy, Galen himself could probably have gotten some start-up funding from venture capitalists with a good enough story.)

Before the new product can be marketed, Stagogen will have to present the FDA with convincing evidence that its product actually works as promised. Your investors sink millions of dollars into Stagogen to conduct the costly and risky studies necessary to take a promising basic science finding "from [laboratory] bench to bedside." They are becoming worried about the company's burn rate; the firm has already gone through $120 million for its initial work on toxicology and pharmacokinetics. A marketing firm charged another $250,000 to come up with the product's new trade name, Lifehorn. (The company pointed out that this would be easy to work into a direct-to-consumer advertising campaign, and could also lead to a synergistic sell-through if the drug were ever marketed over-the-counter.) But there is still no date set for product launch, not to mention the coveted initial public offering. If you want a second round of funding to conduct the expensive clinical trials necessary for the product's further development, you'll need a clear plan for studies that will convince the FDA that your new drug works.

Despite encouraging evidence at the molecular level and a few small studies in mice, you have no proof yet that this will be a useful medication for people who have contracted the plague. You need to demonstrate that your staghorn product works better than those other recent commercial disasters, myrrh enemas and powdered pearls. (The guys who ran those start-ups are now washing test tubes at Merck.) But you have one important advantage over your medieval predecessors: you will be able to make use of a remarkable tool that can distinguish the few therapies that work from the many that do not.

This technology is not a computer program or a laboratory procedure or a high-tech genetic test or a new discovery from the cutting edge of molecular biology. Its potency does not depend on anything material at all: no microscopes, no reagents, no test tubes, no lab animals. It is simply a way of thinking very carefully and clearly about the problem at hand, *a way of asking the question*. It is the randomized controlled trial, or RCT, and in the last fifty years it has transformed the way we understand medications. The RCT is nothing less than the single most important development in the revolution of modern therapeutics, the most powerful intellectual medicine we have—the one that makes all the others possible. It takes a little while to appreciate the enormous power of this tool; like Newton's laws of motion, the concept is both breathtakingly simple and enormously strong. Yet each of its distinguishing characteristics is the product of decades of conceptual evolution.

The single most important element here is the idea of *randomly assigning* patients to receive different treatments. Before the RCT, an experimenting physician might choose to give a new therapy primarily to patients who seemed the most likely to be cured; or to those who would comply best with directions for its use; or to those for whom he felt a special fondness; or to those with the smallest number of other complicating conditions; or perhaps to those who were so desperately ill that an untested new treatment would seem morally justifiable. Yet any of these selection rules would lead to a distorted assessment of its effectiveness.

It took centuries to figure out that the assignment of a patient to the experimental drug or a dummy pill must be done on a completely random basis. What matters most is that there be no human choice in determining who gets which treatment. In modern randomized trials, once a patient has agreed to participate in a study, the physician opens a sealed envelope or calls the study's coordinating center or logs on to the internet to find out whether the next patient in the study has *already* been randomly assigned to Treatment A or Treatment B—in this case, powdered staghorn or placebo. For the sake of our exercise, we'll assume that there is no known effective treatment for the variant of plague we're trying to treat, so there is no ethical problem in randomizing some patients to a dummy pill.

Referring to the patients randomized to placebo as the *control group* suggests the power this design gives us over the data. The French clinical literature uses the word *témoin* (witness) to refer to the untreated subject—an equally compelling image. Giving all subjects some kind of inert pill or injection can control for the placebo response as a cause of any salutary outcomes that might occur, since all subjects would be equally likely to think they were being treated. This also helps in evaluating side effects because of a parallel phenomenon called the nocebo response (from the root for "noxious"), in which a patient experiences new symptoms that are blamed on the treatment, even though it may be a completely inactive substance.

For the power of randomization to work best and the placebo effect to be tamed, it is vital that the patient not know which treatment he or she is getting: both must appear identical. Hence the practice of "blinding"— requiring that the patient be kept in the dark about whether he is getting the experimental treatment or the dummy pill. Good trial form further requires that a study be *double*-blinded, with the experimenter also unaware of who is receiving which treatment. Why can't a dispassionate researcher be let in on the plot? In a sense, the placebo effect can be contagious. Over the millennia, it was not just the patient on the receiving end of the chants, poultices, enemas, or incisions who believed in the effectiveness of these treatments. Their power was also perceived by the chant-singing, poultice-applying, enema-administering, or incision-making healer as well. Some of this surely derives from the delusion of self-efficacy referred to earlier, and some from the innate human desire felt by most of us (particularly those of us who went into medicine) to believe that we are making a difference in alleviating patients' suffering. A new and different reason has been added in the last decade or two, perhaps the most powerful of all: the physician conducting the study may have financial ties to the company whose product is being tested. This provides yet another reason for clinical trials to be conducted with a rigorous double-blind design.

I always thought of the term "double-blind" as benign-sounding, no worse than "venetian blind" or "duck blind." But it has different associations for my colleagues in ophthalmology, apparently evoking images of Helen Keller or Oedipus instead. In submitting a grant proposal to the National Eye Institute of NIH, I was politely but firmly told that in eye research, one describes patients and physicians as being "masked" rather than "blinded" to treatment-group assignment. No such sensitivities arise in plague research, so we can continue to use the conventional nomenclature. Throughout our imaginary clinical trial, both physician and patient will remain unaware of who is receiving the dummy pill versus the powdered staghorn. For the researcher, barring a need-to-know medical emergency, the blinding will come to an end only after the last pieces of data have been collected, protecting us from the possibility that such knowledge might somehow contaminate our interpretation of the clinical outcomes. The patient may never be told at all.

SKEPTICISM AS METHODOLOGY

To understand the power of the RCT, it helps to touch on the work of the philosopher of science Karl Popper. He understood that the real strength of modern science lies in what might be called its negative attitude; we make progress, he argued, by describing a new discovery in a way that enables someone to try to refute it. The history of medicine is littered with insightful breakthrough discoveries that turned out not to be true. The really indispensable ingredient is "the null hypothesis": the assumption that a particular new idea is incorrect. Obtuse as it sounds, the approach is remarkably efficient in making sure that any new discovery passes an intense scientific hazing before it is admitted into the fraternity of true facts.

Such a posture is the opposite of our legal system, traditionally based instead on the presumption of innocence. At least until the post-9/11 USA Patriot Act, every inquiry into a criminal charge began with the assumption that the accused did nothing wrong; it then becomes the prosecution's job to prove beyond a reasonable doubt that the defendant is guilty. By contrast, the genius of modern drug testing comes from its presumption of impotence. The design and analysis of the clinical trial test the assumption that the drug does not work, and it is up to the investigator to demonstrate beyond a reasonable doubt ("statistical significance") that the product is not useless. We could call this the power of negative thinking. It has made all the difference in the world in pharmacology, and explains why so few doctors still prescribe myrrh.

Comparing clinical trial thinking with legal thinking provides other insights into the logic of drug testing. A criminal justice system that starts out with an assumption of guilt could win more convictions, but it would also punish more innocents. Older systems of drug evaluation that began by assuming that a new treatment was effective (often because it Made So Much Sense) gave credentials to large numbers of useless products, some of which were also toxic. Each kind of decision rule imposes its own risks. In the law, assuming innocence means that an occasional guilty person will inadvertently be set free; in medicine, assuming impotence means that occasionally an effective drug will be mistakenly thought not to work. In both cases, society chooses which risk it prefers in order to avoid the greater evils: imprisoning an innocent person, accepting an ineffective drug. The Constitution's protection against double jeopardy guarantees that a guilty person who is mistakenly found innocent can never be retried for the same crime. But in medicine we get a second chance. A drug initially thought to be ineffective can be revisited again and again, subjected to more careful investigation, and eventually brought into the fold of proven therapies with full credentials if it passes muster on a subsequent try.

Beyond any analogy with jurisprudence, this way of thinking about drug efficacy also makes a remarkably good fit with American notions of both government and economics. The ancient view that authority and history are the best guides to therapeutic effectiveness fit well with centralized, nondemocratic governments, and also meshed nicely with economies rooted in aristocratic ownership and entrenched control. By contrast, for our modern approach to assessing new drugs, in principle all that is sacrosanct is the rules of the game—the randomized controlled trial, methodological rigor in its conduct, and generally accepted statistical analysis. As long as one plays by those rules, anybody with a good idea and a new product can, in theory at least, break onto the scene and demonstrate the worth of a new treatment, or demolish the time-honored credibility of an established one.

This way of thinking has had a bracing effect on how we view drugs. Galen's concepts had credibility not because of how well they performed (they did poorly) but because of where they came from and who believed in them. For hundreds of years, this veneration of received wisdom in pharmacology produced a flabby, useless aristocracy of treatments. Like the scions of landed dynasties whose power derived from lineage rather than talent, scientific ideas grandfathered into the canon took up conceptual space and kept out spunky upstarts—intruder discoveries that might have been effective, but just didn't come from the right families. I wade into the free-for-all of this democracy of ideas every time I teach our medical students, or supervise one of the clinical services at the teaching hospital where I work. I may be on the faculty, legally responsible as the physician of record for a ward full of patients, and in practice twenty-five years longer than some of my trainees. But any one of them can challenge my recommendation of a given treatment by citing a clinical trial from this week's *New England Journal of Medicine* that shows the drug I suggested is less effective or more toxic than another. *Veritas* usually trumps *gravitas*. Of course, this is an idealized view. The interplay between pharmacology and free enterprise sometimes brings out the worst rather than the best of each, as we will see in subsequent chapters. But it should be possible to tame those excesses without having to throw out the baby with the snake oil.

The RCT tool can take us far in our quest to determine whether the imaginary Lifehorn works. But even after the clinical trials are completed, our product will still have to pass one more hurdle before it can be approved for use. Understanding this step is crucial for anyone who ever prescribes, takes, or pays for any medication, or knows anyone who has.

Rare is the medication that can transform a moribund patient into a leaping, praising clinical triumph; most of the time the difference between success and failure is far more subtle. What if the clinical trial of our new plague drug finds that 60 percent of patients randomized to get the experimental medication survive, compared to 40 percent of those who got the placebo? Does that mean that the new drug *works*?

If at this point you answered, "Of course it does!" then consider the following: What if there were twenty plague patients in the trial, with ten randomized to receive powdered staghorn and ten placebo? At the end of the study, six of the ten in the staghorn group are still alive (60 percent), with the other four in this group dead of the plague. On the other hand, in the placebo group, four of the ten are still alive (a 40 percent survival rate) and six dead of the plague. Now, take a penny and a quarter. The quarter will be the new staghorn product; flip it ten times and count how often it comes up heads (we'll consider that survival) or tails (death). Then take the penny, which will represent the placebo treatment, and flip it ten times as well. It would not be surprising to find that the quarter had a "survival rate" (landed heads) six, or seven, or even nine times out of the ten flips. But the impact of this observation might be less convincing if the penny had a similarly impressive track record.

The random healing performance of the "staghorn" coin might seem even more powerful if by chance the placebo coin landed heads only two or three times out of its ten flips. Or the findings could have gone in precisely the opposite direction, with fewer heads resulting from the flipping of the quarter—which would not be a surprising occurrence for a plague drug; in the early stages of testing, it wouldn't be unusual to find that a new compound turns out to shorten rather than to prolong life. With your twenty coin flips, you have now conducted a randomized placebo-controlled trial of sorts. (It was not blinded, however. But we'll assume that as the experimenter your knowledge of which coin was which could not possibly have biased your interpretation of whether the outcome was heads or tails . . . except perhaps for that one time that the quarter ended up against the wall in a position that *really looked* like it would have landed heads.)

You and your colleagues at Stagogen have just entered the Alice in Wonderland realm of statistics, in which things are not what they are, but only what they seem to be. In that realm, you can't say with perfect certainty that you are reading this book, only that it is overwhelmingly likely that you are reading this book. Trippy as that sounds, it is the world that must be occupied by all of us who conduct or evaluate studies of medications.

Quantum mechanics, the branch of physics concerned with the behavior of subatomic particles, is usually far from the thoughts of people who spend their days wondering if a given pill is effective. But the way we think about whether drugs work has undergone the same transformation that revolutionized physics decades earlier: probabilistic reasoning. In the old days, which began with Sir Isaac Newton in the seventeenth century and continued until the beginning of the twentieth, classical physics dealt with unambiguous causes and effects: "To every action there is a precisely equal and opposite reaction." Whether it's a hunter firing a rifle or the controlled expulsion of gases from a rocket, we know what should happen each and every time, not "most of the time" or "to a greater or lesser extent." Unless the bullet is a dud or an O-ring is leaking, the force and matter put into the system create an absolutely definable outcome perfectly predicted by the laws of classical physics. In laboratory-based pharmacology, a similar certainty applies to the biochemical reactions that determine a drug's effect: if the experiment is performed correctly and consistently, a given dose of neurotransmitter will always cause precisely the same effect on an isolated frog heart, and the same dose of curare will produce a predictable muscle paralysis every time the experiment is done.

AN END TO CERTAINTY

Once we start to worry about drug effects in typical, real patients, we leave the comfortable world of fixed effects and certainty, and enter the more stressful universe of probabilities. To get a grip on this, think back to the simple version of physics most of us learned in high school, in which electrons spin around their nuclei like well-behaved planets around a sun. The unsettling news that quantum mechanics brought us was this: *We don't really know where any of those electrons actually are.* All we can say is that at any given moment, a specific electron has a certain probability of being in a particular orbit and a certain probability that it isn't there. (This way of looking at the world feels weird at first, but becomes familiar for parents of teenagers trying to determine their kids' location on a Saturday night.) Assessing drug effects in individual patients and populations of patients requires this kind of probabilistic thinking. Thus, we often find that a drug that "worked" in clinical trials may not be of any use in a given patient—and side effects that weren't noted during a drug's development can be common and catastrophic when it comes into widespread use.

For some drugs, the situation isn't so complicated. When my professional ancestors gave morphine to a patient in pain, they didn't need a team of statisticians to tell them whether it worked, because the effect was instantaneous and unambiguous. The same was true for other early medications: aspirin brought down a fever, ephedrine helped asthmatic patients breathe better, an extract from the foxglove plant reduced the ankle swelling and breathlessness of congestive heart failure, then known as dropsy. These compounds weren't called blockbusters then, but they worked so well that no probabilistic calculations were needed to study their effects.

Alas, most drugs don't have this kind of open-and-shut evidence of effectiveness. Hardly ever nowadays can you take twenty patients with a given disease, treat half of them with a new drug, and find that within a week all who received the drug are alive and well, and all who didn't get the drug are still sick or dead. As in our coin-flipping experiment, we need some rules of evidence to decide what level of certainty to insist upon before we decide it's "probable enough" that a given drug is actually better than nothing. Demanding near-total certainty would require years-longer studies in enormous numbers of people, and even this wouldn't provide us with absolute proof in any mathematical sense. Requiring such certainty would also run the risk that some effective drugs could be mistakenly cast aside because the evidence in their favor was compelling but not perfect. By contrast, setting the certainty bar too low would lead us to accept the credentials of some new drugs that were no better than placebo, but just happened to have had the luck of the draw in their favor during inadequate studies (as will often occur in the coin-toss experiment).

Enter the *p*-value, a very little number with the power to determine which drugs can be prescribed and which are rejected as unproven. The universe may operate probabilistically, but governments and regulators have to bite the bullet and say yes or no. Unlike the FDA's zany adolescent days of the 1970s and 1980s, when it tossed around the noncommittal designation of "possibly effective," the agency today usually works in a binary mode—a problem we'll deal with more critically later on. For all new drugs, including the one developed by our hypothetical company, once the data are in the FDA will have to declare either that the product works and is available for use, or that it does not work and cannot be prescribed. Let's assume that when Stagogen's pivotal clinical trial is completed, sixty of the one hundred plague patients randomized to receive Lifehorn survived, while only fifty of the one hundred patients randomized to placebo did. Does that prove that the drug is better than placebo? Or might it simply be the luck of the draw, with Lifehorn no better than a sugar pill?

As you struggle to move your product through the regulatory process, you will find that the FDA follows a convention common in scientific research, one that is as simple as it is arbitrary. As in our coin-flipping experiment, one can take any observed difference in outcomes and calculate how often that result would have happened just by accident. (A crude version of such tables could be constructed by having a hundred undergraduates flipping a hundred coins for a hundred hours, and displaying the results; a real-time process that's more fun to watch can be viewed at several statistics websites listed in the Notes.)

When a clinical trial finds an advantage of a certain percent in a key outcome in patients given a new drug compared to placebo, the FDA asks the statisticians: What is the likelihood that the luck of the draw, chance alone, would have produced this finding? These numbers are readily calculated. By convention, if there is a greater than 5 percent likelihood that chance could have produced the apparent advantage of a new drug over placebo, then the results are written off as a possible fluke. If, on the other hand, we calculate that there is less than a 5 percent chance that a finding of this size could have occurred at random, then the result is accepted as probably real. The p-value simply represents the likelihood that a particular finding is accidental. A p-value of .05 means that there is a 5 percent chance that the observed finding is due to mere coincidence and a 95 percent chance that it is a real effect.

In the case of the Lifehorn clinical trials, it turns out that despite the encouraging-seeming numbers, the statisticians report that the p-value for this difference is .20, meaning that such an apparent advantage had a one-in-five likelihood of having occurred simply by chance. The FDA Advisory Committee on Plague and Pestilential Diseases initially leans fourteen to six against approval of your company's product. When a second vote is taken after recusal of the four members who hold stock in Stagogen or serve as paid consultants to the company, the vote is still thirteen to three against approval.

Was the government correct in concluding that the drug *doesn't work*? Your company's Regulatory Affairs Department arranges a follow-up meeting with the FDA staffers in charge of the Lifehorn application. "This is a travesty!" declares Stagogen's VP for governmental relations, who graduated at the top of his MBA class at Stanford but had flunked statistics as an undergraduate. "The trial data clearly show that sixty of a hundred plague patients survived in the Lifehorn group, and only fifty out of a hundred lived in the placebo group. That's ten fewer deaths in the patients who got our drug. How can you tell me we don't have an effective product here? This decision will deny plague patients throughout the country access to a treatment that could mean the difference between life and death!" (It will also mean a loss of 80 percent of Stagogen's market capitalization when the news becomes public.) But the VP is quite sincere in his question. He had once dated a girl who had a nasty brush with the plague, and he desperately wanted to bring to market a treatment that could help people with this dread condition.

The FDA scientist in charge of the review had been through dozens of such meetings with irate advocates for disapproved drugs. On days when he felt his faith flagging, he did the coin-flipping exercise to remind himself how fickle chance could be, and how many "cures" he would have approved without a clear probability-based standard. He had a ready answer, whose logic has its origins in biblical times. Recall the argument Abraham made to God over the plan to destroy Sodom and Gomorrah. Granted these places were full of sinners, but what kernel of virtue would make it worth saving the cities? What if they contained fifty good people, Abraham demanded. Would God still want to destroy the towns? How about forty-five? What likelihood of goodness, however small, would it take to win divine approval? The outcome is well known; Abraham eventually talks God down to the possibility of just ten good men, for whose sake both cities would be saved. Unfortunately for the townspeople, even this number couldn't be found, and the cities underwent the Old Testament version of urban renewal.

The assessment of efficacy in drug research likewise asks the Sodom and Gomorrah question regularly. What if there is a one-in-three chance that a drug's apparent effectiveness was merely the result of chance? Would it still be worth saving? One in ten? Where should we draw the line?

"Think of what you're asking for," the FDA scientist replies to the Stagogen product team, trying to remain calm. "If we approved every drug with data as iffy as those you produced for Lifehorn, one out of every five drugs on the market would be there by chance, and wouldn't be any better than a sugar pill. But each would still have its risks as well as its costs. What kind of health care system would we have then? One that looks a lot like the Middle Ages. We have to have some standard that we stick to, one that you in the industry can count on when you're planning your studies so you know how to design them. For decades, the rule has been that we reject findings that have a greater than one-in-twenty chance of being the result of mere chance. It may be arbitrary, but that's the standard used by scientists all over the world. Your product got shot down this time, but it's the same standard we'll use on your competitors too. If the drug really works, even a little, you ought to be able to conduct a clinical trial large enough to prove it at the required level of certainty. Come back with a better study of Lifehorn that shows its benefit is 95 percent likely to be real, however small it may be, and we'll be happy to declare your drug effective—even though we know there would still be a one-in-twenty chance that it's useless. This is just the best way anyone has come up with to deal with these questions."

The more we know, the more we understand how little we know—a confession that should ring as true to a drug researcher as it would to a particle physicist or a Zen monk. This perspective is far less comforting than the image of "discovering a cure" pictured in the public imagination. It is hard to think of television's Marcus Welby, M.D., handing a patient a prescription and saying warmly, "Here, take this; it's probably better than nothing." Yet often, this would be a correct assessment.

LEARNING TO LIKE LIKELIHOOD

The probabilistic assessment of a drug's effectiveness looms even larger when we think about the preventive drugs that have become such a major part of contemporary medication use. Before the 1970s, nearly all the drugs we prescribed were designed to treat a particular illness, often an acute one: antibiotics for infection, opiates for pain, bronchodilators for asthma, diuretics or digoxin for congestive heart failure. As we've seen, often both patient and doctor could perceive their effect within hours or sometimes minutes of use—days at most.

It's much more difficult to determine the eventual outcome of a drug that is used to manage a "risk state" like high cholesterol or osteoporosis. The effectiveness of preventive therapies is only partial, and may take years to observe. Over time, cholesterol-lowering drugs reduce the rate of heart attack by about a quarter, with this reduction taking up to a year to observe in many large trials. Although the contribution of these drugs to the prevention of disease and death is substantial, it initially required studies of thousands of subjects observed over years to measure their effect. One example of how the rules changed in my own lifetime: In the 1960s, doctors still hotly debated whether it was worth medicating people who had mild to moderate elevations in their blood pressure; crucial randomized clinical trials published at the end of that decade proved that such treatment prevented strokes, kidney failure, and heart disease, and saved lives—although it took years to see the difference. In the elderly, the issue remained contentious for decades longer; older patients had been systematically excluded from most of the studies that resolved the issue for younger people, even though most hypertension occurs in people over sixty-five. By the close of the 1980s, experiments that specifically enrolled only older people proved that they, too, had fewer strokes and less heart and kidney disease if their high blood pressure was treated.

Managing high blood pressure is surely one of the most useful things a doctor can do. But data from decades of clinical trials prove that we actually have to treat dozens of people for a lifetime in order to prevent just one adverse outcome like stroke. Such dismaying number-needed-to-treat figures are common for all the preventive drugs we use: for osteoporosis, for glaucoma, for elevated cholesterol. The unstated and usually unknown truth is that a large number of the patients we medicate for these conditions would probably come to no harm if we totally ignored them. Of course we must treat them anyway, because we have no way of knowing who will be the one patient among many whom we will help. But it's a statistical kind of healing, nothing like fixing a fractured bone or lopping out an inflamed appendix.

This is probably not the perspective held by all those conscientious patients who take their prescribed medicines with almost religious fervor. Luckily, it is likewise not the view of most of us who care for them: "Honey, I'm going into the office to give drugs to people who in most cases will be no better as a result." As counterintuitive as this may seem, there are many commonsense examples: most people who smoke don't get lung cancer, most unprotected sexual encounters don't lead to pregnancy or AIDS, and most drunk driving escapades don't end in injury. But smoking, unsafe sex, and drunk driving are still risky activities because they dramatically raise the likelihood that these outcomes will occur. Sure, most of the time we put on our seat belts it doesn't prevent us from getting hurt; but we do it (or should) all the time anyway.

The prescribing and taking of medicines to manage risk states require doctors and patients to avoid dwelling on these probabilities too much. All of us get by thanks to a kind of lottery mentality, though this one makes sense because it's based on solid experimental data. In prescribing the risk-reduction medications we use so widely, we act as if each person we treat is the one who would suffer a calamity if left untreated. For their part, our patients who comply with our instructions do the same. As it happens, this belief is usually not true. But it is sometimes true, and it is vital for us all to act as if it were true all the time. We just have no way of knowing in advance who will benefit. The realization is humbling but should not be paralyzing. We plod ahead as we must, ignoring the numbing enormity of the number-needed-to-treat problem. How else could doctors and patients go on? A perfect existential dilemma.

Thanks to the FDA's regulatory clout, essentially all prescription drugs that make it to market fared better than our example did, having succeeded in showing at least that they were significantly better than placebo. The methods of modern drug development and evaluation, coupled with the powers accorded to regulatory authorities in the United States and abroad, make it possible to identify which products have at least some therapeutic utility. As in evolution, the demise of less effective species helps clear the way for the survival and dominance of new, more successful variants. If science and regulation didn't provide us with this kind of selection pressure for drugs, dinosaur remedies would still walk the earth as they did for ages, leaving less room for cleverer new mammal-like treatments.

This raises the question of whether we can do a better job in fostering survival of the fittest drugs. Can our health care systems do more to facilitate the discovery and use of important new medications? The answer is certainly yes, and we will explore this further in later chapters. But first we have to take a detour into a darker, evidence-free zone that remains untouched by the discoveries of twentieth-century drug development. We won't have to visit some preliterate rain forest tribe to see this grisly spectacle unfold. The counterreformation is as close as a store down the block, or the nearest internet connection.

A SLIDE BACKWARD

No quick tour of the intellectual history of drug assessment would be complete without considering the strange turn it has taken in the last decade. The second half of the twentieth century may have witnessed the flowering of modern pharmacology and drug evaluation, but the century ended with a burst of influence by those who reject those disciplines.

With the waning of the trusted family doctor and the growing corporatization of medicine, more and more patients have become alienated from modern health care, turning instead to "natural" remedies to replace or supplement officially sanctioned medications. This impulse is understandable. After all, several of the most effective medications in history had their origins in plants: curare, aspirin, digoxin, Taxol, quinine, morphine. Others, like Saint-John's-wort and sawgrass palmetto, have yielded some interesting clinical trial data suggesting possible effectiveness in treating depression and prostatic symptoms, respectively. Dietary supplements like iron, calcium, vitamins A, C, D, and all the B vitamins can likewise be clinically important, and the element selenium is being evaluated to determine whether it can prevent cancer.

Studied appropriately, some of the substances promoted today as natural therapies might eventually turn out to be useful treatments. But in the 1990s, the manufacturers of many unproven nostrums came to realize that calling a product an herbal remedy or nutritional supplement could also be a lucrative way to evade all the standards set for conventional prescription products. The distinction led to the creation of a new class of medicines, whose makers have managed to exempt themselves from all the carefully constructed requirements of drug efficacy, safety, potency, and purity that were so painstakingly established since the early 1900s.

By the early 1990s, audacious claims abounded for many of these products, usually unsubstantiated by any rigorous evidence that they were true. Standards for dose strength or even accurate labeling of ingredients were either absent or unenforced. The situation resembled the period before the Progressive-era reforms of a hundred years ago. FDA commissioner David Kessler tried to rein in the alternative medicine–herbal supplements industry, arguing that it should be subjected to standards of safety and efficacy similar to those for real medicines. But in a well-financed counterreformation, the industry got itself placed outside the FDA's regulatory control. In 1994 Senator Orrin Hatch thwarted Kessler by championing passage of the Dietary Supplement and Health Education Act, over the opposition of most professional and consumer groups. Written with heavy input from the supplement industry lobby and propelled by generous campaign contributions, the bill was nicknamed "the Snake-Oil Protection Act" by the press. Its logic was based on the idea that if enough people believe in a medicine, then it must work: the Tinkerbell school of pharmacology. The bill sailed through Congress. The rigorous evaluative methods that medicine had used to drag itself out of the Galenic mire and into the modern world now no longer officially applied to a large class of drugs. As long as a product could construe itself as some kind of "supplement" (and this distinction became so vague as to be virtually nonexistent), it did not have to prove efficacy or safety, and was put beyond the reach of most governmental regulation.

Randomized clinical trials do, after all, have some major drawbacks: they cost money to conduct, and they sometimes demonstrate that your product doesn't work or that it hurts people. Far better to avoid doing them and spend the money on promotion. The new law shrank governmental oversight down to an expectation that these advertisements should use terms describing "health" (e.g., "promotes prostate health") rather than illness, and contain a standard disclaimer: "This product has not been evaluated by the Food and Drug Administration. It is not intended to diagnose, treat, cure or prevent any disease."

To see how the law was playing out in practice, my colleague Dr. Charles Morris and I decided to study the issue systematically. He used the most popular internet search engines to seek information on the best-selling herbal supplements, just as a patient might do. This yielded 445 links, most of which were commercial sites or linked directly to one. In a paper published in the *Journal of the American Medical Association,* we reported that among the commercial sites, four out of five made clear unsubstantiated claims for the curative or preventive powers of an herbal product. Over half boldly promoted undocumented medical effects, yet fewer than half the health-claim sites contained the rudimentary FDA disclaimer required by law. Even the emasculated regulations were being flouted regularly. Some examples from these sites:

> [Ginseng] is potentially beneficial for AIDS, radiotherapy, and chemotherapy patients, as it reduces the side effects of toxic drugs by increasing red and white blood cell counts. Dang Shen is given for breast cancer, asthma, diabetes, heart palpitations, memory or appetite loss, and insomnia.

> Echinacea is one of the primary remedies for helping the body rid itself of microbial infections. It is often effective against both bacterial and viral

attacks, and may be used in conditions such as boils, septicemia, and similar infections.

> Q: [I have] high blood pressure (170/190) [*sic*]. Will American ginseng lower blood pressure and if so, how much should one take and how long before results show?
>
> A: While American ginseng will help, we have a combination product that will do a much better job. Look at product #1960, American Ginseng/Garlic/Tien Chi. This is a great product.

> Kava kava . . . is a valuable urinary antiseptic, helping to counter urinary infections and to settle an irritable bladder. . . . Kava kava's analgesic and cleansing diuretic effect often makes it beneficial for treating rheumatic and arthritic problems such as gout.

The last site did not mention that the FDA had issued a warning that use of kava kava can cause massive liver failure; about half the sites promoting this particular product failed to do so, reporting instead that it was both safe and effective. Claims made in print and broadcast media for such herbal products are equally egregious.

The Dietary Supplement and Health Education Act of 1994 may have dealt a blow to science, but it did wonders for the supplements industry, which now sucks about $20 billion a year from the pockets of a nation that can't seem to find enough money to pay for the real drugs its citizens need. During the 1990s, use of herbal remedies increased some 400 percent, and by 2002, two Americans in five were taking some kind of supplement or related nostrum. A few of these were of proven value but many were worthless, dangerous, or both. About a fifth of patients who use prescription drugs concurrently take high-dose supplements or herbal remedies, most of which have never been tested for interaction with active drugs. Adverse events caused by such products now are reported regularly in the medical literature and include bleeding, hypertension, liver disease, heart rhythm abnormalities, kidney failure, and sudden death, among other problems.

At issue here is not the concept of natural versus un-natural medicines, or whether botanical products can preserve vitality and prevent disease. The battle is over the rules of evidence used to determine what works, and how the worlds of commerce and regulation deal with that information. If an alternative medicine treatment is thought to be effective in treating or preventing a particular problem, let's test it in a randomized trial and see how it performs. If it works, let's welcome it into the armamentarium of effective therapies—we can always use more. But if a product doesn't pass that test, it should be illegal to sell it on the basis of an unproven health claim. Creating an alternative pathway to let drugs onto the market without that evidence threatens to undermine the hard-won scientific gains of the last half-century.

It isn't a stretch to think of this rogue perspective as postmodernist drug evaluation. It fits well with other current themes of postmodernist criticism, which depicts most of contemporary Western culture and science as the arbitrary constructs of traditional elites (sometimes referred to as "dead white males"), whose vision of reality is no more valid or legitimate than any number of alternative ways of understanding things. An eerily similar kind of argument is made about medicines in much of the alternative healing movement. Some proponents contend that the scientific method and all of pharmacology constitute just one way of explaining nature, the one that happens to be favored by yet another elite group. According to this view, that perspective has no inherent superiority over other ways of thinking about therapeutics, including herbal medicine, Native American chanting, voodoo, homeopathy, Christian Science, or vitamin megatherapy. It is as if the last fifty years of medical science count for nothing, or never happened.

Like other expressions of postmodernism, the argument is sometimes accompanied by diatribes of cultural relativism run amok: "Your way of treating diabetes, with insulin and pills to control blood sugar, is not inherently more worthy than my way, which involves meditation, prayer, and chewing on roots." At the extreme fringes, periodically a few zealots are put in jail for allowing their children to die of infections or appendicitis or other treatable diseases because they forced them to endure useless alternative therapies at home rather than taking them to a hospital.

Disappointingly, a number of HMOs have embraced a milder version of this philosophy (call it postmodernism lite) by offering a menu of New Age treatments along with the more traditional kinds of medicine and surgery that they make or don't make available. Not a surprising choice: alternative medicine is usually much cheaper than real drugs, and covering it is a good way to enroll younger, hip subscribers who are statistically less likely to take up the time of doctors or require real medical care.

AND SO we have come full circle. The decades that followed World War II saw major advances in the design of drug studies that for the first time enabled us to rigorously tell apart the ones that worked from those that didn't. By the end of the century, humankind had developed the most powerful intellectual tool ever devised for distinguishing medicines with the power to cure from those that were innocent bystanders uselessly adorning a spontaneous recovery, or potential poisons that made patients sicker. This evolution represents one of the finest accomplishments of the human mind, and has given us hundreds of effective drugs.

With literature, the arts, history, and the sciences under attack by the postmodernist revolution, that tool has come under fire as well. A well-traveled back road now bypasses the FDA's painstakingly constructed hurdles for the careful evaluation of drugs; more and more useless and sometimes dangerous products sneak along it into medicine's cultural and commercial landscape. These nostrums are protected from scientific scrutiny by a loathsome alliance of industrial greed and political complicity, cloaked in the newly respectable costume of cultural relativism.

A common theme ties together the estrogen debacle and the current infatuation with alternative medicines. After several decades of defending the intellectual high ground, we have begun to allow the marketplace to usurp the place of evidence in determining which treatments are effective. Scientific validation of what works is increasingly trumped by crass observation of what sells, adorned with cheap pseudo-evaluations of efficacy. These trends threaten to erode the care of patients and drain our already constrained health care budgets.

Over the very long haul, ideas that are correct usually fare better than those that aren't. The scientific edifice of modern pharmacology is still standing, even though several rooms in the basement have been occupied by squatters growing mushrooms. With luck, the rains of time may wash off the graffiti the postmodernists have sprayed on the building, and the geneticists are already drawing up blueprints for a huge new wing to be built on some vacant land next door. But for now, the deconstructionists are widening their control over the lower floors. And the Consumer Products Division of Stagogen has ambitious alternative plans to market an over-the-counter version of Lifehorn through health food stores. A few unpublished reports suggest it may be great for preventing cancer and treating Alzheimer's disease.

PART TWO: RISKS

3: THE FAT IS IN THE FIRE

The flip side of benefit is risk; the former without the latter is about as common as a one-sided coin. Any molecule clever enough to influence one chemical pathway for the better is also likely to have other effects in the complex biologic soup of the cytoplasm. It would be comforting to think of medications as magic bullets that somehow know just where in the body to go, exert their healing action, and then move along: clinical smart bombs that are guided unerringly to their target and obliterate it. As medicine evolves, we have gotten somewhat closer to this ideal but not nearly as close as we would like, or as people think we have. As with our military weaponry, those magic bullets are not always as smart as we're told they are: they often cause important collateral damage, and sometimes they miss their target altogether.

There is a comforting shared myth that by the time the FDA approves a new drug, the product has been studied exhaustively and determined to be a worthwhile new addition, and that all its actions in the body, both good and bad, are well defined. In fact none of these assumptions is correct. The FDA itself does not study any drugs prior to approval, relying on the company that makes the product to generate that information in studies the manufacturer conducts or commissions. The clinical trials that form the basis of approval of a drug may be as few as one or two in number, and may recruit only a modest sample of patients, often younger and healthier than those who will take the drug routinely. That number is usually too small to assess the risk of a side effect that occurs infrequently but could pose an important public health problem once the drug is used by millions.

New drugs are being developed that hold breathtaking promise. But a disturbing insight hovers over the hands of many thoughtful doctors each time we write a prescription: we know much less than our patients think we do about the drugs we use. When a new drug is first marketed, little is proven about its safety and effectiveness compared to existing alternatives, and the situation is often no clearer years or decades later. We have a limited capacity to identify side effects early and reliably, and when a potentially fatal adverse event is detected it may take so long to enforce a recall that thousands of additional patients are put at risk.

Dr. Jacques Lelorier, a Canadian pharmacologist who studies the side effects of drugs, likes to startle medical audiences by beginning a lecture with this slide:

CLASSIFICATION OF ALL SUBSTANCES

1. **Inert compounds**

2. **Poisons**

His next slide divides the category of "poisons" into two subgroups:

(a) **pure poisons**

(b) **drugs (selective toxicity)**

It is a melodramatic but thought-provoking way of making the point. His typology follows the famous dictum of Paracelsus, the sixteenth-century alchemist best known for his observation, "All medicines are poisons . . . the right dose differentiates a poison from a remedy." This is not as terrifying as it sounds; it shouldn't be surprising that intimate tweaking of basic biological processes can have unintended consequences. Often the adverse effect is an exaggeration of the very effect the drug was intended to have, but sometimes the harm seems to come from out of the blue. (A useful aphorism I learned in medical school was "Every drug has at least two effects: the one you intended and the one you didn't.")

The vast majority of prescription drugs used in the United States result in far more healing than hazard. But we still have a lot to learn about this balance and how it can best be made to tilt in the patient's favor. The problem is illustrated well by three drugs for which that balance got badly out of control. The three examples are based on cases in which I served as a pro bono adviser to attorneys working on behalf of patients (or their survivors) who suffered severe illness or death because of drug side effects that were probably preventable. In the course of those legal proceedings, manufacturers and the FDA were required to disclose internal memoranda and other documents detailing the evolution of these problems—material that is normally not available to physicians or the public. Reading them as an expert witness gave me the same sensation that the Watergate tapes produced decades earlier: sometimes things *are* as bad as the most cynical critics said they were. I have reproduced only a small fraction of that evidence here, and not the worst of it. Much of it remains protected under court orders; what follows is material that has for one reason or another been allowed to escape that restriction.

LOSING IT

Drugs to help people diet have a long and generally unsavory history. Ads for them in medical journals caught my eye as far back as the 1970s when as a medical student I was trying to understand what drives physicians' prescribing decisions. I recall one promotional spread that featured a buxom woman wearing nothing but a huge bull's-eye painted on her buttocks and back; its outermost ring was labeled *150 lbs.* and the center *136 lbs.*—a reduction rarely seen with these drugs. The headline promised "CONSISTENT WEIGHT LOSS ON THE WAY TO THE TARGET WEIGHT." One product that stood out at the time had the trade name of Pondimin, from the same root as "ponderous" and "pound"; its generic name was fenfluramine. The drug was manufactured by a company that was eventually merged into Wyeth, the people who sold Premarin for so long without conducting clinical trials of its long-term effects.

The ads for Pondimin resembled those for other silly-drug examples I was collecting in those early years, marked by wonderfully seductive promises and thin-to-absent scientific credentials. They projected an image of safe, reliable, and medically useful weight loss with few side effects. But the clinical trial findings, to the extent that any could be found in the medical literature, were unimpressive. Subjects randomized to Pondimin lost only a few pounds more than did those given placebo, and as soon as the patient stopped taking the drug the weight came right back. Nor was use of this product benign: Aminorex, a similar product used widely in Europe in the 1960s, had been removed from the market there because it caused severe lung damage. During the 1970s, 1980s, and the first half of the 1990s, fenfluramine was a modestly selling, homely product of no great consequence. It didn't work very well, and was approved by the FDA only for "short-term weight loss"—not an appealing goal clinically or cosmetically. And who would want to put a patient on a minimally effective diet drug for life just to lose a few pounds?

Fenfluramine resurfaced with a vengeance in the second half of the 1990s after a therapeutic-image makeover. The drug's stature was transformed when a pharmacologist discovered that if it was taken together with another not terribly effective diet pill, phentermine, the two could act synergistically to produce somewhat greater weight loss. The number of pounds shed remained modest and the weight came back when the drugs were stopped, but this dual-action property was enough of a hook to give the combination new appeal in an overfed, underactive nation. Americans were even fatter in the 1990s than they had been in the 1970s, and there was even more evidence that overweight people were more likely to develop diabetes, high blood pressure, and heart disease. Combining fenfluramine and phentermine became a pharmacological craze, and the cocktail quickly came to be known as "fen-phen." The combination soon led to one of the most prominent therapeutic disasters of the decade.

The FDA requires that in all printed material produced by a company about its drugs, evidence of efficacy as well as risks must be presented fairly and completely so that doctors can make informed choices about whether to prescribe a given product. Yet reports of serious adverse events from Pondimin were coming in to Wyeth but not making it onto the company's official package insert or into their ads. While hardly anyone remembered the European Aminorex disaster of the 1960s (and most American physicians had never heard of it in the first place), it provided reason to worry that similar diet pills could increase the risk of a rare but often fatal lung disease, pulmonary hypertension. In this condition, the blood pressure in the delicate arteries of the lung increases to dangerous levels. In severe cases the patient experiences worsening shortness of breath, heart failure, and death. Even if the Aminorex lesson had been lost, other evidence was accumulating that the newer diet medications could also cause this severe side effect.

Wyeth was keeping track of the diet pill–pulmonary hypertension connection, but doctors and patients did not have access to that risk information. Some of the evidence later came to light in litigation by patients who developed pulmonary hypertension following use of the drug; a Texas law firm representing several of them chose some of the more revealing internal corporate memos and posted them on the internet. According to those documents, as early as June 1994 Fred Wilson, a company official, sent a note to a colleague expressing concern that they had reports on about ten times as many cases of Pondimin-related pulmonary hypertension as their official package insert indicated. "As I mentioned to you last week," Wilson wrote, "I have been concerned that our approved labeling contains only four such cases when in fact, we have 37 reports in addition to those mentioned in the labeling." He initially proposed modifying the label to reflect this new information, but a few days later in another memo he suggested simply leaving the paragraph as it stood but adding the sentence "Additional cases of pulmonary hypertension have been reported." It took over two years more before an accurate presentation of the risk of this adverse event actually made it into the company's official product description.

MODIFYING MEDIOCRITY

Meanwhile, in a laboratory associated with MIT, chemists had begun tinkering with the fenfluramine molecule itself. Like many substances in biology, the drug normally exists in two forms that are nearly identical mirror images of one another, known as isomers. They resemble each other the way the right hand resembles the left; for this reason isomers are referred to as the *dextro* isomer for the "right-handed" version and the *levo* isomer for its mate. Occasionally, one of these will be responsible for most of a drug's effectiveness but confer fewer of its side effects. This is presumably because the target organs are more sensitive to one isomer while the organs in which the side effects occur respond more to the other isomer. Such hopes only rarely pan out, and several expensive searches to isolate isomers of commonly used drugs have produced no meaningful benefit.

Developing a single isomer of a given drug does, however, have one guaranteed advantage: the new compound can be patented anew and marketed as if it were a breakthrough product. This is what happened with the *dextro* isomer of fenfluramine. Riding the crest of new enthusiasm for the fen-phen combination, dexfenfluramine was presented to the FDA with the attractive trade name of Redux. Several companies were involved in the submission, but one main marketing engine was the corporation that made the old fenfluramine, Wyeth. The company hoped that Redux would come to replace the older, no-longer-patented mixture of right- and left-handed fenfluramine that it was selling as Pondimin. Warning that an epidemic of obesity was sweeping the country, Redux backers said that if the drug was approved, it would help slim down the nation's growing death rate from diabetes and heart disease, while generating a solid bottom line for its inventors and manufacturer.

Things were not looking good in 1994 for Wyeth's old or new obesity drugs. Word was circulating that a large pulmonary hypertension study being conducted in France was finding a clear association between the disease and diet pills. In October, one company official wrote to another, "Preliminary results are said to show that there is a relationship between dexfenfluramine and pulmonary hypertension. It is also said to show that other drugs of this class, including fenfluramine (Pondimin), also have an increased incidence of pulmonary hypertension." This was bad news for the still-unapproved Redux: "From all of the information we know right now, it appears that getting the drug approved in the next few years will be a difficult task at best."

Business for the older fenfluramine marketed as Pondimin continued to be brisk, and with the fen-phen frenzy its sales rose handsomely throughout this time period:

1993: $3.7 million
1994: $8.5 million
1995: $48.7 million
1996: $150.1 million

Media reports of the fen-phen weight-loss cocktail had spawned the creation of hundreds of "pill mills"—clinics with minimal medical supervision in which a woman (the patients were nearly all women) could in effect buy a prescription for the drug combo. The better clinics provided some instruction about diet and exercise. The tackier ones (and there were many) just took the money and paid a doctor to write the prescriptions. Annual foreign sales moved up as well, rising from 11,500 tablets sold in 1993 to 148,600 in 1996. Lucrative Pondimin sales were seen as the opening act for the introduction of Redux, which could be the real blockbuster if approved by the FDA. Financial analysts predicted that its annual sales could easily top a billion dollars.

By 1995, the company was trying to deal with an increasing number of reports of Pondimin-related pulmonary hypertension, and at the same time move its newly patented twin through the steps required for FDA approval. Redux had demonstrated only a few pounds' advantage over placebo in its main clinical trial, and growing concern over the lung disease connection wouldn't make the case any easier. The first time Redux was brought before an FDA advisory committee in September 1995, the panel decided that there were too many safety concerns to grant approval. It is very uncommon for such questions to be revisited soon after a decision is made. But following pressure from the company, another meeting of the advisory committee was scheduled for just two months later, in November 1995. No substantial new data had emerged to change what was known about the drug's benefits or risks, but the committee members who attended the follow-up meeting now included more Redux supporters and fewer skeptics. The group decided by a one-vote margin to recommend that Redux be approved for unrestricted use in the United States.

By the end of the month, Wyeth was in negotiation with the FDA about how soon it could market Redux and what it could say about it in the official labeling and subsequent promotion. For especially dangerous risks, the

FDA can require manufacturers to include a highlighted "black box" paragraph that presents important risk information in bold type with a heavy border, to make sure that serious warnings are not lost among the thousands of words of small print that comprise such official descriptions. Dr. Leo Lutwak, the FDA's lead medical officer overseeing the Redux review, was adamant that a black box warning be included in the official description and in all advertising; he was convinced that Redux carried a risk of pulmonary hypertension and was unimpressed with its effectiveness in the first place. The FDA also wanted the company to perform systematic surveillance of side effects once the drug was released for use—a so-called Phase IV study. A drug's first year on the market can be a critical time to assess its side effects, as it comes into widespread use in many more patients than were studied in preapproval clinical trials.

Wyeth had concerns about both requirements. Around Thanksgiving 1995, one of its regulatory affairs officers, Joe Bathish, sent an internal memo to his colleague Fred Hassan about the sales problems that could come up for Redux if the FDA required a prominent warning about pulmonary hypertension. "While we have a very difficult and arduous task of negotiating labeling and Phase IV commitments with the Agency [FDA] over the next few weeks," Bathish wrote, "every attempt will be made to ensure that no 'Black Box' Warnings, restrictions on use or negative statements find their way into the Redux labeling. . . . We will make every effort to neutralize these initiatives." Dr. Lutwak was indeed neutralized. "The management [of the FDA] accepted the company's arguments against the black box," Dr. Lutwak later told the *Los Angeles Times,* "and I don't know why." Lutwak refused to sign the agency's official letter of approval for the drug, and another FDA official had to authorize it in his place. When Redux received its final green light for marketing in early 1996, no black box warning was required.

At around the same time, across the Atlantic the European regulatory agencies were also reviewing initial data from the French study that would be published later that year. They determined that the risk of pulmonary hypertension with Redux was so great that its official description and all advertising would have to include a major warning about this risk.

A LUCRATIVE TIME BOMB

As soon as Redux went on sale, it became clear that, like fenfluramine, it was not being prescribed primarily for seriously obese patients. Instead, its main users were slightly plump women who were striving to meet some anorexic ideal. With so many millions of prescriptions written, there just wasn't enough severe obesity in the land to account for the scale of its use.

Neither the FDA nor the manufacturer saw this as their problem. The agency argued that the task of the regulator is to approve or disapprove a drug, and the task of the manufacturer is to make and sell it. For its part, the company said that the drug was federally approved and appropriately labeled (the details of its participation in that process didn't come to light until later), and that its use was up to the physicians who prescribed it. If doctors and patients were using the drug foolishly, the FDA and the company seemed to argue, it wasn't their fault.

The long-discussed results of "the French study" were published as a major article in the *New England Journal of Medicine* in 1996. In a carefully performed case-control study, a team of epidemiologists led by Lucien Abenheim identified hundreds of patients with pulmonary hypertension, and then looked back to see what medications they were taking before they developed this uncommon disease. The analysis found that people who had taken appetite suppressants had a twenty-three-fold increase in the risk of developing the illness.

By the fall of 1996 it didn't take any special insight to see that something was very wrong; most of the key pieces of information were in plain view. The Abenheim paper was one of the smokiest guns in the history of drug safety studies. On the front lines, clinical experience was making it clear that the weight loss these drugs produced was small and transient, something that could have been predicted from their preapproval trials. After all, the pivotal study on which the FDA had based its approval of Redux showed that even in the tightly monitored setting of a clinical trial, the average weight loss in very obese patients randomized to the new drug was only about six pounds greater than that achieved with placebo. This was unlikely to have any medical benefit and would be just as trivial cosmetically—clearly an underwhelming development. One internal company document summarized a market research study by admitting, "The efficacy of Redux is not impressive, and is insufficient for the needs [of] the patients the doctors would like to prescribe it for."

Nonetheless, use of the fen-phen drug cocktail continued to skyrocket. The six-pound difference was after all an average, and patients were insatiable in their demand for an exercise-free, diet-free way to shed pounds. Millions seemed willing to bet that they would win the slimming lottery and lose much more. And according to the official information that the manufacturer was providing about the drug, it appeared to be a safe gamble to take.

In the fall of 1996 a previously healthy thirty-year-old woman named Mary Linnen had the first of a series of admissions to my hospital. The prior spring, she was preparing to be married; while not terribly overweight, she was heavier than she wanted to be and hoped to look a little thinner in her wedding gown. Her doctor prescribed a regimen of fen-phen. After only a single month of use, Ms. Linnen developed shortness of breath and stopped taking the diet pills. Her breathlessness worsened that fall, especially with any exertion. By then she was also beginning to accumulate fluid in her legs, a sign of heart failure, and had bouts of fainting. On her first admission to the Brigham in November 1996, an echocardiogram revealed that the right side of her heart, which pumps blood into the lungs, was distended and functioning poorly. The pressure in her pulmonary arteries had become abnormally elevated.

Mary Linnen's very brief exposure to fenfluramine had been sufficient to permanently damage the arteries in her lungs, transferring unsustainably high pressures to her heart. She had a steady downhill course punctuated by several readmissions to the Brigham that winter, but there was little that could be done to reverse the damage. She died in February 1997. Not long after, the *Boston Herald* devoted its entire front page to her picture under a gigantic headline: "DIET TO DEATH." Her mother told the paper, "Instead of walking down the aisle before a bride, I walked behind a casket."

The fact that such a devastating side effect could be caused by only a month of fen-phen use was alarming. Within a week of Ms. Linnen's death, two alert pharmacists at the Brigham suggested that we try to get the word out via a letter to a medical journal, warning doctors that this life-threatening complication could follow even brief use of the popular regimen. Our letter was published in the *Journal of the American Medical Association* later that year. In it we wrote:

> Reports of severe adverse events, including fatalities, are increasing with the rising use of these heavily marketed medications. . . . This woman's death serves as a reminder of the potentially formidable risks associated with pharmacologic approaches to managing obesity, as well as the need for more effective post-marketing surveillance.

That same spring, I learned our hospital was considering setting up a diet clinic to meet the increasing demand for drug-oriented weight-loss programs offering fen-phen. This wouldn't exactly be a major medical triumph for the Harvard teaching hospital that had performed the world's first organ transplant, but some saw it as a service the marketplace was demanding that could bring in badly needed revenue to make up for recent Medicare cutbacks. The two pharmacists and I asked to meet with the Medical Staff Executive Committee to point out that this might not be a smart move in light of emerging information about the drugs' risks. The committee agreed, and plans to launch the obesity clinic were scrapped, even as use of these medications continued to increase nationally.

I was drawn deeper into the evolving fen-phen story by a call from Richard Lewis, an attorney in Washington, D.C. Through mutual acquaintances, he had heard that I might be able to help his firm in its litigation on behalf of patients who had developed complications resulting from use of the diet pills. I told Lewis that I didn't do that sort of work; he'd have to find someone else. "Let me tell you a little about my firm," he insisted, and explained that it was a large, established Washington partnership that often took on public-interest cases in which some environmental, civil rights, or other pro bono issue was at stake. Its clients were not a few embittered dieters looking for a huge out-of-court settlement. This was to be a class-action suit that could potentially represent every patient in the United States who had been affected by the weight-loss drug combination. "How this case comes out," Lewis told me, "will help to shape the way that new drugs are tested, marketed, and monitored in the future, throughout the industry."

I agreed to meet him in Boston to discuss the case further with only one condition: I didn't want to be paid for my time. Many of my colleagues on medical school faculties moonlight by serving as expert witnesses, earning up to $750 per hour for such work. But I didn't want even the slightest suggestion that I was an academic hired gun whose opinion could be bought for the right price. I maintained this policy in working on behalf of patients in other cases as well, including those described in the following chapters.

The phentermine half of the fen-phen combination turned out to be an innocent bystander. It soon dropped out of the medical and legal spotlight, leaving attention to focus on fenfluramine (Pondimin) and its right-handed twin, dexfenfluramine (Redux). Lewis sent me several FedEx boxes containing about thirty pounds of documents each. In reviewing them, I began not with the drugs' risks, but with the benefits they claimed to produce. The rationale was simple: all of us—doctors, patients, even lawyers—are willing to incur substantial risk, including the possibility of death, as long as a drug promises a commensurate benefit in a dire situation. This was certainly the case with the early AIDS drugs, and is with many cancer treatments today. As we will see later, how acceptable such risks are has everything to do with the value of the drug's benefits. In this case, it wasn't even close.

The companies that sold the drugs had pointed out that severe obesity *is associated with* (note that phrase) higher death rates and an increased frequency of other conditions such as diabetes and hypertension. They argued that a reduction in these problems among millions of patients would more than offset the occasional rare case of pulmonary hypertension the diet pills would cause, so that the net benefit to the population would be positive. If you want to make a public health omelet, they seemed to say, you might have to crack a few lungs.

But these calculations of benefit turned out to be suspect. First, they considered only the most optimistic estimates of the drugs' effectiveness, and assumed that they would be optimally prescribed in the most favorable clinical settings. The projections assumed several other things as well: that the drugs would be given just to a circumscribed group of patients with severe obesity, that their use would be continued only for patients who showed a clear benefit, that these benefits would result in lower rates of diabetes and heart disease (no one had shown this), and that the duration and consequences of use would be monitored carefully. Thus, the benefit side of the equation required the intersection of multiple best-case scenarios. The risk side against which it would be compared was already established.

It was apparent long before the introduction of Redux that these were all unrealistic expectations. The average five or six pounds of transient weight loss achieved in the closely supervised clinical trials of Redux did not suggest that there would be a major reduction in obesity-related illness, either for individual patients or for society as a whole. This would be even more emphatically true when the drugs were used in more typical settings: everyone knew that most of the patients who would get the drug in routine care would not be morbidly obese, and that the diet and exercise regimens prescribed with the drug would be followed much less well than in the clinical trials, meaning that the actual weight loss achieved would be even smaller. The drugs' modest effects would still evaporate when the treatment was stopped, even if patients continued to diet and exercise. As a result, most patients would have to take them forever to keep the pounds off.

MASSAGING THE DISEASE MODEL

In the 1970s, when I had first stumbled on the Pondimin ads for fenfluramine, most doctors dismissed the product with the following logic: "What good is the drug if the weight comes back as soon as you stop using it?" By the 1990s the diet-pill industry and its academic consultants had succeeded in marketing the view that obesity is simply another chronic disease like diabetes, arthritis, or hypertension. *Of course* the patient has to take medications for her whole life, just as she would need to for those other conditions. After all, the argument ran, we don't dismiss insulin as a bad treatment for diabetes just because the blood sugar goes back up as soon as you stop taking it. But lifelong use of fenfluramine would also guarantee lifelong risk. The benefits would be slight and the risks perpetual.

The clinical trials of fenfluramine and dexfenfluramine had never demonstrated any improvement in health or in survival, but they really never could have. Most of the studies lasted only for a few months—just long enough to demonstrate to the FDA that the drugs produced a five- or six-pound weight loss advantage over placebo that was statistically significant. From the agency's perspective, that was all that had to be shown for the drug to be approved. So where did the promised massive public health benefit come from? It was extrapolated using computer models. But if a reduction in obesity-related high blood pressure or diabetes was to be the mechanism through which those other health benefits would emerge in the future, the trials didn't show that either. Even the trial subjects who lost weight didn't have much improvement in these other conditions. We now understand that the drugs were probably inferior in this important way to older, nondrug approaches like diet and exercise. These low-tech interventions had been clearly shown to improve risk factors like blood sugar and cholesterol as well as take off pounds. They just couldn't be put into a bottle and patented, and so were much less prominent in the marketing-driven discourse about how to manage weight problems.

The blow that caused the fenfluramine drugs' final demise eventually came from North Dakota, and involved a totally different kind of clinical catastrophe. In 1997, an alert technician running tests in an echocardiogram facility in Fargo noticed that she was seeing an unexpectedly high number of otherwise healthy young women with abnormal heart valves. On talking to them, she found that many were taking diet pills. The technician teamed up with Dr. Heidi Connolly, a cardiologist at the Mayo Clinic, to examine the problem more systematically. Their initial report confirmed that pulmonary hypertension wasn't the only problem these drugs caused; diet-pill users were also developing heart valve abnormalities far more often than would be expected in women of comparable age, weight, and health status. The discovery also showed how the insight of just one astute observer can identify an important side effect no one was even looking for.

Their findings were made public in July 1997. A day later, ever alert to emerging public health crises, the FDA issued a statement that there was "no conclusive evidence of a cause-effect relationship between use of the drugs and the development of valvular disease." The agency reminded doctors and patients that diet pills should be used according to the FDA-approved product labeling. At the same time, Wyeth issued a press release noting that "the data from the Mayo Clinic are limited and therefore inconclusive," and again pointed out that obesity itself "is associated with serious health disorders."

But once the report of heart valve damage was published a month later in the *New England Journal of Medicine*, no amount of government face-saving and corporate denial could save the drugs. In September 1997, Wyeth "voluntarily" withdrew both Pondimin and Redux from sale; the newer drug had been on the market for only a year. Dr. Marc Dietch, its medical director, sent a letter to all U.S. physicians. "Even though this new information is not derived from a thorough clinical study and is difficult to evaluate, the company is taking the most prudent course of action," he noted, because Wyeth "is committed to safeguarding the health and well-being of patients and ensuring that health care providers have the latest medical information."

Wyeth continues to pay heavily for its failure to heed the signals of adverse effects more promptly. The legal damages now exceed a staggering $21 billion and counting for the class-action suit brought by Richard Lewis' firm and a spate of others, along with scores of individually litigated cases. This was one of the largest adverse-effects settlements ever for the industry, making Redux at that time the most dearly departed drug in history. The stain on the company goes deeper: in the ongoing mating dance of mergers and acquisitions that continues throughout the pharmaceutical industry, Wyeth is one of the few companies that hasn't been able to get a date. Most observers believe that the huge debt overhang resulting from its double fen-fluramine burdens of Pondimin and Redux makes it too much of a red-ink risk to be worth acquiring. Its market capitalization has plummeted.

A different kind of burden is borne by the millions of women who took Redux and Pondimin. Besides those who developed pulmonary hypertension, thousands of others have damaged heart valves, and it is not yet clear how this problem will evolve as they age. Some have already required open-heart surgery, others will need ongoing medical surveillance, and no one is quite sure what the long-term prognosis for this condition will be.

Why was Redux approved at all? As a prescribing physician, even before the heart valve complication was known I could look at the drug and say, "It's essentially the same as fenfluramine, which we know produces only trivial weight loss, it has to be taken forever, and it poses the risk of a fatal lung disease. I'd rather chew glass than give it to a patient." FDA officials feel that they do not have this degree of latitude. Legally, they argue, their job is not to decide whether a new drug is an improvement over what is already available—just to decide if it's better than placebo over the short term. The health care delivery system or the marketplace is supposed to do the rest. If a manufacturer produces one or two randomized trials of a few months' duration that show that a product works slightly better than a dummy pill in reaching a surrogate outcome, and there is also a plausible story about its benefits outweighing its risks, the agency is under considerable pressure to approve it for widespread use. The pressure can get particularly intense for drugs with enormous commercial potential like diet aids, where billions of dollars in sales are at stake.

In light of the existing evidence about fenfluramine-induced pulmonary hypertension, when the FDA first approved Redux it instructed the manufacturer to begin a large follow-up study as soon as the drug entered widespread use, in which Wyeth was to track how many women developed pulmonary hypertension while taking Redux. Unfortunately, Wyeth's zeal in bringing its drug to market was not matched by comparable alacrity in getting the adverse-effects surveillance program off the ground; the research didn't really begin in earnest until about a year after the drug became available—by then, it had already been withdrawn. This was not unusual; a 2003 report by the FDA admitted that fully half of the postmarketing studies it asked companies to perform had never even been started.

At about the same time that report was released, a new FDA commissioner pleased industry observers by announcing that the agency was redoubling its efforts to speed up the approval process for new drugs, particularly those to treat dangerous medical conditions like obesity.

4: TOO SWEET TO BE TRUE

Irving Motek, a forty-three-year-old baker with diabetes, went to see his doctor for a routine checkup. He had been getting a little sloppy with his diet, and as a result his blood sugar was running a bit high. To address the problem his doctor stopped his old diabetes medicine and began a new one. A few weeks later, Irving felt like he was coming down with the flu; his wife noted his skin had become sallow and his eyes looked yellowish. He became progressively more lethargic, was hospitalized, and found to be in profound liver failure. Two weeks later he was comatose and terminally ill. To survive, he required a liver transplant to replace his own severely damaged organ. Eleven days later a twenty-three-year-old motorcyclist took a curve too fast, hit a patch of ice, and rammed his helmet-free head into the guard rail of the interstate at seventy miles per hour, denting the rail and shattering his skull. On arrival at the hospital the biker was diagnosed as brain-dead and his family agreed to donate his organs.

With a new liver, Irving recovered slowly over two more months in the hospital. He was eventually discharged home in stable condition on a combination of drugs to suppress his immune system; he'd need to take them along with a different diabetes medicine for the rest of his life.

Since 1990, more major drugs have been withdrawn for substantial unexpected safety problems than ever before in such rapid succession. Sometimes this has been the result of premarketing studies that were too small to detect important but rare side effects. Some of the problems may have stemmed from the FDA's attempts to speed up its approval process. But as we saw with Pondimin and Redux, in some instances the disaster was brought on by willful underestimation of a drug's known risks.

This also seems to be what happened with Rezulin, the first in a new class of diabetes medications first marketed in March of 1997.

All of us in medicine would like to believe that the discovery of a new drug is the end product of a disciplined, purposeful search that begins with an insight from biochemistry or physiology and continues over years in the lab: scientists pore over test tubes or rats or printouts of genetic data, and then a dedicated investigator's spark of analytic brilliance catalyzes the final *eureka*. Sometimes it really works this way, but often the origins of a breakthrough drug are much more humble.

Viagra, for instance, was being developed as a treatment for heart disease until a few serendipitous observations came together. In clinical trials, to the embarrassment of both staff and patients, nurses going from bed to bed to measure blood pressures noticed that male study subjects often had large erections. Although the experimental product's cardiac benefits were unimpressive, men given it asked if they could please continue taking the drug after the study ended. (As a heart drug the product didn't show exceptional performance, but its recipients did.) Cardiologists and their male patients sometimes differ on which is the most important organ in the body; although Viagra didn't do much for one it excelled in the other, and was rechristened as a treatment for erectile dysfunction.

Another product that switched identities was minoxidil. It was developed to lower blood pressure but wasn't well tolerated in clinical trials. Many patients who took it complained of an annoying side effect—excessive hair growth. It was later marketed as Rogaine to treat baldness.

Despite the appealing image of the focused, white-coated pharmaceutical researcher so compellingly portrayed in TV commercials, the initial evolution of the diabetes drug Rezulin also owed much to serendipity. An earlier compound called ciglitazone, the first drug in a new chemical class, was being tested as a potential cholesterol-lowering compound. But what it really lowered was subjects' blood sugars, often excessively—a side effect that rendered it useless for its intended purpose. A second reason ciglitazone was not developed further was that it was toxic to the liver, an observation that will be important later. But the experience led to the insight that similar compounds might prove useful in the management of diabetes.

The first product of this kind that made it to market was its cousin troglitazone, trade named Rezulin. (It's much more appealing for a drug to have a name that suggests resolution of a problem, rather than evoking images of troglodytes.) Most other oral drugs for adult-onset diabetes worked primarily by flogging the patient's exhausted pancreas to make more insulin, or by persuading the liver to release less glucose. When all else failed there was always insulin itself. But this novel class of drugs caused the liver to produce less glucose *and* rendered fat cells more sensitive to the effects of insulin, either the body's own or the kind given through a syringe. The physiological rationale for this new double-barreled approach was compelling.

Troglitazone was granted fast-track review by the FDA, a process developed around 1990 after AIDS activists terrified the agency with a massive sit-in to protest the government's inability to approve lifesaving breakthrough products quickly enough. As per usual FDA policy, the manufacturer was not required to demonstrate that Rezulin was better than any existing drug. Studies were conducted in which diabetic patients whose blood sugar was poorly controlled with insulin had either Rezulin or placebo added to their regimens. Not astonishingly, the new drug lowered blood sugar better than placebo did. Its initial approval hinged on premarketing studies involving only about 2,500 patients.

A MISLEADING BEGINNING

Based on this evidence, an FDA advisory committee met in December 1996 to decide whether the drug should be approved for sale. In summarizing the product's safety profile at that meeting, a doctor representing the manufacturer, Parke-Davis, reported that its clinical trials showed that the drug's risk of liver toxicity was "comparable to placebo." The company also had collected additional safety data from other studies, but these were not presented at that meeting. Instead, the Parke-Davis physician said that the rate of liver damage in those other analyses was "very, very similar" to what was reported at the approval hearing, and that he would provide that data to the FDA later on. Based on the data presented that day, the advisory committee voted to allow the drug onto the market. As it turned out, the rate of clinically important liver damage in those early trials had been considerably higher in the patients who had gotten Rezulin rather than placebo. But as a cynical sports commentator once observed, "The rules are defined by what the ref sees."

The company did provide the FDA with the promised data from the additional trials a week after the approval. It revealed a rate of liver abnormalities that was not at all "very, very similar" in the patients who got the new drug; it was substantially greater. But the drug had already been approved and the new information didn't receive widespread attention.

Rezulin's initial approval required that it be used only for patients already taking insulin, limiting its potential utilization and thus its market share. But Parke-Davis quickly sought further permission to market the drug as a stand-alone therapy for diabetes. This would greatly increase the product's commercial potential, but would also expose far more patients to its risks. Backed by a huge marketing campaign featuring its novel mode of action, sales of Rezulin took off. By October 1997, when it had been on the market for just eight months, concern began to grow over a steady flow of reports describing patients who developed severe and unexpected liver damage while taking the drug. In preparation for a meeting with the FDA on October 24, Parke-Davis ran a computer tabulation of all subjects in its early premarketing clinical trials whose blood tests suggested liver abnormalities. But before a company physician reported these findings to the FDA, he tightened the criterion for "abnormal" in patients who got the new product but not for those in the placebo group, obscuring the elevated risk. Parke-Davis then obtained FDA permission to use the lower number of liver cases in its official product warnings, without revealing that the initial estimate had been considerably larger.

Normally, we estimate a drug's potential for liver damage by measuring whether enzymes from that organ leak into the bloodstream. This blood test is a useful indicator of the severity of liver damage: normal levels are reassuring, modest elevations (three times the normal range) raise questions, and much higher levels (as high as ten or twenty times the normal range) are usually a sign of substantial damage. But in reporting these results to the FDA, companies sometimes fold together all abnormal liver tests under the broad category of "greater than three times normal," even if a large proportion of such patients have elevations that were far higher—a clear sign of widespread liver cell destruction. This is akin to asking your child how his day went at school and being told that he had a squabble with the teacher, when in fact he had hacked her to death with a machete. A fair report of the event would have mentioned something about stab wounds and not merely categorized it under the rubric "squabble."

By the autumn of 1997, 135 cases of severe liver damage had been reported in Rezulin patients, including at least five that were fatal. All the cases had occurred in the United States or Japan. Drug safety surveillance is an international field, and news about adverse events in one country is rapidly communicated around the world. Looking back, that period provides a fascinating contrast in how regulatory authorities and companies in different countries can assess the very same data and come to vastly different conclusions.

The drug was approved for use in the United Kingdom a few months later than in the United States. It was sold there under a licensing agreement with the British pharmaceutical firm Glaxo-Wellcome, which did not begin marketing it until September 1997. Within six weeks, Glaxo officials in London became concerned about the rapidly increasing rate of reports of liver damage. The affected patients often had nothing in their histories to suggest that they would be susceptible to this life-threatening problem. It was also becoming clear that stopping the drug when the problem was first detected sometimes was not enough to reverse the damage. New reports of liver disease were continuing to come in from the United States at an accelerating rate. No one could be sure when the tide of toxicity would crest.

The British company concluded that with so many safer options available to treat diabetes without damaging the liver, the drug's risk-benefit relationship was indefensible. In late November 1997 Glaxo notified the British government that it intended to take its product off the market as of December 1, after only three months of sales. Over the next two weeks Glaxo and the Japanese company that had initially developed the product withdrew applications to market Rezulin in twenty-six additional countries from Iceland to Israel, including virtually all of Europe.

TRANSATLANTIC DIFFERENCES

At that moment, in the United States, Parke-Davis was taking a completely different course. On December 1, as Glaxo was removing the drug from pharmacies throughout England, Parke-Davis sent a letter to every practicing physician in America. It reminded doctors to monitor liver function closely in patients taking the drug, and explained that "heightened awareness following the earlier labeling change [recommending more frequent blood tests of liver function] has, as expected, generated some additional reports of hepatic dysfunction." The company admitted that its partner Glaxo had decided to "temporarily suspend marketing" of the drug in Britain "pending their review of worldwide safety data," but added that Glaxo "has experience with only 5,000 patients" on the drug in Great Britain, a number much smaller than Parke-Davis' experience in the U.S. market. This was misleading; although sales in the United Kingdom were smaller, Glaxo's withdrawal decision had been based on liver toxicity data from all over the world, not just events in Britain. Indeed, most of the adverse events on which the decision was based had occurred in the United States.

Parke-Davis' December letter to physicians went on to report that together with the FDA, it had "already completed a thorough review of the worldwide safety experience with Rezulin." In bold type it declared, **"You will be reassured to know that the additional reports received since early November do not indicate a greater frequency of liver injury or potential for serious harm than had been previously estimated. . . ."** and continued, "The FDA continues to find a favorable benefit to risk relationship for Rezulin therapy. . . ." The letter reminded doctors that all treatments for diabetes could cause severe side effects, and ended by recommending close monitoring of patients with once-a-month blood tests to detect liver problems.

During that same week at the end of 1997, researchers at the federal National Institutes of Health were hit with their own piece of the Rezulin crisis. Encouraged by Parke-Davis, the NIH had gone out on a limb by initiating a government-sponsored study that used Rezulin not to treat diabetes but to keep it from developing in healthy patients who appeared to be at risk of *becoming* diabetic. At a cost of $150 million, it was to be the government's largest diabetes study ever. But now NIH was in the awkward position of administering a potentially fatal drug to patients who didn't even have the disease it was approved to treat. The doctors responsible for the trial worried what effect the British decision might have on U.S. physicians who had enrolled their own patients in the study. On November 28, a letter was sent to participating physicians by Dr. Richard Eastman, director of the NIH Division of Diabetes, Endocrine, and Metabolic Diseases. As one of the NIH's top diabetes researchers, he had major responsibility for the design and ongoing conduct of the trial, including the original decision to include Rezulin, as well as the decision now on how to proceed. His letter began by noting that Glaxo's decision to withdraw the drug in England was "apparently a marketing decision, rather than a regulatory decision." The NIH, he reported, "is comfortable continuing with the troglitazone arm of the study despite the decision by Glaxo to withdraw the drug in Europe."

I had known Eastman years earlier, when as young physicians we were both in training at the Beth Israel Hospital in Boston. I recalled that he was a conscientious and talented clinician with a keen interest in endocrinology. I had been proud to learn that my former colleague had risen to become one of the most senior diabetes researchers at NIH. I was not proud to learn that he was also serving as a paid consultant to Parke-Davis at the same time that he was overseeing the design and conduct of the Rezulin study, having accepted over $78,000 from the company through 1997. According to government documents, a lawyer for the Department of Health and Human Services had warned him in 1996 that this represented a conflict of interest, but the relationship was not acknowledged publicly until it was reported in late 1998 by David Willman of the *Los Angeles Times.* Interviewed by Willman, Eastman's immediate superior at NIH said he saw no conflict-of-interest problem. According to the respected journal *Nature,* the university-based chairman of the study also saw no problem, explaining that virtually all medical researchers in and out of government had such consulting relationships with industry. Willman reported that "in his defense, Eastman said that over the last six years he had consulted for five other drug companies" in addition to Rezulin's manufacturer while shaping and overseeing NIH's portfolio of diabetes research. What a defense.

In May 1998, six months after Dr. Eastman's letter of reassurance to physicians, a previously healthy Illinois teacher who had been given Rezulin in the NIH diabetes prevention study developed fulminant liver toxicity. Her illness came on rapidly: despite frequent monitoring of blood tests just as the company required, the problem developed too suddenly to detect. Once discovered, it proved to be irreversible; she was soon dead. Parke-Davis issued a statement that the fatality had nothing to do with its drug, but the NIH concluded otherwise. Her case, and others like it, made it hard to take comfort in the idea that regular blood tests could nip the problem in the bud. This was the same conclusion the British had come to a year and a half earlier when they withdrew the drug from the market. Within a month of the teacher's death, NIH terminated the Rezulin arm of the diabetes prevention trial. But the drug remained in widespread use in routine clinical practice in the United States for nearly another two years.

In October 1998 the Australian equivalent of the FDA refused to give initial approval to Rezulin because of its safety record and doubts that the drug could be monitored closely enough to prevent irreversible liver damage. A similar position was taken by New Zealand's drug review body two months later. Back in the United States, Parke-Davis still continued to argue that careful liver function testing could detect problems in time for the drug to be stopped, preventing major damage. But it was becoming clear to most observers that this was implausible. More reports were coming in of Rezulin patients who suffered liver damage so rapid and devastating that even monthly blood tests could not have spotted it coming. In a number of them, the damage continued apace even after the drug was stopped.

No one who has ever been within a hundred yards of a typical medical practice should have expected that physicians and patients would consistently follow the demanding monthly blood test schedule Parke-Davis suggested. My research unit had taken a look at how well physicians monitored patients prescribed tacrine, a weakly effective drug for patients with Alzheimer's disease. It was also manufactured by Parke-Davis, and also caused liver damage. There, too, the company had told doctors that the damage could be prevented by frequent blood tests to measure liver function. We scanned the records of several thousand patients prescribed tacrine and found that only a tiny fraction were actually getting the blood tests as the company recommended. Later on Dr. David Graham, an FDA epidemiologist, analyzed data from a large HMO to see whether patients given Rezulin in typical practice were actually being monitored as required. He found that by the third month of use, fewer than 5 percent of them were getting all the recommended blood tests. This "monitoring defense" reflected the supine posture often adopted by both drug manufacturers and the FDA throughout the 1990s: "We told you there was a risk, we put it in the official label, so it's not our fault if something bad happened."

Near the end of 1998, another patient enrolled in a different company-sponsored Rezulin study developed rapid-onset liver failure despite regular monitoring; within a month she was dead. But over 2,600 other patients throughout the country were still participating in that study. Parke-Davis had paid physicians a fee of up to $350 for each patient they enrolled. One Parke-Davis scientist asked in a memo, "Do we have to send a letter out to all of the REACH investigators to inform them of this event?" No, responded her colleague at the company, using capital letters to underscore the point. "We have NO REGULATORY OBLIGATION to send a letter to the [study] physicians . . . to send out a letter now would be misleading because we cannot fully explain the case and it would be unnecessarily frightening." The company blamed the death on other causes, and continued to claim that the drug was safe as long as liver function was monitored. In the industry this is sometimes known as "defending the molecule."

In March 1999, over a year after troglitazone had been withdrawn in Europe, the British Medicines Control Agency took a second look at the drug and ruled that it should remain off the market because the evidence showed that it could not be used safely. That same month in the United States, the FDA Advisory Committee on Endocrinologic and Metabolic Drugs was scheduled to meet again to reassess Rezulin in light of the new reports of liver failure that continued to come in. At the time, it seemed clear to many of us that even though the U.S. authorities had failed to grasp the severity of the problem when it first developed, this meeting would provide an opportunity to review all the data and finally come to the right decision. There were by now even more cases of severe liver failure in patients given Rezulin, including several deaths and emergency liver transplants.

Astonishingly, the FDA's advisory committee again recommended that the drug remain on the market. It suggested that its use as sole therapy for diabetes be curtailed, but approved its continued availability for diabetics taking insulin.

On hearing of the FDA decision I remember feeling the sensation people often have in dreams, watching a car or plane or train speeding along and *knowing* it's about to crash. You try to scream but can't make a sound. I recall walking around the hospital that day, asking anyone who would listen, "What the hell are those people *doing*?!" I was able to make some sound, though. I proposed that despite the FDA decision our hospital should stop using Rezulin. The Brigham's Pharmacy and Therapeutics Committee agreed, and we removed the drug from use at our institution.

The FDA medical officer assigned to the Rezulin case, Dr. Robert Misbin, also tried to make a sound. Frustrated at his agency's unwillingness to act decisively, he began a personal crusade unusual for a government worker. He later stated that if he had been aware of the evidence of liver damage already in place when Rezulin was first evaluated by the FDA, he would have been much less willing to see it approved, and would have vehemently resisted accepting its wider use as a first-line therapy for diabetes. Over the coming months, Dr. Misbin vaulted over his bosses' heads and sent anguished letters to congressmen, urging them to act even if the agency would not. In a letter to Representative Henry Waxman, he wrote:

> I have been frustrated in my efforts to convince [FDA] management that the time has come to remove Rezulin from the market. . . . Were this a question of drug approval, FDA would have taken action in six months to meet the user fee goal [of speeding up approvals] mandated by Congress. But since the question is withdrawal of a marketed product, there seems to be no time limit. I am enclosing . . . documentation of Parke-Davis' reluctance to bring to public attention the risk of liver toxicity that they found in their clinical trials.

The "user fee goal" refers to a reorientation of the agency that occurred in the 1990s in the wake of the enactment by Congress of the Prescription Drug User Fee Act, known as PDUFA (rhymes with "palooka"). That law provides for drug companies to pay the agency a fee to have their products evaluated, averaging about a half-million dollars per drug. These funds are then used to pay for the person-time expended by the FDA employees reviewing the evidence. Critics have argued that this can distort the review process, a concern illustrated by the conversation another FDA scientist had with a senior agency official. His concerns about the safety of a particular drug had attracted the ire of its manufacturer.

"You need," his boss told him, "to understand that the pharmaceutical industry is our client."

"That's odd," he responded. "I always thought our clients were the people of the United States."

John Ashcroft was still a senator from Missouri as the Rezulin story was unraveling. In writing to him, Dr. Misbin described a letter he received from a St. Louis physician who claimed that Parke-Davis had omitted data about Rezulin-related liver damage from its reports to the FDA, and that the FDA was ineffective in dealing with the problem. "I believe that [her] complaint about FDA is well founded," Dr. Misbin wrote. "There is little doubt that patients are still experiencing Rezulin-related liver toxicity because of FDA's inaction. In the absence of a threat of Congressional hearing, I see little hope of turning this around until many more patients have died."

A BELATED INSIGHT

One full year after the follow-up advisory committee meeting that again endorsed the continued use of Rezulin, the FDA eventually reconsidered its decision. The committee finally recommended in March 2000 that the drug be taken off the market. More than two years after the same decision was made in England, over $2 billion in sales and ninety-four cases of acute liver failure (sixty-six of them fatal) after its introduction, Rezulin ended its blockbuster career in the United States.

The courts are still considering how much of the Rezulin tragedy was produced by willful malfeasance versus what could be called passive-aggressive surveillance: foot-dragging in following up on signals of a potential hazard. As scores of cases approached trial, the manufacturer's zeal to protect its molecule instead of patients followed what could be called the FDA defense, a gambit seen in many drug product liability suits. In that strategy, a company maintains a bare-bones adverse-events reporting department, staffed on the front lines by people with little or no training in epidemiology or clinical matters. Once its drug is approved for marketing, the company doesn't proactively investigate how appropriately it is being used, or what side effects occur in patients who take it. When reports of those adverse events are nonetheless sent in spontaneously by doctors or patients, the company passes them along to the FDA as required by law, with minimal or no further scrutiny. It's widely known that the FDA division on the receiving end of these reports has traditionally been underpopulated and overworked, partly because of earlier industry opposition to allocating any of its user-fee funds to support those activities. Eventually, if an important side effect does surface, company officials can respond as many have in court, saying, in effect: "We didn't notice a worrisome pattern. We obeyed the regulations and sent FDA all the reports we received. They never made us do a study, or send out a warning, or take the drug off the market. So it's not our fault if anyone got hurt." This is the corporate equivalent of a teenager murdering both his parents and then begging the court for mercy on the grounds that he's an orphan.

How very . . . twentieth century. Case after case of multimillion-dollar adverse-event settlements involving withdrawn drugs have demonstrated that this just isn't going to be good enough anymore. Ignorance of the flaw is no excuse.

In a trenchant postmortem of the Rezulin story published in the British medical journal *Lancet,* Dr. Edwin Gale, an English diabetes specialist, argued that Rezulin had never been a drug of especially great value in the first place. He pointed out that testing it against placebo in diabetic patients was a very low standard to meet. Further, even though safer products from this new class of drug had been introduced in the years following Rezulin's withdrawal, the subsequent clinical experience with them had not borne out manufacturers' claims that they would transform the care of diabetes. "Troglitazone came and went with no demonstrated advantage over existing therapy," he wrote. But because mere advantage over placebo was all that was required for approval, not head-to-head comparisons with standard therapy, "the system did not require the studies that would have allowed us to find out." He continued:

> The regulatory process creates an evidence-free zone at the time of launch of new drugs. Companies need to market aggressively during this period because the countdown on the life of their product licence has already begun. Even the most ethical company will be reluctant to launch studies which might discredit a marketing claim based on weak evidence. . . .
>
> A physician does, however, differ in important respects from a travel agent, or so many of us believe. But who speaks for the clinician? Oddly enough there is no answer to this. . . . Access to information about new drugs is closely retained by the companies, and post-marketing studies are dictated by marketing policy. . . . One lesson from [Rezulin] is that the public interest is not well served by the current system of drug development.

5: COLD COMFORT

The Rezulin disaster occurred in a novel class of drug brand new to the marketplace. A similar problem could never arise in a drug that had been in use for nearly a century and held a trusted place in tens of millions of American medicine cabinets. Or so we'd expect. For decades, phenylpropanolamine, or PPA, was one of the most widely ingested drug products in the United States. Related to the amphetamine class of drugs, it had long been known to have some of the properties of "speed" but in milder form: it reduced the appetite, dried up nasal secretions, and raised blood pressure. The latter property of PPA was known since the early 1900s. By the 1950s, PPA was being used in dozens of over-the-counter (OTC) remedies in two categories, cold remedies and diet aids, and was marketed by numerous manufacturers under myriad brand names. For colds, it was packaged as Dimetapp, Contac, Triaminic, and Coricidin. The trade names for its anorexiant avatar were more poetic: Thinz had obvious cachet, and Dexatrim was intended to sound like dexedrine, the amphetamine whose use had been curtailed because of its addictive properties. Another PPA-containing diet aid lost its marketing appeal with the emergence of a health problem associated with a different kind of weight loss—it had been called Ayds. Its sales plummeted in the 1980s.

The use of PPA increased in the 1970s when the government tightened restrictions on its more rowdy street cousins, the amphetamines. PPA was such an old product that its first use antedated key FDA legislation; as a result, its manufacturers had never been required to prove safety and efficacy as they would if the drug were introduced today. No formal evaluation had ever been demanded until the onset of the Drug Efficacy Study Implementation (DESI) program, the review of grandfathered products and combination drugs that the FDA began in 1962. As the DESI initiative plodded along over more than twenty years, it focused first on prescription-only products; it didn't get to consider most over-the-counter preparations until the 1970s.

By 1979, reports began to appear of otherwise healthy patients who suffered strokes while taking PPA. The authors of one early paper recommended that "withdrawal of preparations containing phenylpropanolamine from general use should be considered in view of their potential for adverse reactions with other commonly used drugs and their doubtful therapeutic value." In 1980 another paper appeared in *Lancet,* reporting an experiment in which PPA-containing diet pills and cold remedies were given to healthy volunteers. A third of the subjects given one PPA product had their diastolic blood pressure rise to over 100 millimeters—well past the level that would warrant a diagnosis of hypertension if it persisted. The authors concluded, "The frequency and extent of the hypertensive response to high-dose phenylpropanolamine-containing preparations suggest that clinical use of such preparations should be reviewed and that their availability without prescription may not be appropriate."

Advocacy groups began to weigh in on the subject. The Center for Science in the Public Interest wrote the FDA commissioner to demand that PPA products be removed from the market:

> Studies conducted since 1978 have demonstrated that currently acceptable doses of PPA can trigger marked rises in blood pressure, even in healthy medical students, and it is known that overweight individuals have a greater-than-average incidence of hypertension, heart disease, and other disorders that could be dangerously aggravated by the drug's effects on the cardiovascular system. All of the data now on public record, including information available through transcripts of the [FDA's] Advisory Review Panel's meetings, suggest that PPA is, at best, only marginally effective in contributing to weight loss, with little evidence that the losses can be maintained past a few months. . . .
>
> It is disturbing that the FDA's evaluation of PPA-based diet aids has been proceeding so slowly. It has been almost three years since the Advisory Review Panel issued its preliminary report on weight-control products. . . . As long as the publication of that Federal Register report is put off, manufacturers of PPA-based weight-control medications will be able to promote their questionable products with impunity. . . . We submit that this evidence demonstrates that PPA-based diet aids are no more than marginally effective and that they do not meet the safety requirements of [the law]. As a result, we call upon the FDA to propose a ban on OTC distribution of these drugs.

That was in 1981.

The most severe adverse effects of PPA were obvious enough when they occurred. Just as diabetic patients hardly ever suddenly turn yellow and die of fulminant liver failure, healthy people with colds or on diets hardly ever have strokes. But several factors complicated the link between PPA and stroke. First, as the manufacturers were to claim vehemently in the coming years, millions of people used PPA in its numerous forms, so any number of unusual outcomes could occur merely by chance while someone was taking PPA: Siamese twins would be conceived, people would have hallucinations, tumors of the pancreas would be discovered, and Nobel Prizes might even be won by PPA users, without any of these events being caused by the drug. This is a common problem in pharmacoepidemiology: establishing a connection between the use of a frequently used medication and the subsequent occurrence of a rare event.

The PPA-stroke story had another complicating wrinkle: tachyphylaxis. This is the body's ability to adapt over time to the effects of a drug—either its intended one or a side effect. In the case of PPA, adaptation to its blood-pressure-elevating effect is fairly rapid. Clinical studies dating back to the 1970s showed that some people experience a marked rise in blood pressure on first using the drug that then subsides over a few days, even with continuing use. The body "figures out the problem" and adapts. This same development of tolerance to a drug's effect is one reason that PPA's sister compounds, cocaine and amphetamine, are so highly addictive. With repeated use of those drugs, users begin to adapt to the high and then crave ever larger doses to get the same rush. Rats put in cages fitted with electrified floors will keep running across the cage to get a fix of speed until their paws are literally cooked. PPA was not anywhere as addictive as amphetamine or cocaine, but it did induce a similar property of tolerance. As a result, if you measure blood pressures in people who have been using PPA for a week, you might miss their transient periods of hypertension. And if you did a study of stroke occurrence in people who were PPA users, you might miss the association if you didn't analyze *when* the stroke occurred in relation to their first use of PPA.

EARLY WARNINGS

By 1982, the FDA had begun to express official concern about the possibility of blood pressure elevation and strokes in patients taking PPA; it ruled that products combining PPA with caffeine and/or ephedrine were a potential health hazard. But ephedrine remained available by prescription, and the amount of caffeine in the PPA combination pills could easily be replaced, intentionally or not, by drinking a few cups of coffee. Representative Mary Oakar held congressional hearings in 1983 to examine the potential risks of PPA. But strong pressure by the over-the-counter drug industry and a lack of countervailing bureaucratic verve prevented the FDA from taking a position on the issue for several more years. This was attributed to the need to gather more information, but very little information was actually gathered during most of this time. The drug continued to be widely sold, with the impasse illustrating the truth of Camus' dictum, "Not to decide is to decide."

In 1985, when the FDA eventually made an official statement on the status of PPA, it expressed concerns about the drug's risks and refused to give it Category I status, the designation for products considered safe and effective. It reaffirmed this position in 1988. Congressional hearings on PPA were held again in 1990 by Senator Ron Wyden. Those hearings again called the product's safety into question; several witnesses argued that it was too dangerous to remain on the over-the-counter market. Clinical reviewers at the FDA concluded in 1991 that a systematic study was needed to define PPA's risks once and for all, but none was initiated. Case reports and review articles continued to appear in the medical literature throughout the 1980s and early 1990s reporting strokes, some fatal, in people who had used over-the-counter PPA for colds or to lose weight.

Safer alternatives had long been available to replace PPA in cold remedies. One was pseudoephedrine, commonly sold as Sudafed, which had also been long used as an over-the-counter decongestant. But PPA was cheaper to produce; such a switch would have increased production costs and could have adversely impacted revenues. When pressure to remove PPA from the market failed to materialize, the companies felt no need to move forward with any reformulation plans. No such easy switch was available for the other commercially successful version of PPA, as a diet aid. However, while PPA did blunt hunger temporarily, like the fen-phen products, it was never shown to be a useful long-term treatment for obesity.

Taken together, these two issues—the availability of other, safer treatments for the sniffles, and the absence of evidence that PPA as a diet aid made any long-term difference—caused the benefit side of the risk-benefit equation to seem weak indeed, especially compared to the possibility that the drug might blow a hole in someone's brain. But consumers were never given a chance to decide that using one decongestant versus another, or having an easier time passing up dessert, might be worth risking lifelong paralysis or death. Virtually none of the labels affixed to PPA products mentioned the possibility of stroke, even in the illegible microprint that passes for fair warning on over-the-counter packages. The *emptor* wasn't even given a chance to *cavere*.

Because the FDA lacks an adequate budget to fund studies of drugs, even the relatively inexpensive epidemiological kind, and no other government agency has the mandate, funding, or will to take on that role on a large scale, the agency has to rely on drug companies to support the research needed to make regulatory decisions. Companies are eager to fund the studies required to win approval of a drug, because unless they can provide data that satisfies the FDA, the product cannot be marketed. But the agency has much less clout when it comes to cajoling manufacturers to support research on already-marketed drugs. It can raise the specter of withdrawal to try to motivate such studies, and the "w" word was indeed whispered about PPA throughout the 1980s and 1990s. But that would have been a hard ruling to make stick because no one had ever conducted a rigorous study to define the risk.

It was not until late 1992 that the over-the-counter drug industry association, under pressure, formally agreed to fund a study to clarify the situation. It would be a case-control analysis: people who had strokes would be compared to similar people who did not, to determine whether the former were more likely to have been recent users of PPA. A draft research plan was submitted in 1993 by a talented team of researchers at Yale Medical School. The study design was the most appropriate one to use for such an investigation, and its details were specified in advance and clarified in numerous communications between the Yale team and the manufacturers' group that requested and funded the research. The lead researcher, Dr. Ralph Horwitz, was chairman of the Department of Medicine at Yale and a highly respected internist and clinical epidemiologist. The project eventually got off the ground in the fall of 1994, and took five years to complete.

By the time the project was finished, the Yale team had contacted and interviewed 2,078 patients, of whom 702 had suffered a stroke caused by hemorrhage into their brains. As they reported in the *New England Journal of Medicine,* the study team found that initial use of PPA for any purpose increased the risk of hemorrhagic stroke by threefold; this rose to a sixteen-fold increase in risk when PPA was used as an appetite suppressant. The OTC industry was quick to respond. The very companies that had funded the research and signed off on its design now complained about the analytic approach that was taken. They commissioned noted pharmacoepidemiologists from great universities to write critiques explaining why the findings might be wrong, and to opine that no regulatory action should be taken based on such "fragile" evidence. They hired well-known physicians to attest to their own experience with the safety and reliability of PPA products, and to develop arguments to reassure parents that it was still safe to use PPA in children. The study's findings were irrelevant to pediatric practice, the argument went, because the Yale study had been done in people over eighteen. (I've wondered about the potential regulatory implications of this argument. Would manufacturers have tried to plea-bargain a settlement in which pediatric products containing PPA could remain on the shelves even if the adult versions were removed? I can see the label now, in tiny illegible type: *This product has been trusted by parents for years to treat their children's nasal congestion. It has also been shown to cause strokes in patients over age eighteen. No such study was ever conducted in children. If your child suddenly becomes paralyzed or comatose while taking this drug, consult your pediatrician immediately or proceed to the nearest emergency room.*)

The industry counterattack failed. By the end of 2000, all products containing phenylpropanolamine were removed from pharmacy shelves. Over twenty years after the initial concerns were raised, a careful epidemiologic study had finally put the matter to rest. The OTC manufacturers immediately replaced the PPA in their cough and cold products with the safer pseudoephedrine, a transition that was made quickly and efficiently. After all, the idea for reformulation had been around for years, but never implemented because it was never mandated. For those who had suffered strokes after taking an over-the-counter cold remedy or diet aid, like Ethel Coryza in the prologue, the FDA's long-delayed decision about the safety of PPA came years too late.

REDUX, REZULIN, AND PPA all represent extreme examples of failures in risk assessment. In each case there was evidence of a willful ignoring of hazard signals as they emerged. Those were the easy cases. It's much harder to analyze the side effects of drugs when there is no intentional foot-dragging or obfuscation. These situations involve no villains or heroes—just fascinating questions and the difference between life and death. In the world of drug risks they are the more common examples, but no less dramatic.

6: GETTING RISKS RIGHT

A twenty-three-year-old pregnant woman suffers from intolerable nau-
sea and vomiting in her first trimester. "It's getting so bad that when
I wake up I can't stand the sight of food, and I feel like puking most
mornings," she tells her doctor. "Isn't there anything you can do?" He
prescribes a widely used antinausea drug, which reduces her symptoms
greatly. The remainder of her pregnancy is uneventful, but at thirty-nine
weeks she delivers a badly deformed baby. The drug her doctor pre-
scribed is later removed from the market because of concern that it
causes such birth defects.

Subsequent research makes clear that the drug poses no such risk.
But it remains unavailable because of fear of litigation.

Each day, all over world millions of people die, recover from illness, develop new symptoms, take pills. Medical interventions and
outcomes are happening all the time. For drugs in widespread use,
it is crucial to evaluate adverse events to determine which of them are
caused by a given medication, and which would have happened anyway.
Enormous numbers of drug exposures and clinical outcomes must be
transformed from mere bits of data into accurate and actionable insights,
preferably instantaneously.

Requiring that drugs on the market be completely "safe" is an impossible goal. The real question is whether a drug's dangers are in some acceptable proportion to the good it does. This fragile balance can fall apart at
any of its seams: the product may have an unrecognized inherent flaw; the
doctor may not prescribe it as its developers intended; the patient may take
too much or too little; expected side effects may occur more often or with

greater severity than anticipated. Much of the work that goes on in my research unit and others like it around the world is aimed at discovering these problems before they make headlines, to take the measure of a drug's risks so that doctors, patients, and policy makers can make better choices in weighing them against benefits.

It is the middle of the night in the Hotel Sheraton Centre, Montreal. A loud buzzer awakens me, followed by a quavering voice. First in French, then in English, he reports that an alarm has been activated in the hotel, the fire department has been called, and all guests are to evacuate. I am in Montreal for a meeting of the International Society for Pharmaco-epidemiology, a group of researchers who study the effects of prescription drugs. I was up late the previous night (pharmacoepidemiologists can get pretty rowdy when gathered together in large numbers) and have to wake up early to chair a plenary session on assessing risk. The young man repeats his message. I feel what most of us feel in such situations, the legacy of too many fire drills in elementary school: "This probably isn't the real thing. They're just going to make us go outside and stand in the cold for twenty minutes. Then there will be an all-clear signal and we'll file back inside. Damn nuisance."

As a child, I wasn't allowed to ignore the alarm; now I can. No one would know. But in the middle of that night in Montreal I wonder, "What if this time it's the real thing? Fires do happen in public buildings, and I'm on the fourteenth floor; if this isn't a false alarm I could be burned alive. But the odds are that it's a false alarm. The buzzer will probably stop soon, and I'll go back to sleep without having to run out into the Canadian night in my pajamas." The buzzer continues. The quavering voice comes back on, repeating his script. I run down dozens of flights of stairs into the chilly Montreal dark.

Some adverse drug effects are self-evident, like morning grogginess after taking a sleeping pill the night before, or lightheadedness following a too-high dose of blood pressure medication. The connection with the offending agent can be less obvious for other symptoms, especially early on in a drug's career: an intestinal hemorrhage that occurs months after starting an analgesic, or jaundice that comes on while a patient is being treated with a new antibiotic. That midnight buzzer gave many of us at the meeting a visceral grounding for the society's session the following morning on measuring risk. Our brief moment of mild anxiety and nuisance provided a low-dose version of what life is like every day for the people responsible for screening and evaluating evidence of suspected drug side effects.

TWO BOXES OF DISASTER

Imagine that you work at the FDA and come into your office each morning to confront two piles of reports. Those in an in-box marked "1" describe cases like the following: A fifty-seven-year-old construction worker in Nevada had been a regular user of inhaled steroids for asthma; a year after being started on a new product, he was diagnosed with leukemia. A twenty-seven-year-old beautician in Seattle was prescribed a drug to treat her migraine headaches; after five weeks of use, she developed weakness in her limbs that was diagnosed as multiple sclerosis. A seventy-one-year-old lawyer in New York City was switched to a new cholesterol-lowering medication and three weeks later ruptured a major abdominal blood vessel, requiring emergency surgery and four units of blood transfusion. A seventy-eight-year-old diabetic nursing home resident started a recently marketed treatment for Alzheimer's disease; within two weeks he had lost circulation in his left leg, requiring a below-knee amputation.

Now, consider a second pile of reports, somewhat smaller, that had also arrived in the previous day's mail. These are in a separate in-box on your desk labeled "2." Here are some of the cases it contains: A thirty-two-year-old teacher in Nebraska was given a painkiller for a sprained ankle, and three weeks later developed hepatitis. A sixty-five-year-old accountant in San Francisco had been treated for rheumatoid arthritis, and was later diagnosed with lymphoma. A fifty-one-year-old factory worker in Chicago found his seasonal nasal congestion did not respond to his usual allergy medication; his doctor diagnosed an upper respiratory infection and added an antibiotic. After six days he developed an irregular heartbeat; in the emergency room he had a cardiac arrest and died.

What distinguishes Box 1 from Box 2? Both in-boxes describe clinical events, often tragic, that occurred in patients who were taking medications. Viewed with the power of hindsight, it turns out that all the events described in Box 1 were random misfortunes, not related in any way to the drug noted on the report form. If we were to give Box 1 a name, we might borrow the title used by Rabbi Harold Kushner for his book *When Bad Things Happen to Good People* (or, if the label was too small for that, *Stuff Happens*).

Box 2, by contrast, we now know contains the kind of initial reports that were the first signals of likely drug-induced illnesses—problems that in two of the three cases resulted in a decision that the offending product was too dangerous to be left on the market. The terrifying reality faced by the people on the receiving end of these reports is that they do not come neatly separated into Box 1 and Box 2. *They are all in the same in-box when they arrive.*

Each day, the case histories that will eventually end up in conceptual Box 1 far outnumber those that will land in Box 2. But that is small comfort given the gravity of the second kind of report. In fact, it only makes the job harder, a little bit like trying to find an AIDS-contaminated needle in a haystack just moments before a busload of schoolchildren arrives to romp through it. The FDA receives more than a thousand such reports every day, and it's vital to figure out which events belong in Box 1 and which in Box 2 while there's still time to do something about it. This is where we must turn to the science of pharmacoepidemiology: usually complex, sometimes arcane, frequently frustrating, always interesting, and occasionally lifesaving.

Pharmacoepidemiology is the study of the uses and outcomes of medicines in large populations of patients. Its first part comes from the Greek *pharmakeuein,* "to administer drugs," which in turn is from the Greek *pharmakon,* which meant "magic charm," "poison," or "drug" (my dictionary lists them in that order). The second part of the word comes from the Greek *epidemia,* or "epidemic," derived from *epi-,* "on or upon," and *demos,* "people." The discipline of epidemiology has its roots in the study of outbreaks of contagious diseases, although it has moved far beyond those origins. One of my medical heroes is Dr. John Snow, a nineteenth-century British physician who was one of the first modern epidemiologists. His work set the stage for the study of how diseases strike populations—a perspective upon which much of modern pharmacoepidemiology is built.

The London of Snow's day was ravaged by wave after wave of cholera epidemics. No one yet understood that the disease was spread when infected patients' stools contaminated the food or water of healthy people. The preferred explanation of the time was based on something known as *miasma*—invisible bad vapors in the air that somehow produced disease. Undaunted by medicine's ignorance of what caused the problem, Snow meticulously noted in which houses cholera victims lived (or died), and which houses had been spared. Inventing the methodology as he went along, he then used utility records to determine the source of each home's drinking water. Victorian London was served by a few large companies that piped water to the homes of their customers. Snow's exercise revealed that the disease's apparently random attack had a great deal to do with which water company supplied a given house. Residences served by the Lambeth Waterworks Company, which drew its supply from high up the Thames, had relatively few cholera cases. But the disease was far more common in homes supplied by the Southwark and Vauxhall Water Company. It drew its water from a part of the river much closer to the city, contaminated with sewage infected by earlier victims of the epidemic.

In linking social phenomena to dread disease, Snow's discoveries had obvious policy implications—even if they didn't fit well with the prevailing scientific notions of his day. In an observational tour de force Snow painstakingly mapped the distribution of one neighborhood cholera epidemic and related it to use of a contaminated public water pump on Broad Street. The pump's handle was removed to stop its tainted effluent from causing any more disease. In a romanticized version of the story Snow, frustrated that his discovery was not being acted upon, goes down to the Broad Street pump by night to rip off its handle himself. It didn't happen that way, but as medical legends go this one is superb. It symbolizes the transformation of an epidemiological insight into the social action that logically should follow it. After all, discovering causes of medical events in large populations ought to bring about changes that ameliorate those risks in individuals. Many of us in this field try in some modest way to follow Dr. Snow's venerable example of science-based activism. These days, we just do it to a more contemporary soundtrack, perhaps the line in Bob Dylan's "Subterranean Homesick Blues" about the pump that wouldn't work when vandals stole its handle.

Since Snow's day, epidemiology has outgrown a solitary focus on the spread of infectious disease and has taken on a much broader scope, using the same tools to study the occurrence and control of all kinds of illness. We now work with computers rather than old city maps, but the intent is the same: to examine the big picture of who was exposed to what risks, and who gets sick—even if the illness is induced by the medical care system itself. As in nineteenth-century England, we can pursue this inquiry even when the underlying biology is not yet understood. After all, it wasn't until decades after Snow's breakthrough discovery that other researchers identified the sewage-borne bacterium that causes cholera.

YIN VERSUS YANG

Learning about drug side effects often requires population-based studies like this. Such epidemiological investigation of prevailing exposures and disease is known as observational research, as opposed to experimental research in which treatments are actively administered by the researcher. The contrast between the two modes of inquiry often takes on the flavor of a battle of cultures, right down to the language used to describe each field. The spirit of *yang,* the positive, or male, principle, dominates the more interventionist experimental approach: the scientist takes command of the situation and manipulates exposures actively through randomized clinical trials or laboratory experiments. This work is described by its practitioners as hard science, often performed in what are called wet labs. By contrast, we observational scientists usually find ourselves following more of a *yin,* negative, feminine path: we generally don't change the situations we study, we just inspect them as thoughtfully and cleverly as we can. Our more macho interventionist colleagues sometimes refer to this work as soft science, and our faucetless research spaces as dry labs.

Following the latest battle in these cultural gender wars, the interventionists have been taunting us that the wimpy observational studies of hormone replacement led to lame and erroneous findings that were blown away when the more powerful tool of the experimental trial was aimed at the question. Shortly after the release of the estrogen clinical trial data, a junior faculty member in my division went to a meeting of experimentally oriented physicians. Knowing that he did research in pharmacoepidemiology, a colleague asked him what he would do now that this field had been proven to be worthless. The estrogen episode will be a burden that epidemiological studies of drug effects will have to bear for years to come.

All the same, when it comes to understanding some aspects of drug effects, the "weak sister" approach often turns out to be the more powerful one. If we think of the conceptually elegant, pristine world of the randomized controlled trial as the Garden of Eden of drug research, then pharmacoepidemiology is the messy world into which all of us are plunged once a drug leaves this state of grace and enters the gritty environment of everyday use. Does the new product cause dangerous bleeding in susceptible patients? Might it get nasty when mixed with other drugs and turn patients' muscles to a dark slurry that goes on to poison their kidneys? Will it cause cardiac arrest in old people? A purist might prefer to test each of these questions in additional, larger randomized controlled trials, in which—now that we know what to watch for—one could administer the drug to tens of thousands of randomly chosen patients to see what happens. But as Adam and Eve learned, we can't go back that way again; the way is barred by angels brandishing flaming swords of ethics, practicality, and economics. So we do what humans have always done since the Fall: we muddle through as best we can, trying to simulate glimpses of the ideal.

But wait a minute. We've seen how reliance on observational instead of experimental findings produced misleading conclusions about estrogens and heart disease. Then I extolled the randomized controlled trial (RCT) as the gold standard for determining whether a drug works or not. At this point we have to add another layer of complexity: *The RCT may be the best way to determine whether a drug works, but it isn't the best tool for assessing a drug's risks.*

As with observational studies, the limitations of the RCT are simply the flip side of its strengths. Consider what's needed to conduct a well-done clinical trial. For ethical reasons, the subjects must volunteer and then give their informed consent to be in a study—there is usually no way around that, nor should there be. This reduces their representativeness; it turns out that people who sign up for clinical trials are in general better educated, less likely to have cognitive impairment or mental illness, more likely to follow medical instructions, and healthier than the average patient with that disease. Even after a patient volunteers for a study, he or she may be excluded because of entry criteria that prohibit enrollment by subjects older than a certain age, or that require them to be free of a long list of diseases or other medications. Exclude the elderly and you're more likely to exclude women, since most old people are women—and you've introduced yet another limitation on how generalizable the findings will be. All this is done in order to have as "clean" a study as possible; purists argue that the evaluation of the drug will be compromised if the study includes people with myriad other diseases or treatments, or those who are more likely to have other medical problems (including death) crop up during the trial.

The physicians conducting these studies are likewise atypical. They are—again, by definition—doctors who engage in research, who practice in settings accustomed to running trials, keeping track of patients, and recording outcomes. Once the experiment has started, patients are likely to be hectored to keep taking their pills and closely monitored for side effects. Add to this the economic concerns of those paying for the trial, nearly always a pharmaceutical company for a drug's early studies. The fiscal clock starts ticking once the original patent is filed at the time of initial discovery, years before the first prescription can ever be sold. As a result, the manufacturer faces enormous financial pressure to quickly complete the pivotal trials on which the FDA will base its approval decision. RCTs are expensive, often costing several thousand dollars for each patient enrolled. So the sponsor will want to keep the number of people enrolled at the minimum needed to clear the required level of statistical significance.

This means making sure the studies are no larger than necessary and last no longer than absolutely needed to make the drug's case. As a result, these trials may involve just two or three thousand people, even less for rare conditions. To get results as quickly and inexpensively as possible, the study outcome may not be the clinical problem it is designed to treat, but a "surrogate marker" instead. For drugs to prevent cardiac disease, for example, the FDA does not demand that the manufacturer show that the new product actually reduces the likelihood of heart attack. Instead, the agency will generally settle for evidence that the drug works better than a placebo in improving cholesterol levels on a blood test. The assumption is that improving that intermediary measure is likely to translate into real clinical benefits years later. The policy is plausible, but brings its own set of problems. One is that drugs to treat diabetes, arthritis, glaucoma, hypertension, and elevated cholesterol, all destined to be taken for a lifetime, often are approved on the basis of clinical trials that lasted only a few months—the time it takes to show an effect on a surrogate marker. If longer-term use results in a side effect, or if improvement in the surrogate doesn't lead to the expected improvement in the real disease, we won't know it from the trial.

All this leads inexorably to the conclusion that we will never be able to learn enough about risks and other outcomes from the studies that are conducted before a medication is marketed. Consider an important side effect like hepatitis that occurs once in every five hundred people who take a drug. The new product is first tested in a randomized trial of two thousand subjects: one thousand are given it and the other one thousand get a placebo. *On average,* we would expect about two in the experimental drug group to come down with hepatitis, and about none in the placebo group. But as we saw in our coin-flipping experiment, that's the idealized rate we'd expect over an enormous number of patients. It's quite possible that there would be three hepatitis cases in the experimental group, or four, or one, or two. And while the likeliest number of cases in the control group would be zero, people get hepatitis all the time without being in drug trials, so the number actually observed could be one, or two, or even more.

Which numbers should earn the drug a clean bill of health, hepatically speaking, and which should delay its release because the product may be unsafe? Recall that this is just one potential side effect out of potentially hundreds. It's true that manufacturers could do a much better job of making their preapproval studies more inclusive and comprehensive, and the FDA could do a much better job of ensuring that this happens. But expecting perfect answers to all these questions before a drug could be used routinely would add years to its premarket testing and millions of dollars to its development costs. Done poorly, this could pose its own risks for the public by delaying the availability of important new products and making them even costlier once they're on the market.

That is the rationale for pharmacoepidemiology. It is simply not possible for any pre-marketing study of a new drug to include enough people of sufficient clinical diversity, and follow them long enough to provide a clear picture of all the important side effects the drug may cause once it is in widespread, lifelong use in typical patients. The problem is particularly acute if there was no clear signal of a given side effect in the pre-marketing studies. Observational studies are inevitable if we are to understand how these drugs perform once they are used in the real world.

This distinction has given rise to an important semantic wrinkle we've ignored thus far: the difference between efficacy and effectiveness.

Although we have used the two terms interchangeably, *efficacy* refers to the way a drug (or any other intervention) performs in the idealized, tightly monitored environment of the clinical trial. By contrast, *effectiveness* describes a drug's performance when used by typical doctors treating average patients in usual settings of care. As we will see, the two are sometimes significantly different.

LET'S RETURN TO the two mythical in-boxes on the desk of the poor FDA official who has to sort out whether a marketed drug caused the problem or was just an innocent bystander. The individual reports taken one at a time are often too fragile to bear the weight of a heavy decision—whether to ban a potentially useful medicine whose manufacturer spent millions of dollars to bring to market, or to keep it in drugstores and run the risk that it could harm many more patients. In talking about this dilemma to physician groups, I often ask how many in the audience ever submitted a report about a suspected adverse drug reaction. Only a few hands ever go up, even in large audiences. I myself rarely do so, and this is my life's work. Only a few percent of unanticipated drug-induced events observed in routine practice are ever reported to the manufacturer or to the FDA.

Why are new drug side effects so vastly underreported? To begin with, a doctor may not even connect the drug with the outcome (for example, an abnormally low white blood count found on a routine test months after a patient started taking a drug). If a possible connection is spotted, it takes a lot for the physician to do the right thing: "I think I'll just fill out yet another form and mail it to the government to let them know I gave a drug to a patient that made him horribly sick." Fear of litigation, growing worries about violating a patient's privacy, and the crushing burden of other administrative paperwork all help keep reporting rates low. As a result, spontaneous reports of suspected adverse drug events are a little like letters to Congress or complaints to large consumer corporations: it's a safe bet that for every document received, there are many more people in the same situation who never got around to sending in a similar message.

Drug companies are legally required to pass along the more serious of such reports to the FDA in a timely manner, and the more responsible ones do so carefully, even if it may spell trouble for their product. Others perform less admirably. In what passes for humor in the pharmacoepidemiology community, the following slide is sometimes shown during a talk on this subject:

TWO VIEWS OF AN ADVERSE EVENT

PHYSICIAN: "This drug could be a real threat to the life of my patient!"

MANUFACTURER: "This patient could be a real threat to the life of my drug!"

To make matters more challenging, these precious nuggets of reality aren't always reliable. A segment on the nightly news about a suspected side effect or a letter to the editor in a major medical journal can precipitate hundreds of "me too" reports, even if the alleged connection turns out to be wrong. If we think of side effects in terms of numerators and denominators (e.g., it will happen to one in every x people who take this drug), then it becomes clear that the spontaneous report system gives us rare numerators of uncertain validity, and no denominators at all. On the other hand, just a few reports of a previously unrecognized complication may be the first sign of a public health crisis in the making, as occurred with the heart valve abnormalities caused by Redux. The needle-in-the-haystack job of the FDA staffer can seem daunting indeed. Surely there must be a better way.

SAFETY IN NUMBERS

There is. Even though it's nearly impossible to conduct a clinical trial that randomly assigns 100,000 typical patients to receive drug A and 100,000 to get placebo, we can try to simulate a "virtual clinical trial," using information about everyday drug use that has already occurred in the real world. If we had enough information on the patients in each group who do or don't develop a particular complication, perhaps we could estimate the side effects that an enormous randomized study would have found. But how to capture that wealth of clinical experience without interviewing hundreds of thousands of patients one at a time? And how can we avoid the mistakes that bedeviled those observational studies of estrogen users?

Technology can help address both questions. To pay for the drugs used by their enrollees, very large health programs like Medicaid and many HMOs regularly receive billing data from pharmacies on all prescriptions filled by the patients they cover. Doctors and hospitals likewise send Medicaid, Medicare, or other insurers descriptions of all the medical services we provide to our patients, along with their diagnoses, so that we can be paid for the services rendered. As described later, in the early 1980s I began to collect the pharmacy billing data sent to several state Medicaid programs because I saw it as a neglected treasure trove of detailed information on the medication exposures of enormous numbers of people. It would of course be necessary to preserve patients' privacy; to do that, we'd assign each person a coded number not linked to any personal identifiers. We could then collect the computerized paid-claims data on all those millions of filled prescriptions and link it to similar paid-claims data on each of these same people, derived from all the bills sent in for their doctor visits and hospitalizations. If we could pull this off while protecting the confidentiality of each person's records, we'd have an enormous database that might become a powerful tool for studying real-world patterns of medication use and its outcomes.

This turned out to be harder than it sounds. The federal Medicare program covered clinical services for all the nation's elderly but at that time covered hardly any outpatient drugs; Medicaid, the state-run programs for the poor, paid for the drugs taken by many of those same elderly but didn't keep close track of the clinical services that Medicare paid for. And of course each government program used a system to identify patients that was completely different from the numbers used by the other. Daunting as the epidemiology was, it soon became clear that the bureaucratic issues would be even tougher.

When I started pursuing this idea in the early 1980s, Medicare and most Medicaid programs saw their paid-claims files as the useless detritus left over as a by-product of reimbursement procedures. Limited by a narrow bill-payer mentality, most of the people running these programs didn't see that they were sitting on gigabytes of valuable data that could be transformed into information to drive a wide range of activities from epidemiological research to quality assurance to cost containment. Some large health systems remain unaware of that potential to this day.

By the early 1990s, we had cajoled data from enough Medicaid and Medicare administrators to amass a huge collection of information on filled prescriptions, doctor visits, surgical procedures, nursing home stays, and hospitalizations, garnered from government programs in several states. The magnetic tapes we were sent contained the paid claims in essentially random order: enrollee 394786025 filled a prescription for digoxin of a given strength on a certain date; enrollee 937523910 got a beta-blocker on another day; Dr. Q removed the gallbladder of enrollee 693721704 at Hospital R nine months later. . . . A seemingly endless and chaotic profusion of medical record chatter. Over the years, a trio of talented Russian-born programmers in our unit transformed the mass of individual paid bills into a sophisticated relational database that we could use to answer queries like these: "Find all the patients who filled a prescription for drug A. Of those, how many had a diagnosis for diseases B, C, D, or E, but not diseases F, G, H, or I, and were later hospitalized with diagnosis J?" Like other research groups, we tried to make epidemiological gold out of the base metal of computerized administrative files.

To see the process in action, imagine the following study: We have the computer scan the filled-prescription files to find all patients taking a particular drug in a given year, let's say an analgesic, and follow those people forward over time. The enormous number of individuals in our files then enables us to identify others who were virtually identical to these patients in every way in terms of their age, gender, race, and all medical diagnoses, but didn't happen to use that drug. We can then turn to the records of hospital admissions to identify all the patients in both groups who were hospitalized with a given adverse event, such as hepatitis, whatever medications they were taking. Each person can then be put into one of the four boxes in the basic two-by-two table below, on which nearly all of pharmacoepidemiology is based:

	HAD THE OUTCOME	DIDN'T HAVE THE OUTCOME
TOOK THE DRUG	Box A: drug yes, outcome yes	Box B: drug yes, outcome no
DIDN'T TAKE THE DRUG	Box C: drug no, outcome yes	Box D: drug no, outcome no

If a large proportion of those who took a particular drug have a given adverse effect, and that problem occurs only rarely in people who didn't take the drug, this will increase the numbers of people in Box A and Box D, and will reduce the numbers in Boxes B and C. To work this through, consider the classical medical school example of spoiled tuna fish salad served at a church picnic one Sunday. By Monday, many (but not all) of those who ate the tuna fish develop abdominal cramps, nausea, or vomiting. Nearly everybody with those symptoms will have eaten the tainted tuna fish the day before, but some might have them for an unrelated reason (a virus making its way around the community, perhaps).

To measure the magnitude of this risk, we would multiply the number of people in Box A (the ill tuna eaters) by the number of people in Box D (the healthy tuna avoiders). We'd then divide that number by the counterexample: the number of people in Box B (healthy tuna eaters) multiplied by the number of people in Box C (ill tuna avoiders). This measures the risk of a specific outcome following a specific exposure. If the product (A times D) divided by the product (B times C) is 10, for example, it means that a picnicker who ate the tuna had ten times the risk of coming down with stomach problems compared to one who avoided the tuna.

It is a neat trick of epidemiology that the logic can work in both directions. Since such analyses used to begin with the outbreak of a disease, people began with the adverse event itself and then looked back to count how many sufferers had a given exposure beforehand, compared to the number of people without the outcome who had the exposure. This analysis, which would have been used by the local health authorities investigating the ill-fated picnic, is known as a case-control study: the cases are those who experience the adverse event; the controls are those who do not. This was the method used by the Yale investigators in Chapter 5 who pinned down the association between PPA and stroke.

Roughly the same math works if we want to study the outcomes that follow use of a particular drug by beginning at the beginning and following people forward in time. We would use our computerized records to track those who took a given medication and similar people who didn't, observing who develops the outcome of interest. (In the church picnic example, that would be the perspective of a demented parishioner who adds spoiled mayonnaise to the tuna salad and then waits to see what happens.) This is known as a follow-up (or cohort) study. In the simplest terms, both approaches make use of the same logic of (A times D) divided by (B times C). In the right circumstances, both will provide about the same answer.

MICROSCOPES AND TELESCOPES

Thinking about risks in populations contrasts sharply with the perspective of an individual physician focusing on a single patient. That is the most familiar agenda of medicine, but it isn't the only way to think about disease and treatment. The tension here is nicely illustrated in a parable I first heard as a medical student. A group of doctors on a hiking trip are urgently summoned to a riverbank, where they see dozens of people floating by in the rapids, thrashing helplessly and close to drowning. One physician after another jumps into the rushing river, grabs a victim, returns to shore, performs mouth-to-mouth resuscitation, then jumps back into the water to drag another person to safety. Abruptly, one of the doctors breaks from the group and runs away.

"Where the hell are you going?" ask his colleagues, appalled.

"I'm heading upstream," he answers, "to find the bastard who's pushing these people in!"

In the circles I hang out in, that upstream-focused hero is an epidemiologist, although my basic science friends like to tell a similar story about their fields.

Patients aren't prone to think of themselves as members of large risk groups with predictable odds that a particular exposure will cause them to come down with a given illness. But this is just what happens in populations, and populations are nothing more than big collections of individuals. More importantly, this is also the best way to think about how to measure and control risk in large numbers of people, whether they are members of a given practice, an HMO, a state or province, or an entire country. The perspective feels somewhat more natural in societies that are more at ease than we are with concepts of community and solidarity. It also fits better in nations with social democratic forms of government, or those where most people have common origins and perceive that they share a common fate. Population-based viewpoints don't mesh particularly well with the atomistic America of the twenty-first century, in which rugged individualism defines the way we think about health as well as about wealth. Most American doctors who worry about "community risk" or "public health" find ourselves swimming as well as running upstream.

Studying the effects of drugs in this *yin*like observational manner requires methods whose subtlety and complexity are more demanding than the leaner and cleaner rules of the randomized study. With all due respect to my trialist colleagues, you don't have to be a genius to divide a population randomly in two and give an active pill to half of them. Obsessiveness helps, compulsivity isn't bad either, diligence is essential, but analytic brilliance isn't always required. But lacking the powerful medicine of random assignment, it takes a lot more cleverness to extract a valid finding from the actionless observation of huge numbers of free-living people.

If we fail to get a handle on some basic difference between drug takers and their comparison group, we may come up with a finding that looks substantial and may even be "statistically significant." It might even be reproducible over and over again when the analysis is conducted in different ways; a result with this reassuring property is described by statisticians as "robust." Yet the insight could still be bogus, as occurred with the multiple replications of the erroneous estrogen heart-protection findings. My colleague Rhonda Bohn and I devised a shorthand name for the scary specter of an epidemiological finding that is both bogus and robust, confirmed by repeated analyses but still fundamentally wrong: "bogust."

Understanding what causes these problems is important not just for those of us who do the research; it's a useful skill for anyone subjected to the increasingly common headlines that begin "SCIENTISTS WARN OF NEW HAZARD FOR PATIENTS TAKING . . ." or "BREAKTHROUGH DRUG OFFERS HOPE FOR . . ." Because the logic and methods of pharmacoepidemiology are still not widely understood, major "discoveries" based on flawed observational analyses still make their way onto the pages of prominent medical journals, newspapers, and prescription pads.

One recurring example is the concept of confounding by indication. This is illustrated several times a year when poorly mentored graduate students discover that patients who take a particular kind of cardiovascular medication are significantly more likely to die of heart failure than patients who didn't take that medication. Of course they are: their doctor prescribed the drug to treat their heart disease. Patients not taking the drug, even if they were perfectly matched with the medication users by age and gender, would be much less likely to have heart disease in the first place. This is a trivially simple example, but the medical literature is littered with specious studies based on more arcane reenactments of this basic goof. One high-profile example of this was an observational study published in the *Journal of the American Medical Association* reporting that high blood pressure patients taking one kind of calcium-channel blocker (CCB) were much more likely to have heart attacks than were hypertensive patients on a comparison drug. The calcium-channel blockers may be overmarketed, overpriced, and not particularly special for most patients, but they probably don't kill you. Tens of thousands of patients and doctors became alarmed about the headlines that followed this discovery, and many people stopped taking their blood pressure pills.

By 2002, the ALLHAT randomized trial made it clear that the calcium-channel blockers didn't carry this risk. The problem was that the stigmatized drugs were also used to treat the angina caused by coronary artery disease. Because of this, doctors were preferentially using calcium-channel blockers in their hypertensive patients who also had heart disease. To make matters worse, the drugs were compared with beta-blockers, which can *prevent* heart attacks, further inflating the apparent increase in risk among the CCB patients. The best solution to this methodological gaffe is to compare drugs across patients *with similar clinical profiles.* Failing that, we must resort to using detailed statistical correction procedures to make the two groups as comparable as possible. This is not easy, and sometimes works imperfectly. It provides another reminder of the awesome power of the *yang* method of the randomized clinical trial, in which one effectively grabs consenting patients by their lapels (or hospital johnnies) and simply *tells* them which drug to take. If the sample is large enough, it is exceedingly likely that each group of patients will be very much like the other one, and all these between-subject differences will be randomized away.

Observational studies work better when the clinical outcome being studied has nothing to do with the disease a drug is used to treat. For example, in the 1990s doctors began to notice that patients taking a certain allergy medication along with a particular antibiotic were developing a dangerous heart rhythm disturbance that sometimes killed them. This was not likely to result from confounding by patient selection, since there was no reason to expect that people taking allergy pills or outpatient antibiotics would be more likely to have severe heart disease. It was the combination that was lethal, and the antihistamine (Seldane) was taken off the market.

A VICTIM OF EXPECTATIONS

Another kind of conceptual trap, and one that also results in erroneous papers and news reports, is the mirror image of confounding by indication. It's known in the trade as "channeling"—the process through which patients with a particular medical condition are more likely to be given drug A instead of drug B. This often happens when a new product is expected to be more effective or safer than its predecessors for particular high-risk patients. We stumbled upon this problem in a study of medications to manage glaucoma, one of the commonest causes of blindness in the United States. When we began our study, the most frequently used glaucoma drug had the side effect of occasionally constricting the airways in patients with lung disease, leading to incapacitating breathing problems. By changing the molecule's structure, researchers were able to reduce the drug's effect on the lungs while preserving its beneficial effect on the eyes.

To study how well this worked in routine practice, we scanned our database of two million people and measured how often patients who took the new drug developed pulmonary complications, compared to glaucoma patients taking the older drug. Contrary to what the pharmacology predicted, we found that people using the newer drug had much higher rates of hospitalization for lung problems than those on the older drug. Was the new product having an effect that was precisely the opposite of what its inventors had intended?

No, the drug worked exactly as it should have. It's easier to see what happened if you take the perspective of the ophthalmologist. The new drug was heavily and appropriately marketed as having a safety advantage in glaucoma patients who also had lung disease. Sensibly, eye doctors all over the country switched their glaucoma patients with lung disease to the new product. Glaucoma patients without lung disease were left on their existing drugs, since there was no reason to make a change. The new drug was indeed less likely to worsen a patient's breathing problems, but it certainly didn't make them go away; it was, after all, a medication for glaucoma. But most glaucoma patients with bad lungs ended up on the new product. They went on having hospitalizations for breathing problems, as such patients are wont to do, while the glaucoma patients without lung disease had relatively few admissions for respiratory difficulty. Had we stopped there, we might have wrongly concluded that the new drug was bad for the lungs.

Deprived of the power to randomly assign patients with both glaucoma and lung disease to the old versus the new drug, we instead tried to simulate a "virtual" randomized trial. We restricted the study to glaucoma patients with lung disease; to define its severity, we tracked their use of emergency room visits and hospitalizations for this problem before the new drug had become available. Once the new drug was on the market, we again measured their rates of hospitalization and emergency care for lung disease. Viewed this way, glaucoma patients switched to the new product turned out to require less medical care for their lung problems than did equally sick glaucoma-lung patients whose doctors left them on the older drug.

A more high-profile version of this paradox initially came up in the late 1980s when Prozac was introduced as the first antidepressant in a new class of drugs, the selective serotonin reuptake inhibitors (SSRIs). Within months, psychiatrists were telling one another stories about their depressed patients who killed themselves shortly after being switched to Prozac. Still other reports described people who went berserk and attacked others after starting on the drug. Concern crystallized around a paper published by a team of Harvard psychiatrists describing a series of patients who committed suicide or homicide after starting Prozac. The new drug's ability to alter serotonin levels in the brain was quite different from the mode of action of older medications. Could it be that raising the levels of this neurotransmitter could also precipitate insanity in some patients even as it relieved depression in others?

At that time, experience with this class of drugs was still limited. The SSRIs had not yet become the subject of adulatory paperbacks, and their use had not yet expanded to premenstrual tension, social phobias, and bad hair days. Faced with how little we understood about messing around with brain chemistry, it made sense to ask whether this new drug, so highly touted as the miracle mind-pill of the decade, might actually make some people terminally crazy. Controversy still persists about this question, and there is evidence that SSRIs can indeed push susceptible individuals, particularly children, into violent thoughts and actions. But for that initial paper another explanation also is relevant.

Imagine that you're a psychiatrist caring for a large practice of depressed patients. With fanfare, Prozac is introduced as a breakthrough antidepressant (which it was), safer (which it was) and more effective (which it was not) than any existing antidepressant. Getting a depressed patient stabilized on the right drug can require months of effort: choosing the medication, adjusting its dose, assessing the response, monitoring for side effects, reevaluating the therapeutic plan, and so on. As a psychiatrist, you will have done this for many hundreds of depressed patients under your care. When Prozac comes along, whom will you switch to this new drug? The stabilized, better-adjusted people who are doing well, back at work, resuming normal relationships? Probably not.

You'll be most likely to try it out on your patients for whom nothing has worked, who are careening close to the cliff of insanity, who have threatened or even attempted suicide, whose behavior has become a subject of increasing concern to those around them. These are precisely the patients who, if Prozac had never been invented, would have been more likely to kill themselves or others in the ensuing months. And they are precisely the patients you are most likely to put on Prozac *nonrandomly* as soon as it becomes available, especially since it's much harder to kill yourself with an overdose of Prozac than with an older antidepressant. This may explain some of the problems seen with users of SSRI-type drugs in observational studies. However, more recent data from clinical trials—some of them initially not revealed by the drug makers or the FDA—now indicate that there may be much more to the problem than that.

Another problem that causes us pharmacoepidemiologists to lose sleep goes by the ungainly name of *protopathic bias*. To put it in terms of an extreme example, this is the misguided thinking that could lead to the conclusion that cherry-flavored cough syrup causes tuberculosis. While no one worries about this as an imminent public health hazard, the same kind of problematic logic can lead to more reasonable-sounding errors whose silliness is not as apparent. Imagine a case-control study in which the cases are patients newly diagnosed with tuberculosis; the controls are patients of identical age, gender, race, and socioeconomic status who do not have tuberculosis. If we look back over all of their medication use in the preceding year, we will probably find that our TB cases had used cherry-flavored cough syrup at a rate dramatically higher than our controls.

What was going on, of course, was that before their tuberculosis was diagnosed, the patients who later became cases had been taking cough syrup to treat the symptoms of the disease's early stages. The bias was protopathic—from the Greek roots *proto* (early) and *pathos* (disease). If we had been able to know precisely when their tuberculosis had started (as opposed to when they were first assigned the diagnosis), we would not have made the mistake. Of course, no one would seriously think that cough syrup causes TB, because we know a lot about what does cause TB, as well as about what's in cough syrup. That is what makes this such a useful example. The same bias continues to appear in analyses of diseases about which we know much less, and medications that may be far less innocuous; this is when such imprecise thinking can become dangerous.

In the PPA-stroke litigation, the manufacturers claimed that the link between their cold remedies and subsequent stroke could be explained away by protopathic bias. According to this logic, slowly developing hemorrhagic strokes initially produced headaches, which patients mistakenly attributed to sinus problems. They tried to treat this with over-the-counter decongestants containing the innocent bystander PPA, but to no avail. Several hours later, the argument went, when the patient is wheeled into an emergency room with a full-blown intracerebral bleed, doctors take a history of recent drug use and the hapless PPA product is unjustly fingered. Neither the FDA nor the epidemiology community bought this argument, but it was a brave try.

REMEMBRANCE OF DRUGS PAST

The problem of *recall bias* is another way that human frailty on the part of patients as well as researchers can contaminate an observational study. It can produce findings that are clear, unambiguous, statistically significant, and completely wrong. The antinauseant drug Bendectin, described at the start of this chapter, provides a poignant case study. Bendectin was widely used in the 1970s and 1980s to treat the nausea and vomiting that often accompany the first trimester of pregnancy. It worked well for this purpose, but reports began to appear of women who gave birth to malformed babies after using Bendectin. Was the drug at fault? In theory, a huge randomized controlled trial could have resolved the question, but here we come up against more evidence of the impracticality of the RCT in addressing certain questions. Imagine the conversation needed to obtain informed consent from a subject in such a trial: "Mrs. Jones, now that you are beginning your pregnancy, we would like to ask your permission to enroll you in a study. You would be randomly assigned to one of two treatment groups. In the first, you would be given an inactive sugar pill to treat your nausea and vomiting, with no chance that this will help your symptoms. If you are randomly assigned to the second group you will receive an active drug that some people believe can cause your baby to be born deformed. Please sign below if you are willing to participate in this trial."

The frying pan thus being unavailable, researchers leaped into the fire. They conducted careful interviews with women (the cases) whose children had been born with deformities. They asked them about every medication taken during pregnancy, as well as about a host of other potentially risky exposures. They then interviewed a large number of women of similar age, medical status, and prior childbearing history, except that these women had given birth to perfectly normal babies; they were the controls. Sure enough, many more of the women with deformed babies recalled that they used Bendectin early in their pregnancies, compared to the women with normal children. The drug was withdrawn from the market, and obstetricians and pregnant women were left for years without an effective treatment for the often disabling nausea that frequently marks the first three months of pregnancy.

This would have been a reasonable policy decision were it not for one important fact: Bendectin almost certainly does not cause fetal abnormalities. More thorough studies eventually showed that the drug had been a victim of recall bias. Prior to the arrival of the epidemiologists, the women who gave birth to deformed babies had spent months ruminating over what might have caused such a tragedy. They obsessively reviewed the illnesses they had had, the traumas they had experienced, the foods they had eaten, and, of course, the pills they had taken while pregnant. Meanwhile, the women who had given birth to healthy children simply got on with their lives. When researchers asked both sets of women whether they had taken Bendectin during the early part of their pregnancies, the women whose pregnancies ended tragically were far more likely to recall that they had, and the women with healthy children were far less likely to do so. In fact, the rate of Bendectin use in both groups was probably about the same.

By the time better studies were completed, Bendectin had been taken off the market. Its manufacturer concluded that even if there were excellent evidence that the drug was harmless, the company would still be sued by patients or lawyers who didn't see it that way. Juries are notoriously insensitive to nuances of research methodology, and famously generous to plaintiffs struck by tragedy, whatever its cause—particularly if the defendant is a large, impersonal pharmaceutical manufacturer. The company saw that whatever the merits of their case, they might still lose a sizable number of legal battles, at enormous expense. Even if they won every suit, the cost of litigation would have exceeded whatever profit they could have realized from continued sales of the drug. Bendectin remains unavailable.

SELECTION FOR SUCCESS

A final kind of bias underlies a host of research papers and articles in magazines and newspapers extolling the virtues of drugs that prevent an astonishing range of conditions, from Alzheimer's disease to depression to death itself—including death from every known cause. This strange property has been studied by Robert Glynn, a senior statistician in our research unit. Analyzing a database of some two million older patients for whom we had coded records of every prescription and every medical encounter over a period of several years, Dr. Glynn measured the death rate in patients who took various categories of drugs, adjusting for age, gender, and a very large number of clinical characteristics. He found that the adjusted death rate in patients taking cholesterol-lowering drugs was dramatically lower than the death rate in apparently identical patients who didn't take these drugs. Part of this was understandable, since a few randomized trials have shown that these drugs can indeed reduce the risk of death somewhat. But the size of the effect he found was substantially greater than had ever been seen in any clinical study. He then went on to find similar reductions in the death rate of patients who took medications for arthritis, and those using certain kinds of eyedrops—drug groups not previously known to have life-prolonging effects.

It soon became clear that this effect was not a property of the drug but of the doctors who were prescribing it. If a patient has terminal cancer, or is in a coma, or is severely demented, or has end-stage disease of any kind, the physician is much less likely to worry about lowering cholesterol, treating arthritis, or prescribing eyedrops. Yes, it was true that patients prescribed these medications were much less likely to die in the ensuing year than those who were not. But this was not because the medications conferred immortality; they were simply markers of being a patient healthy enough to warrant aggressive management of these other conditions. The same flawed logic underlies observational studies concluding that drugs used to treat senility can actually prolong life. Of course they don't; these drugs barely work in patients who are physically well, and they often cause side effects. Doctors are simply less likely to give them to people who are moribund. The error of the association seems clear enough in retrospect, but this has not prevented the publication of studies and headlines attributing similar magical properties to a wide variety of medications. Watch your local paper or the nightly news for the next examples of such breakthrough discoveries.

With all these limitations, why do grown men and women continue to conduct epidemiological studies of drug effects? If the method is so much more prone to bias and erroneous conclusions than the powerful randomized controlled trial, should these other studies be undertaken at all? Granted, they are more practical and less costly than randomized trials, and can be done much more easily and on a very large scale. But is this false economy in light of their greater propensity for bias and flat-out error? Are those of us who perform this research the medical equivalents of the glutton at a Catskills resort who explained that he kept going back every summer because although the food was terrible, the portions were enormous?

The answer has to do with those angels with the flaming swords. It just isn't possible to conduct a new randomized controlled clinical trial for every question we need answered about a drug's effectiveness or side effects. Each new hypothesis would require many additional years of study, and tens of millions of dollars per trial, even if it were practical—and the Bendectin example illustrates how impractical such controlled trials can be even if resources and time were infinitely available. Nor would it be reasonable to delay the availability of every new drug until it had been studied many years longer, or in tens of thousands more patients. That could have its own public health downside.

Like it or not, the lean, muscular, randomized trial is joined at the hip with its occasionally clumsy but often wily sibling, the observational study. In truth, we need them both to get a comprehensive picture of drug effects in the real world. The tool of randomization may be one of the most powerful instruments ever devised to determine what causes what, but it is one that we can't always deploy. All the elaborate methods of pharmacoepidemiology can be seen as valiant attempts to re-create that conceptual womb of the randomized trial after the fact, once we've been expelled from Eden.

Knowing that this kind of research is inevitable makes it both daunting and rewarding, an endless succession of Amazing Medical Mysteries waiting to be solved. As a young boy, I was captivated by Berton Roueche's *Eleven Blue Men,* a collection of true stories from *The New Yorker* describing the work of physician-detectives who confronted inscrutable disease outbreaks and, like Sherlock Holmes, traced each problem to its root—the epidemiologist as clinical crime fighter. This kind of work also has the quantitative appeal of those mathematical riddles that I found so absorbing as an admittedly nerdy schoolboy. The only difference is that with the puzzles I work on now, finding the right answer could have an impact on the health of real people.

I sometimes think that my colleagues at Harvard Medical School who conduct bold laboratory and clinical investigations are a bit like the rocket scientists and astronauts of NASA—performing interventions, sending off space shots, doing experiments with the universe. If that's so, then those of us who do epidemiology research are more like astronomers, destined to sit at our telescopes and observe the movement of the planets and other phenomena over which we exert no control. On good days I realize that it was precisely that kind of observation that made it possible to understand the solar system and to derive the basic laws of physics—insights on which those space shots depend. And new observations made through the Hubble telescope have sharpened our understanding of the universe's very origins and direction. These sciences that can't actually "do" anything possess their own kind of power.

LIVING WITH DUALITY

Because randomized trials and observational studies each have their own strengths and weaknesses, a major agenda for drug research and policy in the coming years will be to figure out how the two approaches can be reconciled. At least since Descartes, Western science has earned its living by dividing up opposites like these, a way of thinking that has served us well but that has its own limitations. If it's reconciliation we want, we'll have to return to our metaphor of *yin* and *yang*. In Chinese art, *yin* often represents the dark side of a mountain, and *yang* its light side. But there are no one-sided mountains, and darkness is not the absence of meaning. It may even be the meaning itself; consider the ink on this page. We've all seen the familiar Asian representation of this theme as a circle with an *S*-shaped line drawn through it, separating a white half from a black half. A small white dot is in the center of the black part, and a small black dot in the white. Some have likened this image to two fish perpetually chasing each other in the dance of life; for our present purpose we can think of it as the experimentalists and the observationalists warily and endlessly circling one another. (The caduceus, that ancient symbol of medicine, is built on a similar theme of two snakes encircling one another along the healer's staff.)

The traditions of medicine are full of such dualities, going back at least as far as Greek and Roman mythology. Aesculapius, the god of the medical arts, was the *yang*ish interventionist, full of phallic traits. He wields the rigid staff encircled by the serpents, and was even said to transform himself into a snake on occasion. He impregnated Epione, the goddess of soothing, and they bore a daughter, Hygeia. She became the *yin*like public health goddess of clean living, lending her name to the tradition of preventing rather than zapping disease. (Another daughter, Panacea, whose name meant "universal cure," was a goddess known for her use of healing herbs. Given the ironic connotation her name has taken on in modern times, this seems appropriate.) All of modern therapeutics can be seen as a family squabble among these competing traditions.

Dualities often contain their own resolution, and as we think about drugs this mythological legacy may help us reach it. Aesculapius' original staff is said to have carried just one snake, not the two we are used to seeing on the modern caduceus. That later symbol is attributed to the god Mercury, who once came upon two fighting snakes and threw his staff between them to stop their battle. They wrapped themselves around it in gratitude, creating a symbol of Mercury's ability to transform hostility into harmony. It may be a stretch, but all those hostile fishes and snakes may have lessons for us about reconciling these two ways of understanding drug effects. If Mercury were a drug researcher, he might remind us that if done well, both experimental and observational approaches are "true." After all, the only reason we do randomized drug trials is to learn about the effects a medication will have in real populations outside the trial setting, something it may predict only imperfectly. And the best epidemiological methods are just attempts to adjust real-world data to simulate the results of a clinical trial that was never done.

Further resolution may lie in those two opposite-colored dots in the *yin-yang* symbol. Their usual explanation is that everything contains a small piece of its opposite at its center. That's fine, but let me propose an additional interpretation. If those are fish, then the dots are their eyes. The best randomized trials are designed when the experimenter can maintain an epidemiologist's eye on the real-world population that will use a drug beyond the artificial constraints of an experiment. And the best observational work requires us to look at data with the eye of a trialist, to see how our findings might approximate that imaginary randomized study no one could conduct. Maybe those fish and snakes are in the chase not to kill each other, but to do what the male and female impulses have always wanted to do: mate. The creation of life requires the union of opposites, just as hearts need their passive diastolic phase as much as the muscular systole if they are to pump properly.

Even with implausibly large budgets, we still won't be able to mount a new randomized trial for every question we need answered about widely used medicines. If we continue to approve drugs based on their capacity to correct surrogate endpoints rather than prevent or treat actual diseases, we will have to have some way to know whether they do for patients what we expect them to do. Or whether some drugs in a given class might achieve their clinical goal much more effectively, or much more safely, than others that also passed the yes/no criterion of better-than-nothing-at-improving-a-lab-test-in-twelve-weeks. Some similar drugs have chemical structures that are drastically different from one another, and we don't always know how these differences may play out in the long-term effects they generate. Even for cousin drugs that differ by just an atom or two, it's useful to realize that so do testosterone and estrogen, and we all know what different effects they have.

This synthesis shouldn't be seen as some quasi-scientific New Age "tantra of pharmacology," a *Taoism for Dummies* fuzzily projected onto the field of medications. Some of the most advanced methods in trial design, epidemiology, statistics, and health services research are currently tackling these very issues with impressive rigor. As we will see in some detail in Part Four, this work can lead us to a new generation of clinical, research, and policy strategies for assessing the drugs we use.

We are left with the realization that we will have to get better at performing and interpreting observational drug studies, since our need for their findings will continue to grow in the coming years. Like it or not, for many of the pressing questions we face there is really no other way to know what is on the other side of the drug evaluation mountain.

7: THE MOST VULNERABLE PATIENTS

One February in a suburb outside Boston, Beatrice Williamson, a seventy-three-year-old widow, slipped on the ice and broke her hip. The fracture was promptly repaired with the surgical insertion of a titanium rod, but healed poorly; she was left wheelchair-bound and could not return to living on her own in her apartment. She hated the idea of moving to a nursing home, but had no other alternative. Her first weeks at the Happy Valley Rehabilitation Center were filled with bitterness and anguish. She kept repeating over and over, "This is not my home; let me out of here. This is not my home; let me out of here." The medical director called in a psychiatric consultant who made a diagnosis of institutional adjustment reaction syndrome. He prescribed Haldol, a major tranquilizer, to manage her restlessness.

Two months later she was visited by her only living relative, a niece from Oklahoma. The niece was surprised to find that although her aunt had been alert and engaging the previous autumn, she now had a blank stare, stiffness in her arms and legs, a tremor in her hands, and general slowing of her movements and thoughts. When the change was brought to the attention of the nursing home doctor, he explained that these were the signs of Parkinson's disease, and wrote a new prescription for a drug to treat it.

For a time, one of my clinical jobs was to evaluate elderly people referred to the Harvard geriatrics program for "one last look" before a family could accept the fact that their parent's steady downhill course had no reversible cause. The children (sometimes themselves in their sixties or seventies) would come into the consultation room clutching long lists of medications the patient had accumulated over the years, the drugs layered upon each other like coral on a reef. A particularly useful exercise was something we called a brown bag session, in which the patient or relative was asked to collect all medications currently being used and bring them in for reassessment. Even when I did this periodically with my own primary-care patients, there would be surprises. Some had stopped taking drugs I had written for long-term use; others were still refilling prescriptions I had intended for one-time dispensing. Still others were sheepishly engaging in what they seemed to think of as pharmacological adultery: "Doctor Avorn, I didn't want to tell you, but I'm also seeing someone else, and he's the one who gave me these arthritis pills." It's unlikely that a patient will know that Celebrex, ibuprofen, Feldene, and over-the-counter Advil are all essentially the same drug, and that taking them together will multiply the risk of side effects but not the benefit.

Many of the pill bottles that would pour out of these brown bags were keeping patients alive, several of them had no discernible effect, and a few were making them sick. The latter seemed to occur particularly frequently with sedative-type drugs, especially the category called neuroleptics, also known as antipsychotics. Old favorites in this group included Haldol (haloperidol), Mellaril (thioridazine), and Thorazine (chlorpromazine); their newer and amazingly expensive cousins included Zyprexa (olanzapine) and Risperdal (risperidone). These drugs had been proven effective when used for their original purpose: treating young and middle-aged people with schizophrenia. I remember one young man I saw with this devastating condition who was convinced that the Martians had embedded wires in his brain to control his thoughts and movements, as part of their plan to create a new race of beings. Soon after he started taking an antipsychotic medication he saw that this wasn't the case; the voices he heard telling him to do weird destructive things fell silent, and he was able to resume a plausible if not totally appealing life.

By the 1970s, it had become common practice to use these drugs to treat agitated behavior and confusion in elderly people, even if they didn't have schizophrenia. There wasn't much pharmacological logic behind the strategy: although we don't know what causes schizophrenia, it probably has something to do with a derangement of function of one of the brain's main neurotransmitters, dopamine. We also don't understand Alzheimer's disease very well, but the best evidence is that a different neurotransmitter is primarily involved, acetylcholine. Despite this, the antipsychotic drugs had one property that made them attractive for dealing with agitated and confused old people, especially in understaffed nursing homes: they were very effective sedatives—hence their other name, the major tranquilizers.

These drugs manage agitation by quieting people down, though there is little evidence that they improve mental processing in Alzheimer's patients the way they literally restore sanity in schizophrenics. But with increasing numbers of patients living long enough to become senile, and more and more of them housed in nursing homes trying to manage large numbers of confused elderly people with the smallest possible staff, the drugs' quieting properties became increasingly popular in these settings. As we saw with estrogens, a drug's everyday use can extend beyond the purpose for which it was originally approved, even if there are no new studies to demonstrate that it works in the new condition. Once a product is on the market, any doctor can use it for any reason he or she deems appropriate. Some studies were eventually done by the drugs' manufacturers so they could legally advertise them for this large-market-share use, but all that was needed was to show the drugs worked better than a sugar pill in quieting agitated behavior in the elderly. Of course they did, as would a double martini or a sharp blow to the head—not that this would make these attractive therapeutic strategies.

THE PRICE OF PEACE

Pharmacology predicted another important outcome of antipsychotic use in the elderly. Years of experience with young schizophrenics made it clear that the drugs' interference with dopamine produced one common downside. They could mimic all the effects of Parkinson's disease, an illness caused by the body's inability to make enough dopamine at strategic places in the brain. Because both the medication and the disease produce a dopamine deficit, the clinical manifestations are similar whether patients develop the problem on their own or because of a drug. To increase the confusion, both syndromes are often referred to as "parkinsonism," as if it were some kind of bizarre neurological cult. More semantically careful doctors describe the non-drug-related disease as being idiopathic, a presumptuous yet simpleminded term describing a disease for which we don't know the cause, a combination of the Latin root for "ignorance" and the Greek root for "suffering."

Whether its origin is idiopathic or drug-induced, people with the syndrome of parkinsonism find that their muscles become stiff, their hands tremulous, their gait unstable, their movements and thinking slow. The disease occurs more commonly in the elderly, although a few atypically young patients have brought the condition into the public eye recently. Muhammad Ali's Parkinson's disease probably was caused by repeated head trauma that damaged an area of the brain known as the substantia nigra (literally, "black stuff"), crucial in the production of dopamine. Other famous patients with less violent occupations, like Janet Reno and Michael J. Fox, developed the idiopathic kind. Not so Mrs. Williamson in the case history above. Her parkinsonian symptoms were likely caused by the antipsychotic drug prescribed to treat her "institutional adjustment reaction syndrome."

These diagnostic subtleties matter, even if both kinds of illness look similar at the synapse and at the bedside. First, a drug side effect should never be labeled a new disease of unknown cause—especially in the elderly, to whom this happens most. Second, it is generally a bad idea to treat a drug side effect by adding a new drug, as long as any good alternative strategy exists. (Reducing or stopping Mrs. Williamson's Haldol would have been a fine first step.) Third, anti-Parkinson drugs are a rough crowd to invite across your blood-brain barrier if you don't have to. Depending on the category chosen, they carry their own baggage of frequent side effects such as movement disorders, hallucinations, nausea, nightmares, and dizziness (for the L-dopa group), or dry mouth, blurry vision, urinary retention, and constipation (for the anticholinergic group), or severe, sometimes unexpected attacks of sleepiness (for the newer dopamine agonist group). Finally, because of the way the antipsychotic drugs affect neurotransmitters, many anti-Parkinson medications don't ameliorate drug-induced parkinsonism much, though they retain full capacity to produce side effects.

A DEMOGRAPHIC TIDAL WAVE

Although people over sixty-five comprise only about 14 percent of the American population, they consume over a third of all medications, making the elderly the most pharmacologically important segment of society. The world is aging; we are living through a time of demographic change unprecedented in human history. Gerontologists report that of all the people who ever lived past the age of seventy, more than half are alive today. As the numbers of the old have risen, the numbers of the young are being relatively contained, at least in industrialized societies. The nation's birthrate declined during the Great Depression, followed by the coitus interruptus of World War II. By mid-century, a rising numerator of older people and a much slower increase in the numbers of births set the stage for the elderly to edge higher and higher as a proportion of the population throughout the industrialized world; that ratio has now reached a level never confronted before by any society. My own generation of postwar baby boomers is about to put its own extra spin on this demographic curve ball. Fifty years later, our mid-century surge of births is becoming a tidal wave of aging. The first of us will hit the beach of age sixty-five shortly after 2010, and few social institutions are ready for us.

For centuries the old were cared for physically and economically by the greater numbers of young people who followed them. That tradition, like so many others, began to erode in the 1960s. The oral contraceptive and the women's movement increased both the capacity and the desire to control fertility, and the birthrate again plummeted. As my cohorts and I prepare to enter the Medicare generation in the coming decade, we look back over our shoulders to find proportionately fewer younger people to support us than any previous generation has had. As America becomes an aging society to an extent never before seen, the resulting demographic shifts are causing tectonic changes in domains as disparate as pension policy, family structure, housing, education, and human services. The impact is nowhere greater than in medicine, and within medicine much of that impact will be focused on geriatric medication use.

Physiologically, just as children are not simply miniature grown-ups, the elderly are not simply wrinkled adults. Even in the absence of any disease, the normal aging process is marked by a series of physiological changes that can have important implications for drug use. Sometimes these changes are misinterpreted by all of us who participate in the care of the elderly: by the older patient, by family members, and by us, their physicians. If we don't think clearly about the transformations that occur with aging, we can badly misunderstand a clinical problem. This is illustrated by the anecdote of an eighty-two-year-old man who presents his doctor with an unusual complaint: "As a young man, when I would get an erection I could take my two hands and grab it, and it wouldn't bend." (He extends two fists as if holding a lead pipe.) "Now, as I get older, I notice that when I grab my erection, it goes like this." (He makes an inverted *U* with his two hands.) "Doctor, can you explain to me why, at my age, my hands should be getting so much stronger?"

More serious misattributions of age-related change are less entertaining, and can create important problems in the way we prescribe for our older patients. Dr. Robert Butler, the founding director of the National Institute on Aging, was among the first to describe the distortions that often taint our perceptions about getting old. He coined the term "ageism" to describe systematic prejudice against the elderly and the clinical and social problems it can cause. Like sexism, racism, or anti-Semitism, ageism is the belief that if I know one small demographic fact about you (your gender, race, religion, or the year you were born), I can deduce your personal attributes.

No television series today would ever air characters who are shuffling black folk, consistently inept women, or perfidious Jews, but the stereotype of the demented old geezer is still found on prime time, as in one of my favorite programs, *The Simpsons*. According to this caricature, the old are prone to confusion, feebleness, forgetfulness, and crotchetiness. They are no longer productive members of society and are just waiting to die. Even positive attributions can reveal our prejudices. Declaring that someone is "very sharp for a person his age" is, on reflection, as bigoted as saying that the black boxing champion Joe Louis was "a credit to his race."

Such ageism can have direct and destructive effects on the way we care for our elderly patients. Alzheimer's disease and other dementing illnesses are indeed more common the older you get, and more ninety-year-olds are incontinent than twenty-year-olds. But the key distinction here is that these problems represent diseases that are statistically more frequent in old age— they do not represent the aging process itself. We can't do anything about how old someone is, but if someone has a disease we can search for a cause, and perhaps for a treatment.

Beyond shaping the way we think about medications in older people, ageism can also determine whether we even get to make that decision at all. One kind of lapse occurs if the medical consultation doesn't happen in the first place. Far too many elderly experience symptoms that could be controlled by drugs—depression, incontinence, joint pains, shortness of breath, erectile dysfunction—but never make it to the doctor because they or misguided family members assume that nothing can be done, that such problems are "just part of aging." Even worse, if the patient overcomes this concern and consults a doctor, it is sometimes the physician who writes off such treatable problems. Dr. Butler tells the story of an eighty-four-year-old woman who goes to the doctor complaining that her left knee hurts when she climbs stairs. After a cursory exam, the doctor dismisses her problem with "That's just something that comes with getting old, dear." "But, Doctor," she objects, "my *other* knee is also eighty-four, and that one doesn't hurt!"

A BETTER HEURISTIC

In talking with medical students and residents about how this relates to their prescribing, I point out that no clinical problem in an elderly patient should ever be dismissed as merely attributable to age and therefore not worth treating. Doing so can cut short the opportunity for conducting a workup that might reveal a medicine that could help. In their careers, they will often hear summaries of patients that sound like this: "The patient has fatigue, forgetfulness, and leg cramps on exercise . . . but what do you expect, she's eighty-six." I suggest to them that whenever an age is given as the explanation for a problem, students should substitute their own and see how sensible the analysis sounds: "The patient was a little disoriented, had some urinary incontinence, and a few signs of depression . . . but what do you expect, he's twenty-three." If that doesn't sound right, I tell them to look for a better diagnosis and a treatable disease, whatever the patient's age. If the cause is a drug side effect, so much the better: there are few conditions in geriatrics that can yield such dramatic improvement, often within days, once the right diagnosis is made.

The connection between ageism and medication use comes down to this: how we conceptualize a situation shapes how we handle it. The positive side of this insight is enshrined in a statement by Louis Pasteur engraved into the entryway of my old medical school dormitory: "Chance favors the prepared mind." Yogi Berra put it differently, but with comparable insight: "If I didn't believe it, I wouldn't have seen it." If a medical student or doctor carries around the mental template of a healthy, well-functioning older person, it's easier to see deviation from that expectation as an anomaly, and try to correct it. By contrast, if the model of "old person" is a shriveled, disoriented nursing home patient lying on an emergency room stretcher, the doctor is less likely to try to discover the right diagnosis or treatment. This framing issue underlies much of the misuse of drugs in the care of the elderly.

The training problem is exacerbated by the growing fragmentation of American families; with each passing decade, fewer of our students come from homes with close contact across several generations. Their first intimate exposure to old people may not come until medical school, when they confront them as cadavers or as acutely ill hospitalized patients, sometimes referred to as "train wrecks." To think clearly about treating elderly people, students need familiarity with reasonably healthy oldsters living their lives and coping with their problems, before they become distorted and obtunded by pneumonia or kidney failure or cancer. Viewing the world from the teaching hospital, it's too easy to forget that most of the elderly are healthy most of the time, or have just one or two manageable chronic conditions.

Many older people owe their lives to their prescriptions, or at least their ability to get out of bed each morning and make it through the day. But they also have a heightened risk of side effects, for multiple reasons. The liver and kidney, our main tools for metabolizing and excreting medications, lose some of their capacity to do so with aging. Several other organs become more sensitive to drug effects, and others grow less sensitive. The relative proportions of fat and muscle change with aging (we all know in which direction), influencing the way drugs are distributed throughout the body as well as the duration of their effects. Because of all these differences, typical doses calibrated for middle-aged patients can be excessive in older people. I once expected that because of this, drugs would be studied particularly carefully in the elderly both before and after initial marketing. Unfortunately for today's elderly and for all the rest of us who are approaching Medicare eligibility, quite the opposite is true.

Far from being heavily recruited into drug studies, older people are often purposely excluded from such trials in the name of efficiency and convenience. Whatever the medication, a thousand subjects in their seventies will have more heart attacks, strokes, hospitalizations, and deaths than will a thousand subjects in their fifties, simply because they would experience more of these events even in the absence of a new drug. The seventy-year-olds are also far more likely to be taking other medications or have other diseases that could interact with the study drug. All this increases the chances that a problem will develop during the course of a clinical trial, making the resulting data messier to analyze. A drug manufacturer must inform the FDA of all deaths and serious medical events that occur in early clinical testing, whether or not they appear to be caused by the compound being studied. As a result, the companies that sponsor most such studies (as well as my colleagues in academia who perform many of them) often prefer to confine trials whenever possible to patients who are younger and healthier.

Our research group tested this question by reviewing all the published clinical trials of drugs used in the management of acute heart disease. Drs. Jerry Gurwitz, Nanada Col, and I looked at the study design for each one to determine whether it excluded potential subjects over a certain age, usually sixty-five or seventy. We found that this was the rule rather than the exception. Another research group replicated the study a decade later in 2002 and found the same pattern. A similar analysis reviewed all the clinical oncology trials funded by the National Cancer Institute. Even though people over sixty-five account for 62 percent of all cancer patients in the United States, this age group was underrepresented by half in the trials, comprising only 32 percent of the subjects in whom cancer drugs were evaluated. Considering how differently older patients can react to medications, this approach to pharmacology leaves many questions unresolved in the very patients for whom we most need those answers.

As first lady, Hillary Clinton became concerned about drug testing at the other end of the age spectrum when she learned that new drugs were not being adequately studied in children. She persuaded Congress to make generous concessions to the drug industry by extending a drug's patent life if its manufacturer tested it in kids. This voluntary arrangement was a bonanza for many companies; pediatric trials that cost just a few million dollars to conduct bought six-month patent extensions that generated hundreds of millions of dollars in additional revenues for some well-marketed drugs. No such arrangement was ever made for testing in the elderly. The FDA has issued limp guidelines requesting that manufacturers include adequate numbers of older patients in their studies, but the requirements are vague and nonbinding, and enforcement is weak.

The agency's timidity here is understandable even if it's not acceptable. Following the pediatric patent extension sweetener, the FDA tried to use its regulatory clout to *require* companies to routinely test their products in children. The drug manufacturers protested, arguing in court that the agency had overstepped its bounds. The courts agreed, and the FDA was forced to back down. It is likely that in the current antiregulatory climate any serious requirement for thorough geriatric testing would suffer the same fate.

It's hard to measure the effect of this weakened regulatory posture on the numbers of older people included in or excluded from premarketing drug trials. I once tried to get this information and was told that the FDA's summary statistics on subjects' ages generally stop at the catchall category "sixty-five and over." As a result, it's difficult to tell how many of the "elderly" in a given study were robust people in their mid-sixties or more complicated, frail people in their seventies, eighties, and beyond—the kind of people for whom we commonly prescribe. As a result, doctors and patients face the paradox that even though the elderly are the most likely to take prescription drugs, the most likely to benefit from them, and the ones at greatest risk from their side effects, they are the least likely to be included in the pivotal studies of those products.

COMPOUNDED PROBLEMS

Problems in medical education make a bad situation worse. Practical clinical pharmacology and geriatrics both receive inadequate attention in most medical schools, even as the use of medications in older patients becomes more and more central to the work of nearly all physicians. Giving short shrift to these disciplines leads to the kind of situation that befell Mrs. Williamson at the start of this chapter: a doctor inadvertently creates a drug-induced illness in an elderly patient, then someone (perhaps a different doctor) mistakes it for a new disease and writes an additional prescription to treat it, missing an opportunity to resolve the initial problem and generating a whole new set of side effects.

Sometimes the misdiagnosed side effect leads to other kinds of misadventure. We often see this with a broad class of medications with properties categorized as anticholinergic. This is a cluster of effects caused by drugs used to treat conditions from runny nose to depression to disorders of cardiac rhythm. Many of these medications are quite useful, but they also interfere with the autonomic processes that work "on background" to keep our intestines moving, our saliva flowing, our eyes in focus, and our bladder contracting (but only on cue). Anticholinergic drugs are one kind that may have been prescribed for Mrs. Williamson to treat her parkinsonian symptoms, and older patients are particularly susceptible to their side effects. But I've never had a patient come in and say, "Dr. Avorn, I'm having an anticholinergic side effect." If the patient is a man and the drug reduces the stimulus to his bladder muscle so it can't push urine past an enlarged prostate, he may fall into the hands of a urologist who will lop out the swollen organ, believing that's the problem ("After all, he's over seventy"). Or a woman's dry mouth may send her to the dentist with a request for new dentures—though no dentures will feel right in a mouth that has stopped secreting saliva. Or the blurry vision these drugs can cause may send a patient to the eye doctor—who will have a difficult time finding any glasses that will help.

Getting a handle on these issues requires knowing what can be attributed simply to being old, as opposed to the specific illnesses that occur in older people. Will the correct dose of medicine for a young person be toxic in a geriatric patient? Might the interaction of aging with a new drug create unanticipated side effects? This is not an easy thing to study, especially in human beings. All of us who have done research on the elderly crave a kind of physiological Picture of Dorian Gray through which we could observe the effects of aging in a concentrated way. If we had that, we might better understand how a drug works differently in a man when he is eighty compared to when he was forty. Unfortunately, such biological models do not exist outside of novels.

One reasonable approximation is the cross-sectional study, in which a measurement is made (say, the response to a particular sleeping pill) in people aged twenty, thirty, forty, all the way up to ninety. Because each age group is studied simultaneously, it is possible to collect the findings and interpret the data in something less than a lifetime. The cross-sectional study has been a boon to the study of geriatric pharmacology, but it has its methodological drawbacks. It's been observed that if you were to conduct a cross-sectional study of aging and ethnicity in south Florida, you might conclude that people there are born Hispanic and then become Jewish as they get older. Nonetheless, cross-sectional studies of aging can tell us a great deal about important differences in how the elderly body reacts to medications, for good and for ill.

In trying to understand more about the problem that patients like Mrs. Williamson had, my first instinct was to go to the clinical literature and read everything I could find on how often antipsychotic drugs cause this kind of Parkinson-like syndrome in elderly patients. But when I first looked, there wasn't much literature to review. The drugs were increasingly used to manage old people with agitation—patients who would be particularly prone to Parkinson-like side effects. But no one had gone back to determine how frequently this side effect was occurring, or at what dosage, or with which drugs. No one had to. It wasn't anybody's job.

So we did the study ourselves. For a project we were conducting in a dozen Massachusetts nursing homes, we had collected information on all the drugs being taken by 850 institutionalized elderly people. We tested for parkinsonian signs in those taking any kind of psychoactive drug—antidepressants, sleeping pills, minor tranquilizers, antipsychotics. Our first finding was somewhat reassuring. Drugs like Haldol, if given in very small doses, were not likely to produce the stiffness and shakiness of parkinsonism. This was important evidence that these drugs could be prescribed safely in such patients, albeit in tiny amounts. But more typical doses of Haldol (anything over one milligram per day) resulted in a threefold increase in the risk that the patient would develop parkinsonian symptoms. We also found that other antipsychotics, then widely believed to be relatively benign in this regard, were causing the syndrome as well when used at higher doses.

If the antipsychotic drugs were causing parkinsonian symptoms in the nursing homes we studied, what was happening on a larger scale? I wondered how often this created the problem I had seen when consulting on patients like Mrs. Williamson. By this time, we had built a computerized database of all drug use and clinical encounters in several hundred thousand older patients, and were ready to try to answer the question in the wider world.

We started by identifying all older patients newly started on a drug to treat Parkinson's disease. These were the cases. As control subjects we identified comparable patients of the same age and sex who were clinically very similar but were not being treated for Parkinson's disease. Then we looked back at all the prescriptions that both the cases and the controls had filled in the preceding months, to learn how many in each group had been taking antipsychotic drugs when they were first diagnosed with Parkinson's.

The study had one final wrinkle. There are three ways a doctor can approach parkinsonian symptoms discovered in an older person taking an antipsychotic drug. First, she can say, "This patient has developed a condition that looks like Parkinson's disease, but it's probably just a side effect of that major tranquilizer I prescribed. I'd better stop the tranquilizer." That's the right answer. Or she can say, "This patient has developed a condition that looks like Parkinson's disease, but it's probably just a side effect of that major tranquilizer I prescribed. I'll add a new drug to control the side effect." This is a plausible strategy in young schizophrenics, but it's a bad one in older patients, who have great sensitivity to the additional side effects these added drugs can cause. It's an especially bad idea if the initial tranquilizer wasn't necessary in the first place, as is often the case.

There's also a third course our doctor could take, the worst one. She can say, "This patient has developed a condition that looks like Parkinson's disease. She's old, so it must be Parkinson's disease. I'd better add a drug to treat it." Armed with this pharmacology, we looked at what hundreds of typical doctors were doing in our database. Sure enough, after we controlled for a host of other characteristics, patients who had been prescribed an antipsychotic drug were far more likely to be put on L-dopa, the drug used for actual Parkinson's disease, which isn't even likely to improve the medication-induced syndrome.

It is tragic enough when a patient develops "real" Parkinson's disease: it can be a cruel, devastating illness for which treatment is still far from satisfactory. How much more frustrating when these symptoms are the preventable consequence of medical attention. Newer antipsychotic drugs are available today that produce somewhat fewer parkinsonian symptoms. But it is still probably true that each day family members are told that while that tranquilizer was useful in managing Granny's restlessness, she's now gotten a new neurological disease that will also need treatment. This drug–side effect combination is but one that I've chosen to present in detail; there are dozens more.

Mrs. Williamson had a happier fate than many older patients in her circumstances. Further discussion with nursing home staff made it clear that she had probably not needed the Haldol in the first place. It was stopped, as was her anti-Parkinson's medication. The dizziness and nightmares caused by the latter went away, as did the tremor and rigidity that the former had produced. A rehabilitation specialist was consulted to see if her ability to care for herself could be improved enough for her to move to a less restrictive assisted-living facility.

Paradoxically, taking care of patients like Mrs. Williamson has made me optimistic about the future of medication use in the elderly. We still have a long way to go, but the field of geriatric pharmacology has at least made it onto the edge of the nation's medical radar, and woeful neglect is one step up from being ignored completely. After decades of inattention, health services researchers are beginning to look at how well we use medicines in older patients, and how we can do it better. Further progress will certainly be driven by us baby boomers. We have seen the medication-related problems our parents and grandparents face, and we don't want to suffer them ourselves. A uniquely self-absorbed and entitled group, we redefined activism as teens and college kids, and as the yuppies of the 1980s we redefined consumerism. We are not likely to quiet down when we confront the medical care system as oldsters in the next decades.

In the coming years, new drug discoveries will target diseases of aging that we cannot treat well today. But even with the medications now available, there are numerous ways we could improve the use and outcomes of prescription drugs in older patients. We will save these for last, echoing the words of the algebra teachers many of us had in high school: "The answers are in the back of the book if you need them."

We will all need them.

OUR FOCUS thus far has been on how benefits and risks are discovered and measured, and how we know what we know about them. In many of these cases, once all the data were in, the decision about whether to use a given drug was fairly lopsided. We now move on to the next level of complexity, a level on which most medication-use decisions by doctors and patients are made. Substantial benefits have been defined, and worrisome risks measured. How are we to compare the one with the other?

8: ENTER DOCTOR FAUSTUS

You are probably going to die of heart disease. I don't mean this in a hypothetical sense. I mean you, the person reading this book. If you live in an industrialized country and you're not presently dying of cancer or another terminal illness, the chances are you're going to die of some form of heart disease. Cardiovascular conditions, particularly pathology of the coronary arteries, are the most common cause of mortality in most wealthy nations, accounting for about half of all deaths each year.

Suppose I offer you a drug that would reduce your risk of heart attack by 30 percent (if you're a man; the effect in women is less impressive). Sounds good, but by now you're wise enough to demand to know about its side effects. Oh, those. The drug can sometimes precipitate an allergic reaction that in severe cases causes swelling of the larynx, and that can progress to respiratory failure and death; the treatment can also interfere with the function of platelets, a component of blood required for normal clotting; it can erode the lining of the stomach or small intestine, and can produce bleeding that is sometimes life-threatening.

Want it?

You're a psychiatrist treating a twenty-five-year-old schizophrenic whose crippling mental illness has not responded to conventional therapy. He's been in and out of state mental hospitals since he was a teenager, and nearly died after a grisly incident involving a train. Now, the patient is living on the streets and hears voices that tell him he has been drafted into a secret international brigade to defend America from a terrorist plot of world domination.

Other doctors have tried nearly all the available medications with results that were transient, disappointing, or both. Treatment-resistant cases like his sometimes respond well to an uncommonly used drug, clozapine. But in some patients that drug can be toxic to the bone marrow, destroying the body's ability to produce white blood cells; this can leave the patient defenseless against infections and may lead to death. At today's visit, the patient calmly asks you whether you think he'd be better off if he never had anything to worry about anymore. You reach for your prescription pad. . . .

Even when a medicine's risks and benefits are well defined, balancing them against each other can be a task of Talmudic complexity. A patient with sudden crushing chest pain who cannot undergo angioplasty would probably want to get the newest, strongest clot-busting drug available to ream out the blocked coronary artery that is causing his heart attack, instead of an older product. By opening the artery more quickly and thoroughly, the stronger drug could save millions more of his asphyxiating heart muscle cells. But what if the newer drug were also slightly more likely to blow a hole in one of his cerebral arteries, reducing much of his brain to the functional status of ratatouille? How to decide?

Such questions must be answered daily by doctors and patients, with scores of new clinical dilemmas turning up each year. In the process, we are forced to confront issues that seem to be part pharmacology and part philosophy: How much risk is acceptable for what sort of benefit? Smallpox vaccine confers good immunity against this often fatal disease, but will predictably cause serious side effects in a small fraction of those who are vaccinated; that is why nations abandoned routine immunization in the 1970s once the disease was (we thought) wiped out. These issues were central to the national policy debate about mass public vaccination in response to a terrorist threat: How large would the probability of infection have to be to warrant an immunization program that could itself sicken thousands of healthy Americans?

On a more mundane level, is using a very effective new drug for severe arthritis worth a small possible increase in the likelihood of developing a malignancy years later? If Viagra can occasionally cause a life-threatening drop in blood pressure, should it still be available to anyone willing to take the chance? Who should be allowed to trade off what risk against what benefit? Just how is that to be done, exactly? Fascinating examples abound. Should such decisions be made on a national level for all citizens by the government, or should individual doctors decide? Or individual patients? Just how good are we at defining the probabilities and severities on which these benefit-hazard trade-offs depend? What should be the proper role of the FDA? The drug industry? Medical schools? Consumer watchdog groups? The questions are pressing, the answers unsettling.

Pharmacology must consort with game theory, decision science, and the psychology of risk assessment if we are to understand how to frame these issues and decide which benefits are worth which side effects. Still other disciplines must then be marshaled to determine how these dilemmas of safety, rescue, and danger can best be communicated to decision makers, whether they are physicians, patients, or policy makers.

As a doctor and drug researcher, I confront questions like these at the level of specific patients as well as the health care system as a whole. But everybody balances risks and benefits in less serious ways dozens of times each day: whether to put your nest egg in the stock market or in a safe but low-yield interest-bearing account; whether you can make it across the street before the DON'T WALK sign comes on and the drivers start speeding through the crosswalk; whether asking that attractive colleague to dinner on Saturday night will lead to a great new relationship or an embarrassing rejection; whether quitting a steady, boring job will lead to a long stretch of unemployment or to the career of your dreams. For all of us, each day brings hundreds of tiny risk-benefit assessments, a veritable slalom course of probability estimates that we navigate well or poorly.

The stories of Redux, PPA, and Rezulin were extreme in the perversity and misbehavior of some of the participants. But once the data were available for all to see, the excess of hazard over benefit was evident. A few pounds of weight loss was not worth the possibility of fatal lung or heart damage; no stuffy nose was worth a devastating stroke; and there were plenty of useful diabetes drugs available that did not cause the sudden death of a patient's liver. Now that we know the frequency of these drugs' side effects, their stories make fascinating case studies in malfeasance and ineptitude, but don't present challenging questions of risk-benefit calculation. Better drugs, still on the market, illustrate the tensions more richly.

Vaccines are one of the clearest examples of slam-dunk benefit-risk relationships, despite their recent histrionic and generally undeserved bad press. Vaccinate 100,000 kids against measles, for example, and a few will develop complications, sometimes severe ones. This is tragic when it occurs, but children as a whole are far better off because measles vaccine is available. The choice of whether to use tamoxifen to prevent a recurrence of breast cancer provides another example of what in skiing might be considered a "green circle" level of risk-benefit difficulty. A patient who takes tamoxifen increases her risk of a new cancer of the uterus at the same time that she reduces the likelihood that her breast cancer will recur. Because the trial that demonstrated this was large and well done, the data needed for this benefit-risk balancing act were quickly available: the number of new cases of uterine cancer caused by the drug was dwarfed by the number of breast cancer recurrences it prevented, and cancer of the uterus can be caught and treated more readily than can a breast cancer recurrence. The use of aspirin to prevent heart attacks, the first drug example at the start of this chapter, is another example of benefit far outweighing hazard, however daunting the latter may sound. But how are we to compare benefits and risks when they are closer in magnitude?

HARDER CHOICES

In the sixteenth century, before the current age of specialization in health care, many doctors also practiced sorcery, astrology, necromancy, and prophecy. One such generalist was Johann Faustus, a legendary character said to have lived in Germany in the first half of that century around the same time as Paracelsus, the man who coined the "All medicines are poisons . . ." aphorism. As depicted in the works of Marlowe, Goethe, Berlioz, Gounod, and others, Faust confronted one of the most famous benefit-risk trade-offs in human history. He arranged with the Devil to gain magical powers verging on omnipotence, in exchange for his soul. This seemed like a good deal at the time, and for years Doctor Faustus traveled around Germany performing amazing acts of magic and building up a lucrative consulting practice. But as the time approached for him to pay up on the risk end of his benefit-risk swap, he grew dissatisfied with the arrangement. These second thoughts led to a colorful death at the hands of you-know-who.

Every drug-use decision is a small Faustian bargain, with risks and benefits that are usually on a far more modest scale. A pharmaceutical manufacturer must decide whether to proceed with the costly and cumbersome development of a new molecule that could be a blockbuster product, a dead end, or a massive liability sink. An experimental subject must decide whether to volunteer for a trial of a drug that could improve her health or cause unknown hazards. A regulator at the FDA must decide whether the new product should then be allowed on the market. A physician must decide whether its promised therapeutic value will outweigh its potential for harm. Ultimately, the patient must decide (sometimes several times each day) whether it's worth taking that drug as prescribed. Since Faust's time, medicine has searched for a way to structure these trade-offs so the decisions could be made scientifically rather than as we doctors often do, by gut feeling. As Dr. Holmes, that nineteenth-century master of the sound bite, once observed, "The gut is not an organ well suited to reasoning."

Let's assume that all the lessons of the previous chapters have been learned well and all the data defining benefits and risks are in—a luxury usually not available when many of these decisions must be made. The task before us now is not one of discovering benefits and risks, but of comparing them. (When we add a third dimension and attempt to relate both benefits and risks to costs, the problem will become exponentially more difficult, but we won't have to face that until Part Three.)

We can start with the easiest kind of balancing act, one that doesn't require us to place gradations of goodness or badness on the outcomes being considered. In this modest way of thinking about things, we can simplistically identify all possible outcomes of treatment, both benefits and risks, as well as the consequences of nontreatment, simply as acceptable or terrible. When this is possible, as long as the numbers are based on solid data from randomized trials, we can tote up the outcomes and determine the best course of treatment.

For a straightforward example of a black-and-white risk-benefit decision, we can return to Tommy O'Rourke, the heart attack patient in the Prologue whose well-meaning ambulance driver took him to a nearby community hospital for an injection of a clot-busting drug instead of to a larger hospital for an angioplasty procedure. How could anyone have determined whether this was the right policy? Let's pretend for now that a heart attack victim can have only one of two outcomes within thirty days: catastrophe (death from the heart attack, or a massive stroke from the drug used to treat it) or disease-free survival. We'll suppose that with no treatment, Mr. O'Rourke would have a risk of x percent of dying from his heart attack, and no risk of treatment-induced stroke. With an injection of the clot-busting thrombolytic drug at his community hospital, his risk of death from the heart attack would go down to y percent, but his risk of a drug-induced stroke would be z percent—for a total risk of catastrophic outcomes of $y + z$ percent—still better than no treatment.

Had he been brought instead to the medical center and undergone emergency angioplasty, his risk of death *and* his risk of stroke would both be lower; clinical trial findings indicate that this approach yields the fewest catastrophic outcomes overall. This is as easy an example as I can think of, and its implications are pretty straightforward. Yet even this obvious way of choosing between treatments has not been put into routine practice in many areas. As you read these words, thousands of O'Rourkes all over the country are having heart attacks and being given clot-busting injections, even if there is a center that could perform angioplasty not far away.

HOW DECISION SCIENCE CAN HELP

As Faust learned, in mythology as in pharmacology the benefits usually appear first; the risks generally don't become evident until later on. Agonizing as his decision was, that choice was in some ways simpler than the ones doctors and patients often face. Its benefits were clearly spelled out contractually, as was the single eternal Side Effect. The stakes may be more modest in weighing decisions about medications, but the nuances are far more complex. For one thing, the probabilities of specific outcomes are much less clear than they were for poor Faust.

Consider birth control pills. They are among the best studied and most commonly used medications on the planet; accurate numbers are available to describe the frequencies of all the outcomes that follow their use. There is one main benefit to consider: the successful prevention of pregnancy. We can restrict ourselves for now to just three bad outcomes: contraceptive failure (i.e., pregnancy), deep-vein thrombophlebitis (blood clots), and pulmonary embolus (which occurs when one of those clots flies loose and lodges in the lungs, a potentially fatal development). With tens of thousands of women enrolled in RCTs of the birth control pill since the 1960s, we have ample data on the likelihood of each of these outcomes. We can pretend for the current discussion that all birth control pills have the same risks and success rates, though they do not.

The basic idea underlying this decision-analysis approach was described decades ago by Professor Howard Raiffa. In an early book, he explained the idea through the example of an oil prospector. The explorer discovers that site A contains 10 million barrels of oil, but sinking a well there would have only a 50 percent chance of striking it. By contrast, site B contains only 6 million barrels, but (perhaps because it's lying just below the surface), there is a 90 percent chance of getting it. The best way to think about the likely output of site A is to "value" it as 5 million barrels (a 50 percent chance of striking its 10-million-barrel lode), and the most accurate description of the likely yield of site B is 5.4 million barrels (a 90 percent chance of extracting its 6 million barrels). The math tells us that a poorer site with a higher chance of a hit is probably a better gamble than a richer site that has a lower likelihood of success. Substitute benefits and risks for barrels of oil, apply the probabilities, and when all goes well (as it sometimes does) we have the beginnings of a guide to therapeutic decision making.

In the case of our oral contraceptive example, as terrible as it is for a healthy young woman to develop a blood clot as a result of taking the pill, when viewed in terms of a large population of women, the aggregate medical risks of pregnancy loom even larger. This can be calculated on a simple spreadsheet; a crude analysis can even be done with pencil and paper. Diaphragms and condoms don't cause blood clots, but they do cause pregnancy, because their failure rate is far greater than that of oral contraceptives and not all those unwanted pregnancies are terminated. Since the pill is far more effective at preventing pregnancy than other available methods, when all these outcomes are considered it turns out that over thousands of women, the number of medical complications caused by unwanted pregnancies in nonusers of the pill will be substantially greater than the complications caused by the pill itself.

Using the same kind of reasoning, recent clinical trial data can provide the information we need to make the best decision for the tormented schizophrenic we met at the chapter's start. In a population of patients like him, the numbers of deaths caused by the potentially fatal drug reaction will be lower than the numbers of additional suicides that would occur if alternative drugs were used. As long as the data are there to plug into such a decision analysis, "running the numbers" in this way can often be a powerful tool for calculating the best strategy when choosing among drugs for a given patient, or between a drug and nondrug alternatives. The problems emerge when no one has ever done the clinical trials needed to generate the numbers needed, or we can't be sure how to value outcomes that are more complex than "well" versus "catastrophic"—problems we'll address shortly.

Even when excellent data are in place and the decision analysis is straightforward, translating this logic into actual practice may be another matter. Clinical decisions don't exist in a vacuum. Like the lines assigned to characters in a play, they take on reality only when brought to life by the everyday actions of real-world doctors prescribing for their patients. That transformation brings with it a new set of challenges and opportunities. To see this interface in action, we can return to poor Dr. Vasily of the Prologue, whose reluctance to use an anticoagulant for atrial fibrillation led to such a miserable outcome. The doctor was a victim of a common contaminant of clinical decision making, sometimes called "last case bias." He remembered another patient he anticoagulated who had a catastrophic bleeding complication, and that unfortunate person loomed larger in his mental reckoning than did the many other patients for whom he had prescribed Coumadin (warfarin) without any problems. We can now examine his fateful decision in a bit more detail.

Anticoagulants are hard drugs to use, for both doctor and patient. The right dose will differ widely from patient to patient; in a given person, a little too much can result in uncontrolled bleeding and a dose that is slightly too low can be ineffective. Even this can change with time: adding other drugs to the patient's regimen can amplify or reduce the anticoagulant effect substantially; the same can occur if the patient's diet changes, or any number of other factors intervene. Constant vigilance by both prescriber and patient are required to keep the coagulation status in its safe razor-thin range. Many patients prescribed warfarin do well once their dose is stabilized, with no greater disability than the need for regular blood tests. But most doctors have also cared for patients in whom things went horribly wrong.

Anticoagulants may be tough to use, but the consequences of not prescribing them can be worse. There was no way to figure out the best way to treat Stan from a theorist's armchair, from a laboratory, or even from studies on animals—many of which turn out to have coagulation systems that behave differently from those of humans. Back when a heart attack was called a coronary thrombosis, many cardiologists believed that it was caused by a simple blood clot blocking an artery supplying the heart. (We now know the mechanism is much more complicated.) With plausible logic, thousands of patients were anticoagulated to prevent these events. Plausible, but wrong. Once randomized controlled trials were finally conducted to test this therapy, it turned out that the patients randomized to the blood-thinner arm of the study bled more but didn't have enough reduction in their heart attack rates to make it worth it. The treatment was abandoned.

Would anticoagulation work any better in preventing the clots that cause strokes? There was only one sure way to find out. Several large randomized trials were designed to address this question; their results were reported in the 1990s. Patients with atrial fibrillation were randomly assigned to take warfarin or placebo, with staggering results. The number of strokes in patients randomized to the anticoagulant group was a full two thirds lower than in the placebo patients. Bleeding events were slightly more common in the anticoagulated group, but this didn't even come close to offsetting the dramatic gains in stroke protection. Warfarin was proven to be a safe and effective way of preventing a catastrophic medical condition that, once it occurred, usually offered little hope of full recovery. Using the same drug to prevent heart attacks was an equally logical concept; it just happened not to be true. These were not insights that any single physician could have come upon alone. The hemorrhages would have been obvious enough, but a randomized trial was indispensable to measure the magnitude of the benefit.

THREE DOCTORS, SAME EVIDENCE

Once the reports of these studies were published in medical journals, the findings had to be implemented through the clinical decision making of individual physicians, and that is where things can get dicey. Let's imagine two colleagues of Dr. Vasily, each treating a similar patient with chronic atrial fibrillation and facing the same benefit-risk trade-off. One, Dr. Reslo, has also read the key studies; assessing the evidence, she decides to commit the patient to a lifetime of anticoagulation. She educates the patient about the demanding regimen, begins the delicate pas de deux of gradually adjusting warfarin doses over several days, has the patient come in to recheck the coagulation status after each dose change is made, and eventually calculates a stable maintenance dose on which the patient is to remain for life. Over the years, whenever the patient needs an antibiotic that might interact with warfarin, Dr. Reslo adjusts the anticoagulant dose while the antibiotic is being taken, checks additional blood tests, and then adjusts it again (with more blood test follow-ups) once the antibiotic is stopped. If a new medication is added for arthritis or diabetes, she again measures the coagulation status, revises the warfarin dose as needed, and repeats the cycle until a new stable dose has been achieved.

If all goes well and both Dr. Reslo and her patient pay close attention to the demanding anticoagulant regimen, the years pass and . . . nothing happens. I have never written in a patient's medical record, "Patient still on warfarin. Did not have a stroke this year. Continue current medications." No patient or family member has ever called to thank me because they or their grandmother remained stroke-free, nor would I expect anyone to. Arduous as the regimen is, it's simply the right thing to do. The sign of its success is the absence of any noticeable events.

Now let's consider a third physician, whom we'll call Dr. Sanger. For the first six years of treatment he and his patient behave in exactly the same way as Dr. Reslo and her patient. But in January of year seven, the following events occur:

> Ten days prior to admission to the hospital, the patient developed a flu-like illness. He remained bed-bound for several days, eating very little and not taking in much fluid. He had nausea and vomiting, resulting in further dehydration. His wife gave him an over-the-counter flu remedy containing a mixture of aspirin, acetaminophen (Tylenol), and several other components. Neither the patient nor his wife were aware of any potential interaction with warfarin, and he took the preparation for three days, during which his anorexia and vomiting worsened. On the fourth day the patient was found by his wife lying in the bathroom in a pool of blood; he was brought to the hospital.
>
> On arrival at the emergency department, his systolic blood pressure had fallen to 80 and he was unconscious. An endoscope inserted into the upper gastrointestinal tract revealed massive hemorrhage in the stomach. Blood tests indicated that the patient was excessively anticoagulated. He continued to bleed uncontrollably despite transfusion of blood and clotting factors. Within twenty-four hours he suffered cardiac arrest and was pronounced dead. Discharge diagnosis: severe gastrointestinal hemorrhage caused by excessive anticoagulation.

Dr. Sanger felt remorseful that the drug he prescribed had contributed to the patient's death. The dehydration caused by the viral infection, along with the interaction between the warfarin and the ingredients in the over-the-counter remedy, had sharply increased the anticoagulant effect of the drug, which the patient dutifully continued to take throughout the course of his illness. His widow tearfully asked whether her husband's hemorrhage had been made worse "because of the blood thinner you gave him." (Of course it had.) A few weeks later, Sanger receives a registered letter from the family's lawyer requesting copies of all of the decedent's medical records.

Let's return to Dr. Vasily. When he detected atrial fibrillation in an otherwise healthy patient, he chose not to pursue the issue further because he was "not a believer" in the preventive use of anticoagulants. He gave Stan a clean bill of health and no prescription. When Stan had his probably preventable stroke, Dr. Vasily was wracked with doubt about whether he had made a mistake in withholding the anticoagulant. But no one in Stan's family asked whether the doctor had caused the stroke that crippled his patient. Strokes happen in older people; doctors don't cause strokes.

Assume that Drs. Vasily, Reslo, and Sanger each had similar-sized practices comprising people of the same age, gender, and clinical makeup. If they were comparable to the patients in the clinical trials, we can make some provocative calculations. After ten years, the patients of Dr. Reslo and Dr. Sanger (who after all took exactly the same evidence-based approach) would have experienced the same number of strokes and major hemorrhages in each of the two practices. The patients of Dr. Vasily, by contrast, would have experienced many more strokes and slightly fewer hemorrhages—far more catastrophic events in all. It just doesn't always look that way on the ground. This is the kind of situation in which formal decision analysis can correctly guide prescribing while one-at-a-time patient assessment could easily lead us astray. But as we will see in the next chapter, there are times when precisely the opposite can occur.

9: IMPERFECT MEASURES

S o far, we've confined ourselves to drug-use choices in which the benefits and hazards were pretty clear-cut—the territory in which formal decision analysis can be a useful guide to practice. But sick people differ importantly from barrels of Texas crude, and the method can cause some serious mischief if applied carelessly. Indeed, some prescribing decisions can emerge from the decision-analysis sausage maker mangled and clinically unrecognizable. It takes a wise clinician or policy maker to know how to proceed when the best computer models clash with the human experiences of illness and care. The problem is toughest when we try to move from the realm of *counting* outcomes to the realm of *valuing* them—even before we start to think about economic issues.

Let's return to our imaginary world in which all randomized trials have been conducted and thorough postmarketing surveillance has identified all risks. In that world we may know the frequency of each of these events, but how can we get a handle on the relative goodness or badness of each clinical state? After all, many medical situations can't be neatly divided into the simplified cure-versus-catastrophe dichotomy we used in the last chapter. A drug that keeps people alive but in a state of disability is surely less useful than a drug that keeps people alive and in excellent health for just as long. Or let's say a drug causes a rash all over the body for a week or two. We might well be willing to take a chance of that occurring if the drug effectively treated a miserable disease like AIDS or cancer, but not if it was a treatment for hay fever. Is it possible to put a number on the awfulness of a given disease, or a drug side effect, so we could calculate these trade-offs more systematically?

To make such analyses possible, researchers have tried for years to devise a scale of badness on which to rank all clinical conditions. Their goal has been to assign a number from 0 to 100 percent to reflect the value of a year of life spent with any given illness: stroke, angina, acne, depression, end-stage renal disease, lung cancer, hot flashes, congestive heart failure, schizophrenia. Fatal events take care of themselves (they result in zero life-years); each remaining year of life with some other outcome could then in principle be "adjusted" by such numbers. A rich but problematic lode of work from other disciplines bears directly on these questions. If we could just get these value weightings right, we could multiply those numbers by the probabilities of ending up in each particular state, as revealed in controlled trials and observational studies. In doing so, we could bring to bear a powerful set of analytic tools developed over the years to guide decisions in other aspects of life. Sometimes this approach works wonderfully well; in other applications, it's a complete bust. We'll look at examples of both.

THE WORLD OF DECISION ANALYSIS

The task of assigning values to clinical conditions often embodies a set of hidden assumptions—about methods, about values—that can sometimes distort the supposedly objective recommendations that flow from these methods. These distortions can be greatest for vulnerable populations such as the elderly and chronically ill. The plausible idea of decision analysis can be pushed beyond its limits, and often is.

It's easy to see how a quantitative method that claims to be both objective and fair could seem to provide a neat road map out of the conceptual swamp of subjective clinical judgment. A by-the-numbers approach to balancing risks and benefits can seem particularly attractive as a replacement for the shriveling professional sovereignty of both physicians and policy makers. Anyone who mistrusts the motives and skills of clinicians or the people who run health care organizations will welcome an approach that promises to reduce the decision-making latitude of both to a standardized set of equations and algorithms. The trend also fits nicely with the movement in the social and managerial sciences to quantify as many variables as possible, in an earnest but sometimes hopeless attempt to imitate the work of the natural sciences. Finally, it meshes neatly with the corporatization of health care; managers who would like to turn all treatments and outcomes into commodities become excited at the prospect of reducing every clinical input and output to a single number. Taken together, these trends have produced a fertile ground for the growth as well as the overgrowth of quantitative guides to medication use.

Medical risk-benefit analysis and its economic cousin, cost-effectiveness analysis, had their beginnings in public works programs and industry, and their methods reflect these origins. In evaluating a proposed activity like building a dam, the good that the project would produce (hydroelectric power, flood control) could be compared with its negative outcomes (harm to the environment, interruption of shipping). Once such benefits and risks were explicitly identified, valued, and projected over time, their sums could in principle be weighed against each other, and the results used to guide decision making. The medical application of these ideas began with counting the number of lives saved by use of a new drug or other treatment, analogous to the number of kilowatt-hours that would be generated by a new hydroelectric plant.

But while a watt is a watt is a watt, the same cannot be said about states of health. Counting "years of life saved" by a given treatment can easily lead down a slippery slope to the next stage: how to value those years of life. Many observers pointed out sensibly enough that a treatment that produces ten life-years of excellent health doesn't really yield the same good as one that results in ten life-years of severe disability. Let's say you have a debilitating illness for which two drugs are available. Drug A would produce a 60 percent chance of cure, but a 35 percent chance of paralysis. Drug B would produce just a 45 percent chance of cure, but only a 5 percent chance of the same kind of paralysis. With neither drug, your underlying illness has a 25 percent chance of killing you within five years. Do you want to take one of these drugs?

Unless you're into consulting Tarot cards, there's a natural desire to try to parse the question rationally: How disabling is the current illness? How severe is that paralysis side effect? If we could somehow put numbers to the burden of these outcomes, we could combine them with the probabilities and approximate the simple oil-well illustration of the last chapter. Do it right, and the numbers could tell you which choice would best maximize your chances of living and minimize your disability. So far so good.

This logic resulted in the concept of the *quality-adjusted life-year (QALY)*—a measure that assigns a number to a year of life in a given state of health, from 0 for death to 1 for perfect health. The benefits of medications can then be analyzed in terms of both the duration *and* the quality of the life that they make possible. Doctors and patients can make better-informed choices; society can pay for treatments leading to the most possible QALYs. When everything goes well, this is just what happens, and this method has been used to illuminate many previously murky medication-use questions.

But there can be problems. How accurately can we assign a number to every possible health state? Even if we could do this, the idea that death is the worst possible state may make sense to some economists but would be contested by many clinicians, patients, and family members of terribly sick people. And should the number be the same for all people with a given condition? What about the ethical assumptions implicit in a calculus that says that a year of life on dialysis is worth only one third as much as a year with functioning kidneys, or that a year of life after mastectomy for breast cancer is worth only six months of "normal" life?

Transforming counting into valuing can also put the health problems of the elderly and disabled at a particular disadvantage. Few interventions in these patients can stand up favorably against programs for the young in terms of numbers of years of life saved. In fact, the very idea of quality-adjusted life-years can put *any* care for the old at a lower premium. Even ten years of life count for very little in this formulation if one has arthritis, emphysema, and renal failure.

FUNNY NUMBERS

The quality-adjusted life-year approach has another, related problem: it often goes beyond the science on which it is based. Quality-of-life adjustment factors are usually calculated by asking healthy people how much less they think life would be worth if they had a particular condition—a strategy required by the underlying theory. But comparing those numbers to data obtained from people who actually have the disease in question raises some disturbing questions about their validity. For kidney dialysis, one survey of healthy persons asked to rank this condition on a scale from 0 to 1 produced a quality-adjusted value of 0.32 year as the worth of one year of life for a patient who had to undergo regular treatments at a dialysis center. But when a sample of actual dialysis patients was asked to perform the same task, the value of a year of treatment rose sharply, to the equivalent of 0.52 year of perfect health. Many of the calculations in this field are based on such flimsy data. Yet the numbers that emerge belie their imprecise origins, taking on an appearance of legitimacy normally reserved for experimental data.

Part of the problem has to do with how these numbers arise in the first place. They often come from asking people questions like this:

> Taking into account your age, pain and suffering, immobility, and lost earnings, what fraction, P, of a year of life would you be willing to give up to be completely healthy for the remaining fraction of a year instead of your present level of health status for the full year? Or, taking into account these same factors, what probability, P, of death would you be willing to accept so that, if you survived, you would have full health rather than your present health status for the rest of your life?

This is not the kind of analysis that we do particularly well as a species. Human evolution put a premium on vision, hearing, pattern recognition, and memory, but making probabilistic assessments has not been our strong suit. Consider lotteries, a kind of regressive tax used the world over to suck resources from the numerically challenged. Each day, millions of people demonstrate in the most compelling way (by giving away their hard-earned cash) that they do not fully understand what concepts like a one-in-ten-thousand chance actually mean. First, the number itself is hard to grasp intuitively. Second—and the relevance to medication use is compelling—even when the meaning is more accessible, say for a one-in-seven kind of odds, people seem to slide into a kind of magical thinking that assumes *their* chance of the rare event is quite different from that of all the other people who are subjected to the exact same odds. At some level, when each of us buys a lottery ticket, we think that we'll be the ones to whom the odds don't really apply—otherwise, why would we ever do such a thing?

To make matters worse, some decision analysts have subjected simply being old to "quality adjustment," even in the absence of any disease. One economist calculated the adjusted value of a year of life at various points in the age span. His initial studies were based in part on a survey of some sixty undergraduates he was teaching, who were asked to assign numbers to various ages to reflect the quality of life at each point. These young men and women, not surprisingly, decided that life-years in the twenties were the best, and those in old age the worst. Citing these responses and quoting Jonathan Swift ("Every man desires to live long, but no man would be old"), the economist concluded, "As a rough and simple approximation, the average quality of life in the years before age sixty-five might be assumed to be constant, and quality of life in later years assumed to decrease steadily, approaching zero at age ninety," a conclusion that would surprise many ninety-year-olds I've cared for. These calculations have then been used to urge a redistribution of health care resources to emphasize the prevention of mortality in the young.

How weird all this can get is illustrated by a recent study that tried to apply patients' estimates of risk and value to assess drugs for impotence. In a paper published in the usually stiff *Annals of Internal Medicine,* two physicians presented a penetrating analysis of the quality-of-life effects of being unable to have successful intercourse. Some of their data came from the Beaver Dam Outcomes Study, a project of the early 1990s that attempted to assign quality-adjustment numbers to a long list of health and disease states; the study was named after the midwestern community where it was conducted. The approach assumes, of course, that a man in the Midwest values his erections about as much as a man in Greenwich Village or

Paris or a retirement community in Phoenix. Other numbers came from a survey of ten healthy middle-aged men who were asked a typical time-trade-off question: *What fraction of a full year with impotence would you be willing to give up if you could have normal sexual function during the remaining time?* Their answer, on average: 26 percent.

If we believe this number, it means that erectile dysfunction reduces the value of each year lived by about a quarter. Orthodox utility analysis dictates that such questions be asked of the community as a whole, rather than just of the people who have a given condition. With this in mind, the team asked the same question of the men's wives. It turned out that for the women, absence of conjugal bliss translated to only a 2 percent annual decrement. In other surveys of men, the downside of erectile dysfunction varied between losses of 5 percent of the year and 40 percent of the year, depending on the population studied.

Combining these numbers, the Beaver Dam data, and other surveys, the authors of the *Annals* paper reported that just being alive and in normal health at age sixty is worth only 87 percent of a year of life at a younger age; having erectile dysfunction reduces that by an additional 13 percent. (Add in some arthritis, high blood pressure, and diabetes, and it's hard to understand why all these older guys wouldn't just throw themselves off tall buildings at the first opportunity.) This research on the utility of sexual function is but one example of the lengths to which decision analysts sometimes go in assigning numbers to conditions that defy enumeration. In other diseases as well, many quality-adjustment analyses of drug effects are based on equally problematic "How good was it for you?" numbers.

My skepticism about this approach deepened further when I discovered the ingenious work on risk and choice by the cognitive psychologists Daniel Kahneman and Amos Tversky. They found that in real life people often weigh odds and make choices in ways that aren't predicted by neat theory. Some of these deviations make sense and others are patently foolish. The sensible kind of deviation was noted as long ago as 1738 by Daniel Bernoulli. This field of research typically discusses outcomes in monetary terms, but the principles apply equally well to the benefits and side effects produced by medications. Here is an illustration of Bernoulli's paradox: Imagine that there are two detachable coupons in the back of this book. Mail me Coupon One and I'll enter you in a drawing in which 75 percent of entrants will win $1,000. Mail in Coupon Two and I'll simply mail you a check for $700, guaranteed. Which coupon would you send in?

Since Bernoulli's day, the overwhelming majority of respondents have gone with the sure thing, even though people who do so will *on average* come out with $50 per person less than those who choose the gamble. Most of us quite plausibly are willing to reduce our maximum benefit if doing so will buy us some certainty. The same applies to negative consequences, in a mirror-image way. In that case, most people would rather accept a state of uncertainty than a guaranteed negative experience, even if their average level of "suffering" would be less with the sure thing. The implications are clear for patient and doctor choices about drug benefits and risks, yet these findings are usually ignored by classical utility theory; this "risk premium" perspective is rarely included in conventional decision analyses of patient preferences.

AN OFFER YOU CAN REFUSE

Other kinds of real-world preferences likewise don't match what the theorists predict, and some of these decisions are less sensible. Consider the following choices:

> Imagine that you have a painful degenerative disease that creates chronic disability and over time will eventually kill you. I have a newly discovered drug to treat this condition, but unfortunately one in ten patients who take it experiences a fatal side effect and dies within the first week of using it. Those who do not die are cured of their disease. Would you take the drug?

> Now imagine that you have a degenerative disease similar to that described above; it creates a comparable state of chronic pain and over time will eventually kill you. But now, you are offered a second drug that has been found to be completely effective in eliminating this condition in 90 percent of patients. The remainder develop a fatal complication in the first week of therapy. Would you take the drug?

Cognitive psychologists have presented versions of these questions, modified from a classic experiment by Tversky and Kahneman, to thousands of subjects. The risks and benefits are of course identical in both formulations. What differs is only the framing—the way the question is set up. The outcome is cast first in terms of mortality, and then in terms of survival. In a famous finding that should serve as a cautionary tale for every physician and patient, respondents offered the scenario with a 90 percent chance of survival tend to opt for the intervention, while many more of those presented with a 10 percent risk of death want nothing to do with it. The findings were remarkably stable in a variety of populations studied. They cannot be blamed on the widespread innumeracy (quantitative illiteracy) for which critics have faulted mainstream American education and culture:

many of these subjects were students of business or medicine at elite institutions, who ought to know a thing or two about decision making in the face of uncertainty.

This area of research has important implications for how patients and doctors evaluate the risks and benefits of drugs. The field of behavioral economics, which attempts to take such psychological dimensions into account, has even won its founders the Nobel Prize in economics in recent years. But medical decision analysis is for the most part still stuck in the classical rational-actor economic world of Adam Smith.

Those of us who spend our entire professional lives thinking about these issues are saddled with the same evolution-challenged brains that everyone else walks around with. A recent meeting of pharmacoepidemiologists featured a talk by Professor Richard Farmer, a heavy-smoking British public health researcher (risk assessment doesn't always begin at home). A man of acid wit, Farmer was discussing the relative chances of developing blood clots in young women taking different kinds of oral contraceptives, and how to weigh them against the risks inherent in other means of birth control. He suggested that such comparisons were too hard for patients to perform on their own.

"Surely," Dr. Farmer observed, "making decisions about contraception based on comparing such very small odds is a task well beyond what can be expected from the public, half of whom are of below-average intelligence."

There was an awkward silence, and when he completed his remarks they were greeted with only tepid applause. During the coffee break that followed, many in the audience expressed indignation over his remark about the intelligence of laypeople, which a number of the attendees felt was nasty and condescending. One woman in the audience had a different take on his comments, and chastised him "for that cruel comment you made about women." (She thought that this was the half of the population he was referring to.) But Farmer was merely attempting some humor with the observation that half of any population will by definition be below average on any measure made in that population, just as the other half will be above average. And he wasn't particularly referring to women at all. His jest apparently went over the heads of many in the audience—in a room full of people who specialize in measuring and evaluating probabilities.

COMPARING BENEFITS AND RISKS becomes even more complex when the treatment is likely to be only partially successful, and its risks may occur much later. This is precisely what happens with the most common kind of drug use: medicines used to manage risk states that are not illnesses in their own right, but whose presence increases the likelihood of future disease. Theory requires use of a time-related discount rate to properly value benefits and harms that will occur far in the future. In this way, preventing a heart attack that might occur twenty years from now (e.g., by using a cholesterol-lowering drug) becomes worth less than preventing a heart attack that would occur tomorrow. Likewise, a side effect that won't strike for fifteen years (for example, a breast cancer caused by estrogen replacement therapy) is supposed to have a level of unpleasantness that is lower than that same breast cancer diagnosed today. How much different? One official answer: 3 percent per year, compounded quarterly. At that rate, a decision analyst might have told Dr. Faust that the net present value of so many years of immediate omnipotence could stack up pretty well against a disbenefit—to use the jargon—that wouldn't kick in for almost two and a half decades. Even if the side effect (necrosis of the soul) is eternal in duration, running the numbers might show that it's a plausible trade-off, if the discount rate is high enough.

The British perform formal analyses to guide the use of drugs and other health care interventions in that nation's National Health Service. Many of them require that clinical benefits and risks and costs be discounted at *different rates*—impossible from an economist's point of view, but quite appealing from a politician's perspective.

A central catechism of the utility dogma is that every human ill must have its value, preferably one that can be expressed with a single number. But many doctors become queasy, as I do, at the prospect of assigning a specific number to each different kind of human misery. (We have drugs for queasiness as well; what value would you assign to it?) My years in practice taught me how enormously variable the experience of illness is from one person to another. I've cared for patients for whom being in a wheelchair was unbearable misery, and others for whom it was a bad nuisance. Should they both be assigned a common number for the disability-related quality of their lives? This variability from patient to patient will often dwarf the differences from condition to condition—differences on which the whole analytic approach rests.

Sometimes despite the best efforts of researchers in this field, the resulting numbers are a hodgepodge of assumptions and projections, cantilevered out from a slender base of real data. Premature extrapolation is the most common numerical dysfunction in this branch of medicine; the problem is hard to talk about openly because its outcome is so unsatisfying and embarrassing for everyone involved. It happens to all of us on occasion. The numbers come quickly if no real-world verification is needed, but the resulting output is too often scientifically sterile, rendering the tool useless.

WARTS AND ALL

It should be clear by now that I have a love-hate relationship with decision analysis as it is used to evaluate medication outcomes. I'm drawn to its potential for bringing a measurable, objective perspective to clinical events that can otherwise seem numbingly ineffable. I sometimes use it in my own research, and as a first-cut estimate it can often provide a useful starting point for some bedside and policy decisions about drugs—even if those decisions end up somewhere else. But as a clinician impressed by the subtleties of human illness as well as the findings of cognitive psychology and behavioral economics, I also worry that orthodox decision analysts sometimes get too big for their quantitative britches in ascribing so much precision to numbers that are so humanly frail in their origins.

The problems with quality-adjusting health states are serious, but many of them are addressable; the field is still young. To begin with, we should expect that every clinical decision analysis that attempts any quality of life adjustment will start out by presenting numbers that are totally *un*adjusted: a year is a year is a year. Grounded in that reality, we'd be able to see how the adjusted result differs, and we could begin to understand exactly which adjustments got us there. These analyses should also present a wide range of quality-adjustment estimates for the most important clinical states being studied, and show how the analysis would change if different values were plugged into the model. If the conclusions are driven all over the map by modest changes in these numbers, the findings may be pretty unreliable.

Taking this to the next step, some have proposed that anyone publishing this kind of research should simultaneously post the program for their decision-analysis model on the internet for all to see. That way, others could tweak it to see what happens if you change the quality-adjustment number used for a given illness. This would also allow readers to get inside the model's black box and see what other assumptions make it tick. But many researchers who develop such models are reluctant to put the fruits of their toil into the public domain.

Making these models both transparent and publicly available could also yield a bonus for patients. If these risk-benefit analyses were made user-friendly, people with a given illness could go to the web and plug in their own estimates of the goodness or badness of specific clinical conditions, to help guide their decision about which course of treatment to pursue. That may sound like science fiction, but an ingenious program started by physicians at Harvard and Dartmouth Medical Schools could lead in this direction. Drs. Al Mulley and Jack Wennberg have put together interactive programs for patients facing therapeutic choices that depend greatly on how a person values different clinical outcomes. Video clips depict patients and doctors explaining the strengths and weaknesses of various treatments and their likely consequences. The patient is then asked to make his or her own judgment about how acceptable each outcome would be. A logical next step would be for a simple program to combine the best available evidence about the likelihood of each outcome's occurrence with *that patient's own values* about the desirability of each, to generate a highly personalized risk-benefit recommendation.

For example, an older man with benign enlargement of the prostate has several plausible choices. He can take a drug to manage the difficulty in urinating that marks this condition. Benefits: no surgery, and the prospect of some symptom relief. Downsides: the drugs often don't work very well, and require a lifetime of pill taking. Or he can opt for surgical removal of his prostate. Benefits: the operation often ends the symptoms. Downsides: surgery hurts, and the procedure sometimes causes impotence or incontinence. Finally, he can engage in "watchful waiting": taking no action now and reassessing later if the symptoms become worse. Benefits: no pills, no surgery, no complications of treatment. Downside: it doesn't make the peeing any easier.

Having walked through this choice with many patients, I can see the value of a computerized adjunct to the medical consultation. It could place the benefit-risk trade-off in accessible terms, enabling a man to calibrate the choices to his preferences. Some men I've cared for have said, "Doc, getting up every hour at night to pass my water is driving me crazy. I'm not worried about the impotence; my wife died years ago. A diaper wouldn't be so bad if I dripped a little. Call the surgeon." Others have said, "I don't want to risk ending my sex life, and the idea of wetting myself disgusts me. Maybe those symptoms aren't so bad. You got a pill I could try?" In such a program, the probabilities of each outcome could be updated regularly as new data emerge or new treatments are introduced.

As this young field matures in the coming years, one of its main agendas will be to understand when the approach can be applied well and when it is likely to be useless or misleading. Rather than embracing decision analysis as the single solution to all clinical questions, we will need to rigorously define when it works poorly as well as when it performs splendidly. Only after doing this hard and sometimes debasing work will we be able to apply the method's strengths where they will help, and avoid relying on it when doing so could cause confusion or harm.

10: WHOSE RISK IS IT, ANYWAY?

You've been appointed to an FDA advisory committee considering whether a drug should be approved for routine use. The product was first discovered through screening large numbers of medicinal plants consumed by indigenous peoples. It has stimulant properties that produce a sense of alertness and well-being at even small doses; its use for these purposes by aboriginal peoples drew the attention of industry, where scientists succeeded in identifying its active ingredient and producing a more potent formulation of the original herbal preparation.

In clinical tests, subjects consistently report that the product relieves stress and curbs the appetite, suggesting a supplementary use as a possible treatment for obesity. However, epidemiological studies of longer-term use uncovered two important side effects. The first was that with continued use the compound becomes highly addictive, making it difficult to stop treatment once it is started. The second was that long-term users were found to have sharply increased susceptibility to developing several kinds of cancer. The product's manufacturer disputes the latter effect, arguing that the data "merely show an association, but do not prove a causal relationship."

Would you recommend approval of this drug? If so, would you allow it to be sold over the counter, as the manufacturer requests?

The second product being evaluated by your hypothetical advisory committee is the male hormone testosterone. It is being proposed for widespread use as a "lifestyle drug" for older men. Data presented to the committee based on twelve-week randomized clinical trials convincingly show that men given testosterone increased their muscle mass, reduced body fat, reported a general increase in energy and quality of life, and had an improvement in sexual functioning. The studies met all the usually applied criteria for the demonstration of efficacy and safety.

As the findings are presented, the investment analysts observing the meeting from the public gallery begin to dash off e-mails through their wireless palm-tops to the home office: "Approval likely; increase company rating to a strong buy." But then they hear the following interchange among panel members:

DR. C.: *Wait a minute. How do we know whether chronic testosterone use might not have long-term side effects? This is a powerful male hormone; it could stimulate prostate cells and cause them to become malignant, or turn on an undetected prostate cancer and trigger its growth.*

DR. L.: *And what about cardiovascular effects? We still don't fully understand why middle-aged men have so much more heart disease than middle-aged women, but testosterone could play a role here. Do we really want to risk increasing the rate of coronary artery disease or stroke in these patients?*

MR. M., THE COMPANY'S VICE PRESIDENT FOR REGULATORY AFFAIRS: *Gentlemen, you raise interesting points. But with all due respect, isn't this just vague speculation? The FDA would never approve a product based only on possible beneficial outcomes; we'd be asked to produce the data. Shouldn't risks have to pass the same evidentiary hurdle? It sounds to me like the hazards you worry about are all in the realm of theory, not clinical facts.*

DR. L.: *Of course we don't have long-term data in humans; we haven't approved the drug yet!*

DR. P.: *I have a different concern. Should we really be approving feel-good drugs like these if there's any risk at all? Tampering with a person's physiology so he can have a better sex life or look trimmer at the beach is not what medicine should be about.*

MR. M.: *Excuse me, Doctor, but is it really for this committee, or the federal government, to decide what risks a person should incur to derive what degree of pleasure? Isn't that a choice that should be between a man and his doctor?*

DR. L.: *Nonsense. We do that all the time. Do you think the nation would ever allow someone to consume a product that can cause cancer just because it makes them feel good temporarily?*

MR. M.: *Well, we let people use tobacco. Is this any different?*

For some pharmacological substances, the benefit-risk calculation is performed by national authorities for the country as a whole instead of by doctors for one patient at a time. Despite years of experience to the contrary, cannabis has often been judged by courts and federal agencies to be unacceptably dangerous, useless, or both; it remains illegal in many parts of the country to use, prescribe, or even possess these benign little leafy products. By contrast, psychoactive chemicals of the alcohol family are considered foods rather than controlled substances or medications. Despite the fact that they account for more drug-induced illness than any substance other than tobacco, those powerful medicines are ubiquitously tolerated, their use encouraged by lavish direct-to-consumer advertising campaigns by large, respected corporations.

In the case of tobacco, the "indigenous medicine" in the vignette above, former FDA commissioner David Kessler famously reminded us that it is little more than a delivery system for the addictive substance nicotine: its benefit-risk profile makes leeches and purgatives look like wonder drugs in comparison. Being in possession of other stimulants, like speed or cocaine, can land you in jail; still others, like Ritalin, are labeled as medicines available by prescription only. And a somewhat less addictive upper that's been assigned to the food category will just cost you just a few dollars at the nearest Starbucks. From the viewpoint of pharmacology, each of these products is a chemical that triggers specific effects and adverse events when ingested. Culture defines some as prescription medicines, some as accepted recreational products, some as illegal banned substances, and some as nourishment. In politics and policy, perceived benefit and risk are shaped by cultural consensus; even the definition of what is or isn't a medication lies in the eye of the societal beholder.

COMMUNICATING ABOUT HAZARDS

The notorious Tuskegee study didn't produce much useful new medical knowledge about syphilis, but it did change the way we think about patients' rights. It reminded us again of the importance of requesting the informed consent of patients in medical research, as well as those undergoing routine medical care. We now expect that people in both settings will be told of the main pros and cons of an offered treatment, to enable them to decide whether to enroll in a clinical trial or to accept a given course of therapy. But when it comes to routine use of medications, informed consent is like British royalty: it is the object of much ceremonial activity and occasional veneration, but often has little impact on actual decision making.

Ideally, a patient's choice about any medical intervention would follow a discussion with the doctor about its hazards and its benefits as well as possible alternative treatments. Spurred and sometimes gored by our colleagues in the legal profession, we usually make sure that such agreement is obtained before performing an invasive procedure such as surgery. The formality of this form-signing is often a patient's best opportunity for dialogue with the physician about what might go wrong. But even for operations, the ritual is sometimes conducted almost automatically, with many surgeons commanding an intern or nurse to "go and consent the patient." (This idiom, another annoying instance of the verbing of nouns, says a lot about the extent of the dialogue that may occur, and who is doing what to whom.) Researchers have interviewed patients immediately after they provided informed consent for invasive procedures, to gauge their understanding of the risks and benefits they just acknowledged. The findings of such studies have been profoundly depressing.

Of course we have to do this before major surgery; it would be ethically and legally unthinkable to omit the process, however often it falls short of its intent. But what about informed consent for prescriptions? Not in the clinical trial context, which is a very different matter, but in routine practice? In general we don't bother, and it is instructive to ask why. Many of the drugs we internists use are at least as risky as some of the minor procedures our more invasive colleagues perform, so it can't be just a matter of danger. It's more about tradition: if the skin is pierced or a bodily orifice entered, you get consent, and if it isn't, you generally don't. In reality, it would be difficult to "consent" a patient adequately before prescribing most of the medications we commonly use. As we have seen, the available data for a given drug often tell us merely that it's better than nothing. Head-to-head comparisons of different drugs for the same condition are appallingly rare. As for side effects, there may be dozens of them, with widely varying severity and frequency.

The most commonly consulted source for risk information is the ponderous *Physicians' Desk Reference,* where its depiction may be both overwhelming and useless. The *PDR* uses an odd format for describing side effects. Its 3,500 pages of tightly packed small type comprise the FDA-sanctioned listings that each manufacturer provides for its drugs; most descriptions are thousands of words long. Confusingly, risks can appear under one or more of several headings: Warnings, Contraindications, Precautions, and Adverse Reactions. Nausea might be listed as having a 4.7 percent frequency in patients who took the drug in controlled trials, and lightheadedness 5.6 percent. But patients given the placebo in those trials may have had a rate of 4.8 percent for nausea and 5.5 percent for lightheadedness, making any association with the drug unlikely. Even when the rates are expressed in comparison with those seen for placebo, there is virtually never information about the frequency with which the same symptom is caused by other drugs that might be possible alternatives.

Some companies will list an enormous number of problems that have occurred in users of a given drug, whether or not there is good evidence that the drug caused them. The rationale here seems to be CYA, which does not stand for "Concidental, Yet Attributable." A pharmaceutical company liability lawyer once explained the strategy to me: "If an adverse event is mentioned in the official labeling and then it occurs in a particular patient, the company's in the clear because it can say, '*See? We told you that could happen!*'" As a result, the physician or patient who looks up a drug in the *PDR* is often overdosed with an unusably long catalog of maladies, many of which have an extremely low signal-to-noise ratio. I asked the lawyer whether that approach might dissuade doctors from prescribing a drug with so many listed problems. "That's not a real issue," he answered. "Everyone knows no one actually reads that stuff carefully. It's mostly useful in court." Some companies provide more usable risk information in these listings, dividing side effects into those that occur in 10 percent or more of patients, 5 percent or more, 1 percent or more, and fewer than 1 percent. This helpful practice is not required, nor is it common.

THE BARRIER OF LANGUAGE

Such formal "labeling" has been the fig leaf that both the FDA and the pharmaceutical industry have sometimes relied on to cover the sin of improper use. As we saw earlier, both sides have contended that if these official listings depict risks accurately, they ought to be off the hook if untoward reactions occur. This explains the fervor that accompanied negotiations over the depiction of side effects for the Redux diet pills and the diabetes drug Rezulin. The label is printed as a package insert that accompanies the product when it is shipped to drugstores; it is then usually thrown away by the pharmacist, who rarely passes it along to the customer. The information is also contained in tiny type in ads directed at doctors or consumers, and we all know how often that is combed through carefully. It also appears in the *PDR*. For decades, lawyers and regulators have drawn comfort from the mere existence of these words on paper, even as they knew they were rarely read. It was a little like the warm feeling some people derive from the inscriptions inside a St. Christopher's medal worn around the neck, or a mezuzah on the doorpost of a house. Just knowing the words are there confers a mystical sense of protection for believers.

Reliance on the package insert talisman as the governing document of risk-benefit responsibility left the FDA and the pharmaceutical industry with an argument that could have come straight from the National Rifle Association: "Drugs don't kill people; people kill people." The culpable people, of course, were we doctors and occasionally our patients. According to this view, the manufacturers and the agency that regulated them were no more to blame for drug disasters like Rezulin and fenfluramine than the box-cutter industry was for the attacks on the World Trade Center and the Pentagon. But does the responsibility of industry and government for how a drug is used really end once the ink is dry on the package insert?

By century's end, juries and courts became less tolerant of this defense. Was Wyeth free of culpability because it ignored the fact that its products were used by millions of women who were not medically obese, and because it then followed up signals of dangerous adverse events with ham-handed indifference? Judges and juries didn't think so. The Rezulin case was another turning point. The company argued that if doctors had measured liver function tests monthly they could have spotted drug-induced liver damage in time to reverse it. Did that shift all responsibility for problems from the company to the doctor? We can leave aside the evidence that the company knew this may not have been enough to protect patients. Even if it was, everyone knew that doctors weren't likely to follow these demanding blood test recommendations. After Rezulin, it became harder for a manufacturer and the FDA to claim that as long as the labeling was adequate, it must be the doctors and patients who were the problem.

Although the FDA must approve the content of all these dense labeling descriptions, its standards for intelligibility are so minimal that even an informed user can easily succumb to semantic vertigo. A few years ago the agency announced it would begin requiring manufacturers to produce more accessible and coherent descriptions of risks, benefits, dosing, and precautions. The idea was well received by physicians and the public but wasn't popular with some manufacturers; the initiative has not gotten far.

All this makes a challenging situation even more difficult for doctors and patients. Let's say I want to treat someone's heart condition with a drug that can sometimes cause impairment in kidney function, potentially dangerous elevations of potassium levels, liver failure, a loss of the capacity to make white blood cells, and an allergic reaction that can lead to obstruction of the airways, suffocation, and death. The description applies to the ACE-inhibitor class of drugs. Used by tens of millions of patients, they are a well-tested, valuable, and quite safe group of medications that prolong life for patients with several kinds of heart disease. They are also very useful and reliable in the management of blood pressure—all in all, a mainstay of modern pharmacology. Dozens of excellent drugs used to treat hypertension and heart disease—nearly all of them, in fact—have a pedigree of *potential* disaster that can sound this scary or worse. Do I have an ethical obligation to describe each of these side effects to the patient, and in what level of detail? What about my legal responsibility? Forcing patients to sit through such a litany of possible catastrophes might even cause harm in its own right if it discouraged them from taking the medications they need, thus worsening rather than protecting their health.

In my own practice, whenever I tried to review such a list of possible horrors with a patient before starting a new treatment, the response was always the same: "Whatever you say, Dr. Avorn. I trust your judgment." This wasn't because I had infallible therapeutic acumen, nor because my patients were unusually passive or gullible. It's just that this is the most common patient response when these rare conversations do occur. *Of course* drugs can cause terrible side effects. Our patients expect that we will know all about this and avoid exposing them to unnecessary dangers as we care for them. With that faith, they will daily ingest several complex chemicals as we command in order to rearrange their most basic cellular functions. This trust is humbling and a little terrifying. In its extreme form, it explains why one of my patients with abject seriousness used to call me Dr. God, and why another would sometimes ask to kiss my hands at the end of a visit. They (and the other, less demonstrative ones) believed that I possessed all the information needed to make these decisions unerringly. If only I did.

A provocative Canadian book, *Mad Cows and Mother's Milk: The Perils of Poor Risk Communication,* offers some revealing lessons about how we talk to each other about health risks. Its case studies are not about medications, but they demonstrate how inept presentation of any risk information can produce inappropriate reactions to those risks. The authors point out that those of us who derive and analyze data about hazards see the world quite differently from the people who consume that information. We work with numbers that are probabilistic, and often think of risks in terms of populations; but our audience is more likely to make decisions that are intuitive, and to think in *yes/no* terms about their own personal situations. We wonder whether the inevitable risks of an intervention are low enough to be acceptable in comparison with the equally inevitable risks of a competing alternative. By contrast, our patients want to know whether a particular drug "is safe" or isn't. Finally, we are often cavalier in our manipulations of quality-adjusted life-years, discount rates, and time trade-off methodologies, thinking of them as the mathematical distillation of everything that matters about benefits and side effects. But whatever the numbers say, individual patients usually have their own ideas about how bad it would be to die of breast cancer versus a heart attack (in the case of estrogen replacement therapy), or how disruptive a blood clot in the legs would be compared to an unwanted pregnancy (in the case of birth control pills).

Successful risk communication requires more than just getting the numbers right. It isn't only that the subtlety and details of academic analyses may be beyond the grasp of many people. It's that when it comes to their own values and preferences our patients are the experts, not us. In balancing the hazards and benefits of a given prescription, we must learn about their perspectives as much as they need to hear about ours. We can't expect patients to get training in risk communication before they get sick and need a prescription. But we doctors can and should be expected to know about it before we start writing them.

BRIDGING THE COMMUNICATION CHASM

Helping someone to really *get* ideas like risk or probability of benefit can be a little like trying to explain traffic lights to a color-blind person. I include myself here, since even after years of thinking hard about such issues, I still don't intuit them well. I've merely developed a passable prosthetic sense of such things. The majority of doctors and patients resemble the color-blind driver in that we may not see the redness of a red light or the greenness of a green one; we've just learned that you stop when the one on top is lit, and go when the bottom one is on. This works fairly well at most intersections, but can be dangerously confusing if the light is a single flashing one, or just an arrow. Imagine that variations in the light's size, hue, and intensity also mean different things, and we've begun to approximate the challenge in communicating a complete sense of a drug's risk or benefit to doctors and patients. Just what *does* it mean for a drug to increase the risk of a particular kind of cancer by 35 percent, or to prevent one in three heart attacks? (And what if there were one drug that did both?)

Those are precisely the kinds of numbers that emerge from the computer in epidemiologic analyses as an odds ratio or a relative risk. But those numbers require interpretation. If the cancer whose likelihood is increased is very, very rare, then a 35 percent or even a 200 percent increase in its occurrence may be of almost trivial importance. For example, a 75 percent increase in a one-in-a-million risk becomes about a 1-in-571,000 chance—still pretty tiny. On the other hand, a drug that produces just a 20 percent reduction in the risk of a common event (say, a heart attack in a man with elevated cholesterol) can be a real boon.

Such confusion took on national prominence when the results of the estrogen replacement trials were published. As we know, the drugs increased the risk of breast cancer, blood clots, stroke, and heart disease, but also reduced the risk of colon cancer and of hip fracture, and blocked the uncomfortable symptoms of menopause. How could these competing risks and benefits somehow be put together? It was often done poorly. For some women, stopping the hormones may cause an immediate return of hot flashes, insomnia, and vaginal dryness. Some HRT advocates argued that the increase in risk of breast cancer was only one in several thousand patients, and somehow as a result not worth the discomfort of menopausal symptoms.

Here is where decision analysis can help both doctor and patient in clarifying the consequences of this choice by putting some tangible numbers onto it. Breast cancer is one of the commonest cancers (one in eight of all women will have it in her lifetime), so any increase in that risk will be applied to a fairly high baseline rate. In a population of ten thousand women who take an estrogen like Prempro for five years, forty extra women will develop breast cancer. The clinical trial data also tell us that in the same time period there will also be thirty-five extra women who have heart attacks, forty extra women who have strokes, sixty-five extra women who develop blood clots in their legs, and forty extra women whose clots migrate into their lungs, a potentially fatal condition. Adding all this up, we can calculate that two out of every hundred women who take HRT for five years will have one of these very serious complications caused by their prescription. For most doctors and patients, putting the risks in these terms makes the right choice clear. But even when these numbers are spelled out this way, some women have told me that they still prefer to continue taking their estrogens indefinitely. "I don't care about statistics," one patient told me. "I don't like the way I feel when I'm off HRT. It's my body, and I don't care about theoretical risks, or probabilities of things that may or may not happen years from now. I want to go back on estrogen." Is it a patient's right to do so? And what rights and responsibilities does her doctor have in this regard?

STRAIGHT TALK

The trade-off between gender-based symptoms and the risk of death is not limited to women.

Edgar Schwanz is a fifty-six-year-old pipe fitter who has had insulin-dependent diabetes since his twenties. It has left him with heart disease (first heart attack at age fifty-one, second at age fifty-four), mild kidney impairment, and retinal disease that has reduced his vision to 20/200. His diabetes also led to angina that causes chest pain when he exerts himself too much, for which he takes another daily medicine as well as

rapid-acting tablets for use during these attacks. On a routine visit, he
asks his doctor to write him a prescription for a new medication he has
seen advertised on television.

   His doctor explains that the drug is not medically necessary and with
Edgar's medical condition, it could precipitate a new heart attack or
even death. Edgar explains that he has done his own research about the
drug on the internet, and agrees completely with the doctor's assess-
ment. But he still demands the prescription. The doctor refuses, and a
heated argument ensues.

Patients may differ with their doctors about whether a particular drug is
worth its risks even when there is no disagreement about probabilities or
outcomes. Such clashes of personal values are often overlooked in discussions of drug effects. This case study isn't a hypothetical thought experiment concocted to advance our examination of benefit-risk trade-offs; it's a
real clinical conundrum doctors face every day. Once again, the drug is Viagra. During its first years of use, case reports described cardiac patients
who had heart attacks or episodes of dangerously low blood pressure while
using the drug; some of these events were fatal. The men were often elderly
and had other medical conditions like diabetes and vascular disease, which
may have caused their erectile difficulties in the first place. Many of them
had not had sexual relations in years, and were in poor physical shape. The
manufacturer argued that Viagra made it possible for them to have an experience that had been beyond their grasp (or perhaps only within their grasp)
for years; some of them simply exerted themselves to death. Viagra didn't
cause the deaths, Pfizer argued; sexual intercourse caused the deaths. Viagra may have led to the sexual intercourse, but did that make these events
drug side effects?

   Counterintuitively, Viagra works by making certain muscles go soft—in
this case, the muscles in the arteries that allow blood to flow into the network of blood vessels in the penis. Engorged with blood, the penis stiffens.
A different class of drugs also works by making the blood vessel muscles go
limp: nitroglycerine (not the explosive variety, but a medical formulation of
the same compound). Nitroglycerine is a mainstay of treatment for angina,
the chest pain that occurs on exertion if too little blood is reaching the
heart. But if a patient takes nitroglycerine along with Viagra, blood vessels
all over the body can relax excessively, causing a potentially lethal drop in
blood pressure. The penis may remain proudly erect, but the entire patient
becomes flaccid.

   Mr. Schwanz did not disagree with his doctor about the possibility of
such a pharmacologic *Liebestod;* he understood the basic concept, he knew

that he had to keep taking his nitro to manage his heart disease, and he agreed that Viagra would therefore increase his risk of a drop in blood pressure, heart attack, and death. But he wanted the drug anyway.

> *Look, Doc,* I imagine him saying, *I know it can react with my nitro and raise the odds that I might drop dead in the middle of—everything. But this diabetes has taken away so much of my life already. Sex was one of the only things I really could still enjoy, and now I'm losing that too. I know what the Viagra could do for me, I know how it could hurt me, and I've made my choice. You're my doctor, and I need you to write that prescription.*

There's no easy answer here. Patients with erectile dysfunction often have to take medications for heart disease as well—the two conditions often coexist. The official labeling for Viagra explicitly states that it should not be used in patients who are taking nitrates of any kind. ("Your Honor, please remind the defendant that I did not ask him what the decedent did or did not ask for; I simply asked him to read to the jury the section clearly labeled 'Contraindications' on page 2423 of the *Physicians' Desk Reference.*") But who has the right to make such benefit-risk trade-offs when the data are not at issue? Who's the better doctor: the one who allows a patient the autonomy to make his own choices about benefits and risks, or the one who refuses to be pressured into a prescribing decision that could lead to a fatal outcome? The resolution plays itself out in myriad ways. Some pharmacy computer systems will not allow a druggist to dispense Viagra to a patient who also has a prescription for nitroglycerine. A drug benefit program in one state will cover Viagra in such patients only if the prescribing physician affirms that he or she is aware of the risk and approves use of the drug. This raises a moral as well as a clinical dilemma.

I was drawn into this controversy when the same large health care system that allowed doctors to override the Viagra-plus-nitrate prohibition was considering ending its coverage for lifelong HRT use, in order to protect women from the long-term effects of estrogen. "So older men get to enhance their sexual function even if it could kill them," I asked, "but you're not going to let older women use their hormone pills to deal with their symptoms?" On the distaff side of the gender boundary, strikingly similar questions come up over long-term estrogen use. In one corner we have Dr. S., who says, "I refuse to collude in the use of a drug hyped to enhance a sexist stereotype of perpetual girlishness, especially since it also causes an unacceptable rate of terrible complications." In the opposite corner is Dr. T., who retorts, "I respect my patients' autonomy, particularly a

woman's right to choose what chemicals she wants to put into her body."
Who's the better feminist?

At its best, prescribing is about balance and negotiation. This is what
traditionally made the practice of medicine such an intricate and demanding task, and such a quintessentially human one. Yet for better or worse,
weakening of the professional role of the physician and the regulatory
authority of government has moved some of these issues into the realm of
personal license. Viagra is now readily available on the internet, with no real
physician risk-benefit adjudication required. Similar developments resolved
the two hypothetical policy dilemmas with which we began this chapter.
The tobacco industry successfully rebuffed the FDA's attempts to gain control over its drug-based products, so the "indigenous herbal stimulant" that
is both addictive and carcinogenic remains readily available in corner stores
throughout the nation. Testosterone was allowed onto the market years ago
as a prescription-only drug for the treatment of a rare endocrine condition,
hypogonadism. It was never approved to enhance sexuality or improve
vigor in men without this disease, but doctors are free to prescribe it to anyone. Its use is rising sharply for so-called lifestyle indications despite concerns about the risk of cancer, heart disease, and blood clots such use might
bring about. The drug's virtues are now touted in "educational" materials
that might as well be titled *Masculine Forever*. It is as if Congress had
passed a law guaranteeing men the same right to hormonal self-harm that
women have had for so long—a kind of glandular affirmative action. The
struggle to juggle risks and benefits continues, providing us with endless
opportunities to relearn old lessons.

11: A BALANCING ACT

Binary processing of information made the digital age possible. By expressing everything in terms of zeros and ones, total *NO*s or absolute *YES*es, electronic circuits have given us PCs, e-mail, ATMs, digital cameras, and satellite TV. But binary logic is not a good way to think about medications. Nonetheless patients, doctors, and especially the FDA often structure questions about the benefits and risks of drugs in terms of YES/NO answers to two questions. For the first question, "Does it work?" an answer of NO simply ends further consideration of a given product, as it should (unless the compound portrays itself as a dietary supplement and slithers into the marketplace beneath the regulatory radar). A YES answer allows the product to be prescribed; but that should just be the start, not the end, of its assessment. The second question, "Is it safe?" usually cannot be answered in a YES/NO manner, but only in shades of gray; those shadings will make sense only in terms of the darkness or lightness of the efficacy answer.

Hazard is an inherent part of any effective medical intervention; the goal is not to deny risk or try to eliminate it, but to embrace its reality, understand it, respect it, and control it. Freed from the impossible belief that all drugs must be totally safe, we can be open to dealing with their inevitable dangers. Managing those dangers is becoming a central agenda for practitioners, manufacturers, and regulators, and we are beginning to learn how this can be accomplished. The FDA is starting to think more in terms of risk management, and physicians, who for generations did it intuitively, are developing more precise tools to bring this approach to the bedside.

DIFFERENT PATIENTS, DIFFERENT BALANCES

At the Brigham, we confronted a striking example of this balance with the arrival of a new drug known as Activated Protein C (APC). It was developed for patients with an often-fatal condition known as septic shock, a catastrophic complication that sometimes develops on the heels of a serious bacterial invasion. Once a severe infection takes hold, the body's inflammatory responses may kick in with a vengeance, precipitating a cascade of reactions that go on to become a full-blown and potentially lethal syndrome in itself. These defensive molecules begin to take their own toll on the liver, kidneys, and other organs; in their manic zeal to destroy the enemy they wreak havoc on the body like billions of chemical Robespierres, producing a new disaster that can be more life-threatening than the original problem.

For centuries, septic shock defied all attempts to block its death spiral. Antibiotics would be prescribed, but once the inflammatory reign of terror kicked in, defeating the underlying infection didn't help much. New kinds of drugs were invented to block the inflammatory process itself, but didn't work in clinical trials. Giving anticoagulants earlier in the disease process seemed physiologically clever, but didn't pan out. The mortality rate from septic shock remained stubbornly high. That is why so much excitement greeted the announcement in early 2001 that a medication with a totally new approach to the problem had been found to reduce the death rate in these patients—the first time any treatment had been able to do this. It didn't combat the infection; it didn't reduce the inflammatory reaction; it wasn't a conventional anticoagulant. Rather, it blocked a specific point in the coagulation cascade—that self-reinforcing chain of biochemical reactions that causes blood to clot. Its manufacturer, Lilly, gave the new product the inelegant generic name of "drotrecogin alfa activated." It's much easier (as intended) just to use the trade name, Xigris (pronounced *Zye*-gris, which rhymes with the river in Iraq). Unwilling to be semantically bullied into using brand names, my colleagues and I chose instead to call it by its chemical nickname, Activated Protein C, or just APC.

Like many major clinical trials, the one that tested APC had a cute acronym: PROWESS, for PROtein C Worldwide Evaluation in Severe Sepsis. Before the advent of APC, 30–40 percent of patients who developed septic shock died. The same pattern was seen in the study patients randomized to the placebo group: 69 percent lived and 31 percent died. But among the patients randomized to receive the drug, 75 percent lived and 25 percent died. Unlike the situation with our mythical drug Lifehorn, the difference here was statistically significant, and the FDA approved the product for use. But in the trial, some of the treated patients developed serious bleeding, sometimes in the brain. That wasn't surprising for a drug that interferes with the clotting mechanism, and seemed like a downside worth accepting in exchange for the increased survival rate the new product made possible.

The study results were scheduled to appear in the *New England Journal of Medicine* in March 2000, but the editors took the unusual step of releasing the report a month earlier on the internet. This is done only rarely, primarily when a study's results could have such important implications for practice that any publication delay would be unacceptable. But this drug hadn't yet been approved by the FDA, and so wouldn't be available for routine use until many months later, making the scientific rationale for such a splashy early release unclear. Activated Protein C immediately became a compelling case study in the need to balance substantial benefit with significant risk. (At a projected price of $6,000 to $8,000 per patient it also brought the cost dimension vividly into play, but we won't tackle that piece of the puzzle until Part Three.)

It will help here to reflect again on how drugs differ from cars. The weight of my old Volvo is an inherent part of its nature. It also has a color that defines it, and an engine with a fixed number of pistons, valves, displacement, and so forth. These properties of my Volvo are immanent— they "live within" the car and relate directly to its performance. Activated Protein C also has some inherent properties, such as its molecular structure. But what really determines how APC *performs* is how it interacts with particular kinds of patients. In this respect its properties do not lie exclusively within the molecule, but rather in the interplay between that molecule and a given sick person.

This is a little like the number of miles per gallon my Volvo gets. Any car will rack up more MPG on the highway than in city traffic. It's the same car using the same fuel, but it behaves differently in different contexts. Such context-dependent definitions of performance are modestly important when it comes to cars. But in pharmacology, it can be the name of the game. Because a medication's benefit-risk relationship is not a one-size-fits-all property, different patients will experience different manifestations of that balance depending on their clinical situation.

Initially, it seemed from the PROWESS study that APC would offer its own kind of Faustian bargain: you can reduce the patient's risk of dying from a frequently fatal condition, but the price you pay is a small increase in the risk of devastating hemorrhage. Faced with a moribund patient, it didn't seem as if there could really be any other choice.

As it turned out, there was. My division at the Brigham and Women's Hospital is responsible for assessing new medications before they reach the market, to help guide the way our institution will use them once they become available; some other examples of this work will appear in Part Four. Dr. Michael Fischer headed up the APC evaluation for our group, beginning with a close reading of the only readily available material about the drug, the paper describing the PROWESS trial. That was just the start. He then went onto the internet and searched the FDA website, where anyone can access transcripts of the advisory committee deliberations about each new product. He uncovered an important "story behind the story" about APC that FDA staff had noted, but that was not reported in the original paper. True, the death rate was lower in PROWESS among patients randomized to APC rather than placebo. But an additional insight became clear only after someone at the FDA slogged through page after page of the raw data submitted by the company. The original journal article reported that the drug behaved the same in all subgroups studied, but that turned out not to be true. The reduction in mortality was seen in only half the patients—the ones who were the sickest. The other half, although they all had septic shock, were just as likely to die whether they got APC or placebo. Yet the rate of devastating hemorrhage caused by the drug was the same for all patients who were given it. As a result, the sickest subjects had a significant reduction in their risk of death in exchange for a small increase in the risk of hemorrhage, a trade-off we'd all be willing to make. But the less sick patients just incurred the bleeding risk with no mortality benefit, a trade-off none of us would accept. Same drug, same dose, same diagnosis—but stratifying patients by the severity of their illness determined whether the risk-benefit relationship came out favorably or not.

Working with colleagues from other departments at the Brigham, the team Dr. Fischer led developed guidelines for APC use to help doctors determine whether a given patient was likely to be in this benefits-exceed-risks group. We used the hospital's computer system to guide this decision in a real-time manner, as described later. In the future, as thinking about drug safety moves beyond excessively simple categories of effective/ineffective and safe/not safe, we will be seeing many more analyses of drug effects stratified by the clinical situation (or the genetic makeup) of a particular individual.

RISK MANAGEMENT

If *risk stratification* is how we identify which people are most likely to come out ahead when they take a given drug, *risk management* is the implementation of strategies to minimize problems once the drug is being used. It is an approach that the FDA has only recently begun to embrace enthusiastically. Prior to 2000, the agency still lived in a mostly binary world of drug approval. Before a drug was registered for general use, no one could prescribe it, except in very constrained circumstances such as an approved clinical trial; that's as it should be. But once the drug was judged effective and safe enough to approve, any doctor in the country could use it however he or she saw fit, in any dose, for any reason, in any patient. If new problems were detected once the product was in use, the FDA might ask the manufacturer to send out a mass mailing to tell doctors about it; after that, the agency would usually wince and bear it, up to a point. If the problem finally got bad enough to flip a product into the intolerable side of the *yes/no* universe, it would be taken off the market.

The need for a more subtle approach was brought into sharp focus for both industry and the FDA with a drug called Lotronex (alosetron), introduced in 2000 as a treatment for irritable bowel syndrome.

Sally Trotter planned her life around bathrooms. Since she was a young woman she had been plagued by irritable bowel syndrome, or IBS. The condition caused bouts of abdominal pain and diarrhea that struck without warning, sometimes three or four times a day. Now forty-two, for years she had had to avoid long car trips, hikes, or any other activity that put her more than a few minutes away from the nearest toilet.

A succession of doctors had written her off as neurotic. IBS produces no telltale lesions on X-ray or endoscopy, and there is no blood or stool test or any other objective measurement of its existence. But talk to a patient who has it, and the medical history is as compelling as that of anyone with severe asthma or bad angina.

Sally eventually found a gastroenterologist "who believed that I really had an illness." Together, they tried a succession of diets, relaxation exercises, prescriptions, and over-the-counter medications, even acupuncture. Nothing really worked, and Sally thought she'd have to live with daily cramping and paroxysms of loose stools for the rest of her life.

In 1999, her doctor told her a new drug was coming to market that might make a difference, called Lotronex. He enrolled her in a clinical trial, and both were pleased to note that her daily pain and diarrhea subsided, and then ended altogether. He wrote her a prescription for Lotronex as soon as it was approved by the FDA, and for the first time in years Sally was able to plan her days without regard to plumbing.

Evan Mellet was cursed with a different kind of colon. Now in his late thirties, he had suffered from irritable bowel syndrome since he was about eighteen; like Sally he had daily bouts of abdominal cramping. But Evan's IBS was marked more by severe constipation than by diarrhea— though on occasion he had both. He described this as "a geyser breaking through cement"—a metaphor that he, but no one else, liked very much. When Lotronex became available his doctor prescribed it to Evan as well. The studies had shown that Lotronex worked well in female IBS patients with diarrhea. But since nothing else had ever worked for Evan, the new drug seemed like an option worth trying.

After six weeks on Lotronex Evan's chronic abdominal cramping became much worse, and his rare stools stopped altogether. When the pain became unbearable his doctor admitted him to the hospital and per-formed an emergency colonoscopy. It revealed that a section of his large intestine seemed to be starved of its blood supply. When Evan's pain worsened further and he began to have some rectal bleeding, a surgeon reviewed the video of the endoscopy and decided that an operation was urgently needed. He removed a segment of nearly dead gut in a long operation that was followed by a succession of postoperative complica-tions.

Four weeks later, Evan was discharged home. His abdominal pain continued as before, but his doctor refused to prescribe any more Lotronex, which he considered the cause of his hospitalization.

Once Lotronex came into widespread use, other cases like Mr. Mellet's began to appear, then more. Deaths occurred in some IBS patients following similar episodes of colon ischemia. As annoying and sometimes debilitating as IBS was, it had never required surgery, and it was never fatal. Should a drug that could kill a patient ever be used to treat a disease that never did? By 2000, the FDA realized it needed more debate on the risk-benefit issues surrounding Lotronex. After years of underfunding, understaffing, and low morale, its own pharmacoepidemiology group needed some outside rein-forcement. I got a call from the agency asking me to attend the next meeting of its Advisory Committee on Gastrointestinal Drugs. I was eager to see at close hand how the FDA approached a problem like this.

Over the next few weeks I was reintroduced to the inner world of the FDA, a world I hadn't visited since the completion of a grant I had received from the agency back in the 1980s. Its staffers sent me several pounds of manuals, guidelines, ethical standards, and forms to sign in order to enlist as a Special Government Employee, the status required for me to partici-pate in the one-day meeting. I learned about the FDA's lenient policy on conflicts of interest that could occur when its outside advisers have financial ties to a company whose product they are reviewing. In sum: such ties are perfectly permissible, as long as they are described in a statement. (I had nothing to declare.)

The agency would reimburse me for my hotel stay near Washington the night before the meeting, but government regulations prevented them from mailing me a check; the agency had a policy requiring direct bank deposit of all reimbursements. The Fidelity account I used didn't qualify, so I had to set up a new bank account. To prepay my airfare, I was sent a computer punch card, the kind used for data processing back in the 1960s. When I presented it at the airport ticket counter, the first five people I showed it to had never come across one before and didn't know what to do with it. "I've only seen those in books!" one exclaimed.

Like most FDA hearings, the Lotronex meeting was held in a motel near the agency's headquarters in Rockville, Maryland. A series of tables formed a large rectangle in the center of the room where I and the other Special Government Employees sat. The rest of the room was filled with representatives of the drug's manufacturer (Glaxo-Wellcome), investment industry representatives, and a few journalists. There were also some irate patients who had flown in to represent the consumer's perspective and to oppose the possible withdrawal of the drug.

The meeting came down to the old Sodom and Gomorrah question we've seen previously: How many cases of severe, even life-threatening events would it take to make this drug too dangerous to keep on the market for anyone to use? How are these events to be weighed against the good the drug could do for patients with never-dangerous but often-annoying IBS? The patient testimonies were compelling. Some reported that before Lotronex, they had been unable to leave their homes because of frequent diarrhea. Now they had their lives back; they didn't want to see the one drug that worked for them taken off the market. We learned from the FDA and the manufacturer that there was only sparse information on the frequency of the adverse effects caused by the drug. Both groups had records of the spontaneous reports sent in by concerned doctors, but everyone knew that for every report sent in, there are somewhere between ten and a hundred events that never get reported. It was not clear what to make of some of the sketchy reports of extreme abdominal pain that had not been adequately diagnosed; after all, this was a drug used to treat abdominal pain.

We were operating in an information-poor environment. I pointed out that someone had to gather more facts much more systematically before it would be clear what to do. All we had were anecdotes on both sides of the question, and as a wise colleague once observed, the plural of "anecdote" is not "data." Others felt the same way, and that ended up as the group's recommendation. After the meeting broke, I asked my FDA contacts about the next steps and whether I should initiate any research back in Boston to help work up the problem, perhaps using our databases of drug use and medical outcomes in two million people. They said no, but thanks for coming.

The ensuing months were not kind to Lotronex. Reports continued to trickle in describing IBS patients taking the drug who developed constipation so severe they had to be hospitalized. There were additional reports of colon ischemia; in some patients it resolved when the drug was stopped, but others had to have surgery to remove damaged sections of intestine. A few more deaths occurred that were attributed to the drug. The FDA decided that the risk-benefit relationship was becoming indefensible and had the drug withdrawn from the market.

The story did not end there. IBS patients across the nation became irritable; angry letters were sent to Washington. Many of these were from individual patients who felt their medical care had been hamstrung by a meddlesome government. Critics would later contend that some of the loudest protest came from patient self-help groups funded by pharmaceutical manufacturers; the patient groups denied that this was their motivation. The company argued that the agency had overreacted, and contended that the small number of tragic events were not proven to be caused by their product. Glaxo further charged that the FDA's decision was itself generating considerable harm by denying needed therapy to patients who had no other recourse. In a nearly unprecedented move, the FDA agreed to consider allowing Lotronex to reenter the marketplace, but only if a careful risk management program could be designed and implemented.

This was a sea change in thinking and policy for the agency. It marked a leap beyond the binary thinking that had heretofore classified nearly every drug as either too unsafe to use, or safe enough for unfettered use. The newer FDA position was quite plausible from the perspective of anyone who had ever taken care of a patient, yet from a regulatory standpoint it was novel. Restriction of use had been previously employed as a risk management strategy only for a very small number of other drugs. Two of them had similarly been removed from use and then allowed back on the condition that their use be tightly controlled. One was clozapine, the bone-marrow-destroying antipsychotic drug we met in an earlier chapter; it often worked in schizophrenics when nothing else did, but could sometimes demolish a patient's ability to make white blood cells. Clozapine had returned to use under special circumstances: the patient had to have a blood count each week before a pharmacist could dispense the next week's dose. Unlike Rezulin's liver toxicity, clozapine-induced bone marrow damage could be detected before the problem was irreversible, making this an effective if cumbersome risk management strategy.

Another back-from-the-dead drug was thalidomide—the very product whose use in pregnancy during the early 1960s helped bring on the modern era of drug regulation. To the surprise of nearly everyone, three decades later thalidomide turned out to be useful in treating AIDS and leprosy, among other conditions. Strict provisions were established to make sure that once it was reintroduced, it never passed the lips of any woman who was or might become pregnant.

A third drug on the FDA's very short risk management list had also caused terrible problems when taken by pregnant women. It was Accutane (isotretinoin), the first really effective treatment for severe acne—not just stubborn zits, but scarring, disfiguring pustules that can mutilate a face. Accutane transformed the lives of thousands of miserable adolescents, but it soon became clear that its success could lead to tragedy. Many of the girls so treated went on to become pregnant, but then miscarried or gave birth to badly deformed babies. Unlike the case of Bendectin, the fetal anomalies were proven to have been caused by Accutane. How could the FDA, which had won its modern regulatory clout in the wake of the thalidomide tragedy, possibly leave Accutane on the market?

But no other product worked nearly as well as Accutane in treating disfiguring acne, and nontreatment was not an appealing alternative. Faced with loss of a uniquely effective product, its manufacturer, Roche, created a comprehensive education-and-packaging plan that warned in English and Spanish against use in women who might become pregnant, with vivid graphics for those who couldn't read either language. The program was well designed, but some women taking Accutane still became pregnant, a source of continuing concern. How many Accutane pregnancies are too many? The exact answer depends on how many person-years of facial disfigurement one would be willing to trade for what number of miscarriages, abortions, and fetal deformities. There may be someone who would try to come up with an equation to define this relationship, but I'd rather not meet him.

The Lotronex problem emerged against this background of a few isolated risk management programs that had been developed for a tiny number of hazardous but worthy drugs. But the background also featured debacles like Rezulin, which badly undercut the credo of "Don't blame us; we got the labeling right." As a condition of reapproval, the FDA told Glaxo it had to develop a plan that would (a) ensure that physicians understood how to use the drug; (b) guarantee that patients were aware of its risks and accepted them; (c) track how well the drug was being prescribed; and (d) identify adverse events proactively, comprehensively, and promptly. I was asked to help in the development of the program, and welcomed the chance—not because irritable bowel syndrome is a fascinating medical problem, or because Lotronex is a remarkable drug. Rather, it presented a good opportunity to help the FDA and the industry take one more small step beyond the simplistic binary view of drug approval and use. If we could make this idea work for Lotronex, its risk management program could become a useful model for many more drugs in the coming years. This effort is still in progress, and will require new kinds of nonadversarial thinking on the part of both the manufacturer and the agency if it is to succeed. It reminds me of the biblical phrase about the lion lying down with the lamb, and then of Woody Allen's famous coda: "—but the lamb won't get much sleep." I'm still trying to figure out who's the lamb.

RE-AIMING OVER TIME

Just as a drug's benefit-risk balance isn't a fixed number living inside the pill, it's also not static over time. No good doctor starts a medication and continues it mindlessly forever, sealing the patient's destiny the moment the first prescription is written. Because drug hazards aren't determined by some kind of immutable pharmacological Calvinism, ongoing decisions the doctor and patient make together can offer many chances for redemption; and risks can be contained throughout the life of a prescription. The technical term for this kind of varying relationship is "stochastic," from the Greek *stochos,* meaning "target," "aim," and also "guess." Over days, months, and years of constantly reassessing how the patient-drug relationship is going, this aiming can be fine-tuned again and again, turning up the volume on the benefits, tuning down the risks. But this presupposes a stable ongoing doctor-patient relationship; it works much less well in a world of replacement-part medicine.

Doctors have known about risk management for years, even if we never called it that. Consider the way we've used steroid drugs since the 1950s to manage some chronic diseases. These drugs damp down the body's inflammatory response when it runs amok and produces diseases like asthma and rheumatoid arthritis. In asthma, the body's immune system becomes paranoid and releases a host of invasion-fighting substances that tighten the small airways in the lungs. Steroids call off the demented chemical troops and open up the airways, stopping the wheezing and eliminating the terrifying sensation of suffocation. Similarly, in patients with rheumatoid arthritis the body turns on itself and attacks hands, wrists, and knees from the inside. Steroids resist the attack and literally cool off joints that are hot, red, and swollen. Pain is diminished, mobility restored.

The problem is that in doing so, steroids can also derange a patient's metabolism and normal immune function, thin the bones, predispose to ulcers, and cause fatty deposits to form in an odd distribution over the body. Until recent decades, when more modern replacements became available, doctor and patient would typically work together to titrate the steroid dose: once the symptoms were controlled, we could reduce the amount taken until the symptoms returned, then ease the dose up again. In a way, each patient became his or her own bioassay of the drug's benefit-risk balance. For most chronic diseases, this kind of teamwork between experienced physician and patient leads to an ongoing dialectic of increasing the dose (or adding a new drug) until the side effects become unacceptable, then reducing the dose (or subtracting a drug) until the symptoms become unacceptable. Risk management, one patient at a time.

SYSTEMS APPROACHES

Classical pharmacology is hard enough to master, but risks and benefits that vary by person and over time in the same person—it's almost more than the human mind can handle. The problem is made more intractable by the minimal exposure most medical students get to these issues, and the brief time that's available to spend with patients during an office visit or a hospitalization. But the health care system itself can enhance decision making as well as impede it. To see this, we can return one more time to the anticoagulant warfarin. (Despite its potential lethality, the drug's name doesn't bespeak a military origin; it was developed at a midwestern medical school with funds donated by its graduates—the Wisconsin Alumni Research Foundation.) Warfarin, often marketed as Coumadin, presents a clear example of the arcane but crucial distinction between efficacy and effectiveness.

In efficacy trials of warfarin, the study team will make sure that subjects come in at regular intervals for the required clotting tests, and uses these results to adjust the dose to keep the level of anticoagulation in just the right narrow range. This hematological ballet is harder to perform in the real world. Busy physicians not guided by a study protocol may omit a particular blood test, or get it later than planned. Patients (that is, average sick people, rather than those who volunteer for a medical study) may fail to show up for the test, or may not change their dose as directed. Drs. Jerry Gurwitz, David Bates, and I looked at the problem in elderly patients living in nursing homes. We were dismayed but not astonished to find that anticoagulation levels were way out of control in many patients taking warfarin—far more than one would have predicted from the way the drug was used in clinical studies. Nearly all serious bleeding complications occur when this level drifts beyond its target range; such catastrophes happen far more often in typical practice than they do in randomized trials. Which rate represents the "true" risk associated with the drug? Answering the benefit versus risk equation now becomes even tougher: for a given molecule used in a given patient at a particular point in time, this relationship will depend heavily upon how skillfully the drug is used by both physician and patient.

There are several ways the health care system can act as a powerful lever for enhancing the effectiveness of drugs and reducing their risks. A drug like the antipsychotic clozapine may at first appear too hot to handle because of its potential for fatal side effects. But when the problem is viewed from a systems perspective, we can find ways to tame the drug and take advantage of its impressive effectiveness while defanging its lethality. Just set up a system in which the pharmacist must be presented with a recent blood test report before the prescription is refilled. In the case of the blood thinners, many medical centers have established anticoagulation clinics that do nothing but manage warfarin blood tests and make dose adjustments. These clinics, typically staffed by nurses or pharmacists, devote all their attention to managing patients' anticoagulant status, and they do it well: the drug's safety profile is much better in these settings than it is in the more chaotic world of typical primary care. Our trio of hypothetical doctors who each confronted the decision about whether to use warfarin in a patient with atrial fibrillation would have had very different notions of how safe the drug was if they had access to such a service.

NEW TECHNOLOGIES TO THE RESCUE

One of the best ways to put a benevolent thumb on the benefit-risk scales is through better science. New discoveries have enabled us gradually to replace therapies that have poor benefit-risk relationships with innovative ones that have better properties. Pharmacology in the twenty-first century continues to try to discover more forgiving treatments: antibiotics that won't induce as much bacterial resistance; anticoagulants that won't increase the chance of major hemorrhage; antihypertensive medications that won't drop the bottom out of a patient's blood pressure. Pharmacogenetics promises to help us know in advance which patients' genetic makeups will make them particularly susceptible to a particular side effect, as well as predicting who will be most likely to benefit from a given drug.

The steroid example is relevant here as well. For asthmatics, it became clear by the 1980s that taking the medicine by inhalation instead of in pill form made it possible to use much smaller doses, and concentrated its effects in the lungs rather than sending it helter-skelter to all parts of the body. In the last decade a completely new class of drugs emerged: the leukotriene inhibitors. These were developed to replicate the beneficial effects of steroids in blocking the inflammatory process while avoiding their downsides. Most recently, still another approach using monoclonal antibodies was introduced to help asthmatics who require near-toxic levels of the older drugs to control their symptoms. Exploration of the benefit-risk balance of those drugs is still in its early stages.

The late 1990s and early 2000s also saw the introduction of several new kinds of drugs for rheumatoid arthritis, known as TNF inhibitors. These biotech products work wonderfully well in many patients while avoiding steroid side effects. Yet the new drugs may increase susceptibility to malignancies and infections. The lesson we keep learning: technological fixes can push the risk-benefit balance farther in the patient's favor, but rarely do they make it go away completely.

THE FACT THAT so much of a drug's effectiveness and safety depends on how it is used is good news, because it opens the door to numerous opportunities to maximize benefit and minimize risk. We physicians can learn to match drugs, patients, and doses more astutely, and if doctor-patient continuity isn't rent asunder by daffy coverage systems, we can reassess these decisions frequently over time. Patients can provide feedback on their symptoms and adverse events to help inform those decisions, and can take their medicines appropriately instead of haphazardly. The benefit-risk balance can also be tilted for the better at higher levels of health care system organization. Risk management can occur nationally as well as at the bedside through mandated programs that begin immediately upon drug approval, as with Lotronex. Other infrastructure fixes can help tame dangerous drugs and monitor their effects in additional ways.

To drive our automotive analogy into the ground: The world of prescription drugs has many biochemical Volvos—reliable, useful, and safe enough to reduce the risk of harm to the user, even in an accident. Rarely, a product will appear that's more like a pharmaceutical Pinto: inherently dangerous, likely to crash and burn even with normal use. But most drugs are more like midsize Chevrolets. They work reasonably well, and their safety has everything to do with how they are used. The same Chevy can be all utility and no risk when driven by the legendary little old lady schoolteacher, but turn into a hazardous killing machine in the hands of her drunken teenage grandson. The better we understand this, the more we will be able to get beyond simplistic YES/NO regulatory decisions, to focus on those vitally important border zones where drug, patient, doctor, and system interact. For most drugs, that's where the real action is.

PART THREE: COSTS

12: LIVE CHEAP OR DIE

It is time to visit the odd landscape of prescription drug economics, to try to understand how a drug's price relates to its benefits and its risks. Far too much pharmaceutical policy debate has focused on those expenditures without considering them in light of a drug's effectiveness and safety. Now that we've paid these key dimensions their due, we can turn our attention to costs, the 800-pound gorilla in the medicine cabinet.

Much of the work done in my research group comes down to analyzing the encrypted zeros and ones that describe medication use and outcomes in hundreds of thousands of patients, stored on scores of magnetic tapes or in our computer's terabyte of disk space. This work can sometimes feel like boxing with ghosts. That sense of insubstantiality hit a peak years ago when we were reviewing data from several state Medicaid programs that cover the costs of health care, including prescription drugs, for the poor. We were evaluating the outcomes of a project we had devised to "de-market" several overused medications, described later in Part Four. My colleague Steve Soumerai and I noticed that in one of the states we were studying, New Hampshire, the use of drugs we had targeted was dramatically lower than it had been in the previous year. That was what we were trying to achieve, but prescribing by physicians in the control group in that state had also dropped sharply, and they hadn't participated in the experimental program at all. More confusing still, the reduction in prescribing occurred for *all* drugs on the market, not just the ones whose use we were trying to curtail. What was going on?

We reviewed all the data extraction procedures with our programmer; she had implemented them exactly the same way as in the other three states we were studying. The data from the other three Medicaid programs—Arkansas, Vermont, and the District of Columbia—looked fine, with no unexpected dips. We phoned our contacts in New Hampshire Medicaid to see whether they might have copied their tapes incorrectly, or perhaps forgotten to send us a few of the huge nine-track reels we needed (it was the 1980s). They double-checked, then triple-checked; everything had been done correctly on their end. This was when I wished I had a mouse to biopsy, a patient to send for a blood test, or even a roomful of paper records to review by hand to get to the bottom of the problem. But all we had was a stack of magnetic tape reels with their implacable zeros and ones, and the numbers just didn't add up. It didn't seem possible that prescribing in an entire state program had simply gone down for a whole year. The number of enrollees had not changed, and it was unlikely their health had improved dramatically during that time. It looked as though we had a major problem on our hands. That turned out to be true, but not in the way we thought.

Bill Pareto had moved to New Hampshire when he turned sixty-one because he liked rural life and low taxes; he enjoyed them even more after he retired from his job as a machinist. Years of smoking had left him with bad emphysema and heart disease, but he had a good family doctor who helped him manage his symptoms, along with the diabetes and high blood pressure that had been with him since middle age. Bill's drug regimen was based on a delicate combination of seven medicines his physician had fine-tuned over a decade of tinkering and adjustment: digoxin to regulate his heart, insulin to control his blood sugar, nitrates to contain his angina chest pain, a diuretic to prevent him from retaining water, a pill to lower his blood pressure, and a bronchodilator and a steroid inhaler to keep the wheezing down. His wife, Ellie, helped him keep his medicines straight; she used to joke that she was his own personal pharmacist.

Ellie died of cancer when Bill turned seventy; that made it harder for him to live on his own, and he moved in with his son and his family. The den became his bedroom, and although the house wasn't big, the move made it easier for them to look after him. Bill's daily pill routine was complicated, but it worked, keeping him feeling fairly well and out of the hospital. He didn't have much of a pension, but he qualified for Medicaid and that covered his medical expenses, including all those prescriptions.

After Bill turned eighty he started to get a little forgetful and occasionally lost his urine. It became more difficult for the family to care for him, but they were committed to keeping him at home. His daughter-in-law quit her job at the local supermarket so she'd have more time to tend to him as well as to her small children.

One day Bill got a letter from Medicaid explaining that to contain its costs, the program would be limiting its payment for his prescriptions to a maximum of three drugs a month. A similar letter went to every drugstore in New Hampshire: for each Medicaid enrollee, the state would cover only the first three prescriptions filled each month; no subsequent ones would be reimbursed. Unless the pharmacy wanted to give the drugs away and absorb the cost themselves, they'd be obliged to enforce the new "cap" policy. Immediate objections were voiced by the state's nursing homes, which housed many Medicaid patients. The homes' owners said they just couldn't care for these frail patients with that tight a limit on medications, and they weren't about to pay for all the extra drugs on their own. So the state exempted nursing homes from the cap policy.

Neither Bill nor his son could afford the hundreds of dollars required to pay for his other four prescriptions out-of-pocket every month. Reluctantly, the family decided to admit him to a nursing home so he could stay on all his medicines; the decision broke their hearts. Once Bill was institutionalized, the Medicaid program resumed covering all his drug expenses, along with an additional $30,000 a year for his nursing home care.

The real cause of our apparent data glitch became clear when I got a phone call from a public interest lawyer in New Hampshire. She was looking for a physician who could testify in a class-action suit her firm was bringing on behalf of patients in the state's Medicaid program; someone told her that a Dr. Avorn at Harvard would be a soft touch. "You're not going to believe this," she said, "but last year someone in state government decided to save money by limiting everyone in our Medicaid program to a maximum of three prescriptions a month. Doesn't that seem crazy?"

It turned out that our numbers problem reflected a real statewide reduction in the use of prescription drugs throughout the entire New Hampshire Medicaid program. The first Reagan administration had just begun, and word had come from Washington that state programs getting federal assistance had better tighten their fiscal belts. New Hampshire had never exactly been a welfare magnet; traditionally conservative, the state prided itself on its very low taxes and a state budget that was puritanically frugal. The motto stamped onto every New Hampshire license plate, "Live Free or Die," was meant to reflect its attitude toward rugged individualism and personal liberty. But as I was drawn into this issue, it began to seem more like a statement about the state's policy toward the poor. Even its nickname, The Granite State, came to sound like a description of its approach to human services as much as of its geological endowment.

"How could anyone think this was a good idea?" I asked her, recalling the many patients I was caring for at the time who needed five or seven medications a day just to last until suppertime.

"They looked at the expenditures and somebody calculated that the average number of medications was only about one per patient per month across the whole program," the lawyer explained. (They were averaging in all the young mothers and children in Medicaid, who used few if any prescriptions.) "So they figured tripling that would be plenty." The lawyer described a few case histories to me, similar to the situation Mr. Pareto faced. Young women and kids aside, the other bump in the Medicaid demographic comprised frail elderly patients like Mr. Pareto. The bureaucrats' averaging reminded me of the mythical laboratory rat sometimes described in introductory statistics courses. You could put its front half in a freezer and its rear in an oven, but it could still have a "normal average body temperature." Of course, no scientist would ever actually do such an experiment on a rat. But there were no ethical prohibitions in place to prevent zany policy experiments using an entire population of poor people.

I told the lawyer I'd be willing to testify if that would help, but added that perhaps we could be of greater use by documenting the consequences of this really dumb plan. The attorneys already had anecdotal evidence from distraught patients forced to decide whether to skip their heart medicine, blood pressure pills, insulin, meat, or rent; she told me such bleeding heart stories hadn't been enough to move the conservative legislature into rethinking its policy. Soumerai and I had more than anecdotes: those millions of zeros and ones on the Medicaid claims tapes (none were missing, of course) reflected every single prescription filled by every participant in the state's Medicaid program over a span of several years, including the fateful year of the new cost containment policy. Moreover, we could link all that information about filled prescriptions with data we were getting about those same people from a separate source, the federal Medicare program. This could provide the other half of the story, since Medicare pays for and records all physician and hospital bills for virtually every American over age sixty-five. Once all personal identifiers were encoded to protect people's privacy, we could track every doctor visit and hospitalization of these patients, before and after the start of the new prescription restriction.

Still better, I was planning to add to our library of zeros and ones a new set of data from people enrolled in Medicaid and Medicare in New Jersey; after their personal identifiers had been encoded, those tapes would provide valuable information on similar patients in a comparison state. There are more pharmaceutical companies based in New Jersey than anywhere else in the solar system, so it was unthinkable that its state Medicaid program would impose any kind of restriction to limit the purchase of prescription drugs. For our purposes, that would provide a stable program to compare with the New Hampshire experience—what's sometimes called a "natural experiment." We couldn't have done a randomized trial of the drug-limit policy by assigning Medicaid patients to the previous policy or to the stupid new one—and what ethics review board would ever permit such a study? But we could, in the best tradition of epidemiology, approximate what such a trial would have found through a carefully designed observational study comparing the two states.

DECODING A DISASTER

We began spinning the New Hampshire tapes to address this question, a project on which Dr. Soumerai took the lead. Rather than consider the entire Medicaid population, including its large numbers of young mothers and their children, we had the computer identify patients who had been using multiple medications for chronic illnesses before the new policy took effect. This was the actual cohort at risk—the people who had the greatest chance of getting into trouble from the restrictions. For those over sixty-five (and most of them were), we then linked their drug use information to the Medicare data to learn more about the totality of their medical conditions.

The findings were astonishing. The data Soumerai produced showed that in New Hampshire, as soon as the Medicaid monthly "cap" was put into place, patients had substantial drops in their use of vital drugs. Surely such reductions would make clear the folly of such punish-the-sickest cost containment. But we wanted to go further and find out what actually happened to these patients. We turned to our New Jersey Medicaid data and identified a large group from that state who were nearly identical to the New Hampshire patients we were studying in terms of their age, gender, medical conditions, socioeconomic status, and baseline drug use. We could use the coded numbers representing patients to track all medication use, health care encounters, and deaths in both programs, to see if the fates of medically similar people differed across the two states.

Defenders of the cap policy had argued that it probably wouldn't harm anyone. Some of them even pointed to papers I had written stating that the elderly are often overmedicated; what better way to cut down on the overuse of drugs in this population than to limit the dollars society made available to pay for them? If someone really needed a lifesaving drug, they argued, surely the patient would be able to prioritize which prescriptions to fill, or pay out-of-pocket, or find some family members or a charity to help out. And if some were so ill that they needed that many drugs each month, maybe it was better for society for such frail people to be cared for in nursing homes anyway. Preventable hospitalizations? Needless deaths? There was no reason to expect that, we were assured. But no evaluation had been planned to measure the consequences of the new policy. Sick old people are hospitalized and die all the time, we were told; no sense in blaming Medicaid policy for that.

Having documented a significant drop-off in the use of these vital drugs and published our first results in the *New England Journal of Medicine*, Soumerai and I were eager to see whether the reduced drug use affected the health of these patients. We needed funding to pay for the additional programming and data analysis and computer resources, as well as our own time to do the research. The federal agency that had supported the first stage of the research, the National Center for Health Services Research, was chronically short of funding. At best, it would take at least nine months from the submission of a proposal until more grant support would be available—if it was funded at all. We wondered whether the pharmaceutical industry might be willing to provide arm's-length financial support for the follow-up project more quickly. We knew we'd be protected by the language Harvard requires in any contract with a corporate research sponsor that would guarantee our right to perform the study however we saw fit, and to publish our findings with total freedom.

There were some precedents for such industry support. Most of the large drug companies had joined together to create an organization called the National Pharmaceutical Council, which awarded grants to researchers to conduct studies of medication policy. With some trepidation, Soumerai and I went to visit NPC headquarters just outside Washington, D.C. It was an odd meeting. We explained that although paying for prescription drugs was a key aspect of health policy, not enough research had been done on the impact that drug coverage had on other health care use—and there were almost no studies about coverage of the poor. If our hunch was right, this would be the first large-scale analysis to demonstrate rigorously that public payment for medications for the poor (or the lack thereof) could influence patients' clinical outcomes as well as their use of other health care resources. That was an article of faith for many inside and outside the pharmaceutical industry, but there was surprisingly little hard evidence about the magnitude of such an effect, or even whether it existed. The abrupt curtailing of prescription coverage in one state could provide a golden opportunity to study this relationship.

"Weren't you the ones who did that 'anti-detailing' research?" the NPC director asked, referring to our project that de-marketed overused drugs, described later in Part Four.

"Yes," I answered, "but that was a different study. Now we're trying to understand the problems that patients run into when their drug coverage is taken away." This took a while to explain, as his assumption seemed to be that there were basically two kinds of people who did drug policy studies: the bad kind who were anti-industry "enemies," and the good kind, who would discover whatever you asked them to find as long as you left enough cash on the dresser in the morning.

His next question was, "What do you expect the results to be?"

"We can't be sure," I replied, "but clinically I'd expect that if you take away heart medications from cardiac patients, and insulin from diabetics, and inhalers from asthmatics, then bad things will happen to them."

"Is there a chance you might find no difference in the results?"

"Of course there's that chance; that's why we want to do the study. But I don't think it's likely."

"Would you publish your results either way, even if there was no difference in health care outcomes?"

"Yes, we would."

"Let me get back to you on this."

The National Pharmaceutical Council declined to fund the study.

CALCULATING THE DAMAGES

Eventually, we persuaded the federal Health Care Financing Administration to give us a grant to cover the costs of the next phase of the research, but it took a long time for the funding to arrive. When the final analyses were completed, we found that although our study patients in the two states had been nearly identical in the months before the policy, once the limits were applied the New Hampshire Medicaid patients ended up in nursing homes, hospitals, or cemeteries significantly more often than the similar New Jersey Medicaid patients, who retained full drug coverage. As for the cap policy, after about a year the New Hampshire authorities came to their senses and replaced it with a new cost containment policy that instead required only a one-dollar copayment for every prescription filled, but with no monthly limit on the number of drugs. Substantial revenues were collected in this way with considerably less damage to patients. When the cap policy was abandoned, the survival curves for the two states became parallel again: the rate of institutionalization, hospitalization, or death in New Hampshire Medicaid patients once again was the same as in the comparable patients in New Jersey Medicaid, but with one important difference. Nearly all those extra patients in New Hampshire who were put into nursing homes because of the cap policy stayed there, incurring the human and economic toll of institutional life every year until they died. Our follow-up paper was published in the *New England Journal of Medicine* four years after the first one.

It has always been hard for our medical neighbors to the north to live in the shadow of the internationally renowned clinical and research centers of Boston. But now their state had achieved a certain fame of its own. Policy makers and students of prescription drug reimbursement still refer to "the New Hampshire experiment" as the clearest evidence to date that dollars spent or not spent on prescription drugs can have an important impact on the rest of the health care system. In the end, the study provided several lessons.

The first one is obvious, but still pervasively ignored: mindless across-the-board limits on reimbursement for medications may appear to save money on one small part of the balance sheet, but can have important negative effects that pop up elsewhere in the health care system, as well as in patients' lives. This myopic focus on only one line item at a time has been dubbed the "silo mentality" in health economics. Our papers made a clear case for the folly of simplistic limits on drug coverage by health insurance programs, particularly those for the poor. Nonetheless, in the years following those publications, new cap policies restricting the monthly number of drugs reimbursable by Medicaid were put in place in several more state programs, as if our findings had never been published or read. In my dreams, the bureaucrats who thought up that original policy are ridden out of New Hampshire on a rail. In the nightmare that follows, they keep turning up in other states, doing more of the same damage.

A second important point of these studies is that major changes in health care delivery programs must be evaluated rigorously to determine their outcomes on patients. This is rarely done. The spastic shifts in payment policy in both the public and private sectors of the U.S. health care system represent some of the largest medical experiments ever done on humans. But these experiments are done without the informed consent of the patients experimented upon, are generally devoid of any adequate experimental design, and lack even the most rudimentary follow-up assessment.

A further lesson of the New Hampshire fiasco is that policies, like drugs, don't always work the way you expect them to. We later discovered that the New Hampshire cap restriction had been designed to make it possible for patients, pharmacists, and physicians to work together so that a doctor could write extended three-month prescriptions for three drugs each month, instead of the normal one-month supply. In theory, a patient could have been covered for as many as nine drugs at any given time. However, this aspect of the policy wasn't communicated with the same alacrity as the "limit of three" rule. As a result, hardly anybody took advantage of it.

The final step in our analysis of the New Hampshire policy was to estimate the excess costs the state government had to pay for the additional nursing home bills incurred by the many patients like Mr. Pareto who were institutionalized primarily because they couldn't afford to pay for their drugs at home. Once we did the math, it turned out that the program had hardly saved the New Hampshire Medicaid program any money at all.

It has been nearly two decades since we published those papers, but they remain distressingly current. I still receive calls from colleagues in drug-benefit programs all over the country who want to talk about our old findings. The caller is usually trying to fend off a similar "cap" policy that someone wants to implement in a particular Medicaid program or HMO or employee benefit system. With rising pressures on drug expenditures, particularly in impossibly stressed state budgets, the calls are becoming more anguished as a new generation of managers becomes willing to try anything to contain medication costs. This is not reinventing the wheel; it is reinventing the flat tire.

13: FILLING THE PIPELINE

In the years since that early New Hampshire experience, many more health care programs in the public and private sectors have grappled with the escalating costs of drug coverage, and many more people have found themselves unable to pay for the medications their doctors prescribe. Policy changes still leave important gaps in coverage, and we remain unable to implement a plan to cover the medication expenses of all Americans as comprehensively as nearly every other industrialized nation has. While the costs of pharmaceuticals are rising all over the world, the problem is much more acute here. Some of this has to do with the prescribing decisions that we physicians make; we will explore that aspect of the problem in Part Four. But much of the difficulty also stems from what drugs cost; it is now time to stare unflinchingly at that gorilla.

The industry's position defending its high U.S. drug prices might be called the Research Ultimatum. It argues that the income from those high prices is necessary so the money can be plowed right back into research to develop new products. According to this view, the discovery of new medicines depends primarily on work done by the pharmaceutical industry; all those other countries that limit drug prices are depicted as foreign free riders who unfairly share in the fruits of research paid for by American consumers. The ultimatum is this: the industry warns that if it doesn't continue to enjoy its rich cash flow and stellar profits, it won't invest as much in new research, and the pipeline of desperately needed new medicines will run dry.

The pharmaceutical industry does invest heavily in drug development: the annual R&D budget listed by the industry's trade group is now greater than the amount spent annually by the entire National Institutes of Health on biomedical studies of all kinds. The moment in the 1990s when this occurred marked a milestone in the shift of American medical research dollars from the public to the corporate sector. Much industry-based research is of high scientific quality and contributes directly to the discovery and availability of new medications. This is in part because the companies have been able to attract talented scientists away from university settings, lured by the availability of copious funding and the freedom of not having to continuously submit grant proposals to support their laboratories. Many of these scientists are first-rate researchers, and the quality of their work is often excellent, although their focus is constrained by the need to generate marketable products. And their ability to communicate freely about discoveries is often limited by an obligation to protect corporate intellectual property. But there is more to the story.

Because the origin of therapeutic innovation is such a vital concern for everyone, it is crucial to understand to what extent that research ultimatum is valid and to what extent it's hyperbole. The industry claims that the issue is pregnant with portent for the future of medicine. But for many scientists, its logic just leaves stretch marks on our credulity, and fails to deliver on most of the policy implications it implies.

True, nearly all new medications are eventually brought to market and commercialized by pharmaceutical companies. But it's essential to go back and trace the origins of the breakthroughs that made them possible. As with most scientific developments, it isn't always easy to document an exact genealogy, as I learned in working as an adviser to the Congressional Office of Technology Assessment on a report, *Pharmaceutical R&D: Costs, Risks, and Returns,* which tackled this complex issue before that agency was eliminated.

A vast and costly foundation of basic biomedical research is supported by federal funding, primarily from NIH. In addition, scores of philanthropies such as the American Heart Association and the Howard Hughes Medical Institute also fund basic studies that lead to new drugs. Drawing on this rich lode, the pharmaceutical or biotech industries identify early discoveries with commercial promise and may then perform considerable additional work to transform these findings into potentially useful products. Some basic research is also done within the research-intensive companies themselves.

A number of analyses have traced the role of publicly funded research in the development of medications that were later privately patented by manufacturers. For some drugs, like AZT, the first successful drug to treat AIDS, or alglucerase for Gaucher's disease, the key initial discoveries and developments occurred within the NIH itself. Despite this, the companies that commercialized these discoveries were able to charge dearly for the drugs once they patented them; in the case of alglucerase (Ceredase) the price tag initially came to over $200,000 per patient per year. Other drugs built upon seminal publicly supported developments in biomedical research, but important aspects of their development and clinical evaluation were accomplished (and paid for) by the drug companies that eventually marketed them.

In thinking about the fairness of drug prices, it would be useful if we somehow could parse out the relative contribution of research done with public monies in the nonprofit sector, versus the additional applied research performed by a specific company. The year 1980 was a watershed moment in the evolution of public policy in this area, when Congress passed two pieces of legislation to encourage the transfer of federally funded medical discoveries into private hands. The National Institutes of Health later contended that in view of the taxpayer-supported origins of so many treatments, such arrangements with private companies should lead to "a reasonable relationship between the pricing of a licensed product, the public investment in that product, and the health and safety needs of the public."

But by 2001, the pharmaceutical industry had successfully argued against the viability of this reasonable pricing requirement. According to Michael Gluck of Georgetown University, advisory panels persuaded NIH that rapid commercialization was the most crucial issue in moving discoveries from the laboratory to the bedside. It was less important, industry contended, whether the fruits of such research were affordable for patients, or whether the companies involved paid a fair share of licensing fees back to the taxpayer. They saw NIH's proposed quid pro quo as problematic, because "a reasonable pricing clause would inhibit technology transfer and the development of new health care products." In both 2001 and 2002, the House of Representatives tried to restore the reasonable pricing requirement for drugs developed with federal support, and in both years the Senate removed it.

MODERN ALCHEMISTS

The origin of one major blockbuster drug group vividly illustrates these tensions. In the 1980s and early 1990s, Professor Donald Young and his colleagues at the University of Rochester were studying the fundamental causes of pain and inflammation. A common culprit in both processes was the prostaglandins, a family of chemicals originally discovered in the prostate gland, but now known to play numerous vital roles throughout the body. Limiting the body's production of prostaglandins could reduce pain and inflammation, an insight that had led to the development of drugs like ibuprofen (Motrin). But prostaglandins also have helpful effects, like protecting the lining of the stomach. Because of this, inhibiting their production with these drugs can sometimes lead to ulcers and gastrointestinal bleeding. In studying this problem, the Rochester team made a pivotal discovery: there are two separate enzymes responsible for prostaglandin-related effects, Cox-1 and Cox-2. The latter is the mostly evil twin, mediating pain and inflammation, while the former helps to preserve the stomach lining, among many other things. The researchers discovered that selectively blocking just the Cox-2 enzyme would relieve pain and inflammation without inhibiting the protective effects of the Cox-1 enzyme. To round out their work, the Rochester scientists developed a new biochemical screening method to evaluate potential drugs and identify which ones would inhibit the Cox-2 enzyme selectively.

Those studies led directly to the development of a new class of drugs, the selective Cox-2 inhibitors or coxibs, designed to reduce pain and inflammation as effectively as older products like ibuprofen, but with somewhat lower risk of gastric bleeding. The discovery gave rise to two blockbuster products, Merck's Vioxx and Pharmacia's Celebrex. Annual sales for this new drug class exceeded $6 billion by 2003, before concerns about their cardiovascular side effects became widespread. The University of Rochester had the foresight to file patents on the discoveries made by its faculty members, covering the treatment of pain by selective inhibition of the Cox-2 enzyme as well as the test they devised to identify new drugs that could do so. The university expected that companies developing products based on these discoveries would pay it royalties on sales of such drugs; as a nonprofit institution, it planned to recycle those dollars into support for additional research and related activities at its medical school.

The manufacturers saw it differently. They noted that Pharmacia and Merck had taken the process to the final step and developed the actual drugs based on these discoveries, and therefore owed the university nothing. A federal judge sided with the manufacturers and invalidated the university's claims. He acknowledged that the medical school researchers had made a pivotal contribution by discovering the selective inhibition of the Cox-2 enzyme and developing a test to identify drugs that could do so. However, they had not actually produced the drugs themselves. In his ruling, U.S. District Court Judge David Larimer wrote, "While the court does not mean to suggest that the [university] inventors' significant work in this field is on a par with alchemy, the fact remains that without the compound called for in the patent, the inventors could no more be said to have possessed the complete invention claimed . . . than the alchemists possessed a method of turning base metals into gold."

It would come as a surprise to my university-based research colleagues that a federal court has determined that what we do is intellectually akin to alchemy. True, a drug patent is most cleanly defensible when it describes a specific product that has been synthesized and shown to have a particular effect. But what of the seminal biological discoveries that led directly up to that point? Is this the same patent law that allows companies (and, yes, universities) to patent strands of naturally occurring DNA they have isolated, or rats of a particular genetic makeup, even in the absence of practical products? The Rochester decision dealt a blow to medical schools throughout the country in their efforts to help support their programs with royalties from products their research made possible.

As for the products in question: years of clinical research and experience have confirmed that the coxibs are no more effective than older drugs, despite massive ad campaigns that subtly imply otherwise. And while the coxibs do reduce gastric bleeding somewhat, this advantage appears to be modest. Then, of course, came the findings that these medications can increase the risk of heart attack and stroke. But until these risks were proven, extravagant marketing aimed at patients and doctors made these among the most profitable drugs ever sold. Those of us who work at universities may not be very good at turning ordinary things into gold, but others clearly are.

By the time of the federal court decision, Pharmacia and its coxib drug Celebrex had been acquired by Pfizer, which found itself engaged in another legal battle. Two new impotence drugs were coming to market; although they were novel molecules, each blocked the same enzyme as Pfizer's Viagra. Pfizer sued both manufacturers, contending that it had patented the concept of inhibiting that enzyme and therefore owned all rights to any subsequent application of the discovery. The irony of this argument was not lost on the University of Rochester's attorneys.

CORPORATE WELFARE

Like the courts, Congress and the executive branch also intervene heavily to protect the pharmaceutical industry from the downsides of drug development work. Such subsidies go far beyond support for NIH, where public dollars pay for the costliest part of drug R&D—its high-risk basic science component. Research conducted by the drug companies themselves is also partly underwritten by government (and hence by taxpayers) in the form of substantial tax benefits. It is not just that all of a manufacturer's research costs are deductible expenses; the federal government also provides a generous R&D tax credit that allows companies to deduct up to half their research costs from their federal tax debt. (This benefits only the larger companies that are profitable enough to be paying taxes; smaller start-ups with huge research expenses but little or no profit can't take comparable advantage of these credits.)

One striking example of the lucrative and generally unreciprocated generosity shown by NIH to the industry was development of the cancer drug Taxol, marketed by Bristol-Myers Squibb. The General Accounting Office traced Taxol's evolution from its earliest development to its position as the best-selling oncology drug ever. The report noted that even before an agreement was signed with BMS, and continuing into the first two years of that agreement, "NIH [paid for] most of the clinical trials associated with the drug. The results of these trials were critical for BMS to secure FDA's approval. . . ." The GAO estimated that through 2002, NIH invested $484 million to fund Taxol-related research.

A 1996 agreement provided that in exchange, BMS would pay NIH royalties at the rate of one-half of 1 percent of its worldwide Taxol sales. (One can assume that the BMS executive who negotiated that deal received a hefty bonus that year.) Those sales totaled more than $9 billion through 2002, but by that point the company had paid NIH only $35 million in royalties, $10 million short of even the paltry sum agreed upon. The federal government also continued to underwrite Taxol in other ways, with Medicare paying the company nearly $700 million for patients' use of the drug during 1994–1999 alone. "NIH made substantial investments in research related to Taxol," the GAO reported in its understated conclusion, "but its financial benefits from the collaboration with BMS have not been great in comparison to BMS's revenue from the drug."

It isn't clear how well NIH has assimilated this lesson. A few months after release of the report, its director announced a sweeping plan to reorient NIH priorities. The new vision called for committing more NIH resources to support early-stage studies of drug development. The plan would deemphasize research initiated by university-based faculty in favor of more central governmental planning to direct funding into particular areas, and the fostering of more partnerships with the private sector.

FOLLOW THE MONEY

When it comes to American economic policy in the early twenty-first century, the era of big government may be over for welfare mothers, Medicaid patients, veterans, and the uninsured, but big government is alive and well for large companies, many of which have been remarkably resourceful in soaking up the federal dole. When the ideology of family assistance was in its heyday, it led to both useful and counterproductive results. In the same way, there are better and worse kinds of corporate welfare. Taxpayer and private-sector subsidies of companies that reward the discovery of vital new medicines can be a benign and useful kind of federal charity if properly reciprocated, although its advocates prefer to avoid words like "government subsidy" and "welfare" in favor of more politically correct terms like "free market" and "avoiding the tyranny of price controls." But these policies act in the public interest only when they actually lead to important research advances. An overly permissive pro-industry agenda can not only create bad public policy, but also weaken these businesses themselves over the long term. This has begun to occur.

The National Institute for Health Care Management is a health policy think tank supported primarily by the nation's Blue Cross and Blue Shield plans—insurers that have been hit hard by rising drug expenditures. In a study of innovation in the pharmaceutical industry, NIHCM examined the drug companies' contention that high costs lead directly to more discoveries. It reviewed all 1,035 of the new drug applications (NDAs) submitted to the FDA during the period 1989 through 2000. For each application, the FDA determines whether a product will undergo rapid priority review or a standard evaluation. A drug is given priority review if compared to drugs already on the market it appears to be more effective, have fewer side effects, result in better patient compliance, or have efficacy or safety advantages in a new population of patients. A drug is given a standard review only if none of these attributes is present. NIHCM researchers divided the new drug applications into 361 new chemicals (new molecular entities, or NMEs) and 674 existing molecules, most of which were "incrementally modified drugs" (IMDs). They found that only 15 percent of all new drug applications were for new chemicals that the FDA considered worthy of priority review; another 9 percent were IMDs that represented important improvements according to the agency's criteria. Thus, only about a quarter of all new drugs reviewed by the FDA during this period were deemed by the agency to have important advantages over existing products, and three quarters did not.

The NIHCM analysis had two additional disturbing findings. Because the nation's expenditures for prescription drugs more than doubled during the 1995–2000 period, the report measured the proportion of the increase attributable to expenditures for breakthrough drugs versus less innovative "me too" products. It found that two thirds of the increase in expenditure for new drugs during this period was accounted for by products that the FDA rated as noninnovative (although their marketing programs apparently were). To see if there was a time trend in this pattern of less-than-revolutionary drug development, the report divided the period studied into two halves: 1989–1994 and 1995–2000. From the first period to the second, the greatest growth was in the number of products that were just incrementally modified (up 82 percent), compared to a much smaller increase in the number of innovative new molecules (up only 10 percent).

The analysis considered only drugs developed by the large established drug manufacturers collectively known as Big Pharma, and did not include products developed by smaller start-ups such as the newer biotech companies, where innovation arguably occurs at a faster pace. But all sources of innovation were taken into account in one recent analysis that tracked the number of patents cited in descriptions of new drug products through 2002. The number of references to discoveries made by U.S.-based drug companies showed a steady erosion over the last ten years, despite enormous profits and unprecedented sums attributed to research at those firms. Another disturbing trend is evident from a very simple measure: the number of new drugs approved by the FDA each year. That figure reached a high of fifty-three products approved in 1996. Since then, despite quicker evaluation procedures at the FDA and the availability of more revenue-driven capital than ever before for companies to pour into research, that number drifted down to a mere seventeen new drug products approved in 2002.

What accounts for this detumescence in the innovative vigor of the large pharmaceutical companies? The industry was just responding rationally to the legal, regulatory, and economic pressures of a marketplace that had become perverse. Its decades of effective lobbying had been successful: laws designed to encourage and protect meaningful innovation had been turned into a system that rewarded trivial pseudo-innovation even more profitably than important discoveries. In many companies, corporate leadership and power had shifted away from the scientifically and clinically based divisions and toward the sales and marketing divisions. With the ascendancy of promotion over hard data in driving doctors' and patients' drug choices, it became even more attractive for companies to generate unremarkable, expensive products that are superbly promoted.

The contention that the companies require huge profits in order to recycle those dollars into the development of needed new products is also under attack by a growing army of critics armed with pocket-protectors and calculators. A recent study of the economics of the drug industry was performed by analysts at the Department of Health and Human Services—not exactly a hotbed of anticorporate radicals. In studying the nine largest American drug companies, they found that a hefty 31 percent of total revenues were used for sales, marketing, general expenses, and administration. Profit consumed an additional 20 percent of revenues, and research and development accounted for just 13 percent.

This R&D figure, of course, also includes the substantial sums required to perform and evaluate the small chemical manipulations done primarily to extend a drug's patent, as discussed below. The clinical benefits of such molecular masturbation may be trivial, but the cost of that activity is not, since it must include all the expensive toxicology studies, clinical trials, and regulatory compliance requirements that a real innovation would entail.

EDGAR HAS ALL THE NUMBERS

The HHS analysis mirrored the findings of other researchers who obtained corporate data from a powerful ally in Washington. A well-informed source known as EDGAR, deep within the Securities and Exchange Commission, provided access to details of the companies' financial activities that most of us never get to see. EDGAR is no socialist mole; it is the acronym for the Electronic Data Gathering, Analysis, and Retrieval system of the SEC. For any publicly traded company, EDGAR can let you know where the financial bodies are buried. At no charge, he'll provide access to all the annual and quarterly financial reports and other disclosure documents that corporations are required to submit to the federal government. And he'll spill everything he knows to anyone with an internet connection.

The advocacy group Families USA used EDGAR to review the financial reports submitted to the SEC by nine of the largest U.S.-based pharmaceutical companies (the firms it studied differed from the HHS investigation by only one company on each list). Like the HHS analysis, the story EDGAR told about the flow of dollars in the pharmaceutical industry didn't completely match the story the industry tells about itself. As in the government study, Families USA calculated the proportion of revenues each company reported for three broad categories: marketing, advertising, and administration; profit; and research and development. Their analysis produced similar results: of the $168 billion in total revenues these nine companies reported for one recent year, the largest share (27 percent) was spent on marketing, advertising, and administration ($45 billion); next came profit, at 18 percent ($31 billion); and then research and development, at 11 percent ($19 billion).

There is a certain logic here: if a company spends too much of its research budget to develop new products that are tweaked but basically unimproved versions of existing drugs, it will have to spend even larger sums to market them to convince doctors and patients that they really are "new and improved." The consequences are unsettling: several large pharmaceutical companies face uncertain futures because they don't have enough new product in their pipelines. The current reward structure in the marketplace induced many to spend too much money and effort on developing, promoting, and defending molecules of minimal worth, rather than devoting more of their R&D investment to truly groundbreaking medical research.

The trend here is not encouraging. According to analyses done by the Health Research Group, during one recent year the companies' expenditures for advertising were rising at a rate of 32 percent annually, while R&D expenditures increased at less than half that rate. Self-serving television commercials aside, the trail of dollars depicts an industry heavily focused on promotion and its own bottom line, rather than an enterprise that successfully transforms a sizable portion of its revenues into the discovery of new breakthrough medicines.

A GROWTH SECTOR

The interplay between science and business is particularly intense in the world of cancer drugs. In May 2001, after a remarkably short review time of just two and a half months, the FDA approved a new leukemia treatment trade-named Gleevec. The drug worked at a novel site in the cellular machinery, had a dramatically high cure rate, and produced surprisingly few side effects. The development of Gleevec was widely hailed as an example of effective collaboration between university researchers and the pharmaceutical industry in which the manufacturer, Novartis, worked closely with academic colleagues to bring a breakthrough drug to market. Those closer to the process have told a somewhat different story.

For decades, basic scientists had been trying to define exactly which events inside a cell trigger the deadly transformation into malignancy. Work leading up to the discovery of the innovative approach on which Gleevec capitalized had been going on for decades at MIT, the University of California at San Francisco and at San Diego, the University of Chicago, and the Salk Institute. Basic researchers at those institutions were trying to find a way to inhibit a particular "signaling protein" named BCR-ABL that turned on uncontrolled cell division. Earlier work at the University of Pennsylvania had demonstrated that patients with one rare kind of blood cancer, chronic myelogenous leukemia (CML), had an abnormal chromosome that seemed to play a pivotal role in causing the disease. The team named it "the Philadelphia chromosome"; other investigators read their papers and speculated that this might be a promising target for a new line of attack.

Dr. Owen Witte was one of the basic scientists whose work led to the discovery of Gleevec; his research was funded by the Howard Hughes Medical Institute, an enormous medical philanthropy created from the fortune of the reclusive businessman. The problem was that CML strikes only about five thousand Americans each year. Dr. Witte recalled that despite the scientific promise of the new approach, "because CML does not affect large numbers of people, it was very hard to interest companies in developing inhibitors specifically for BCR-ABL."

The account in a Hughes Institute publication depicts an industry reluctant to sink much money into this work because in spite of its scientific importance, curing such a rare condition would bring only limited financial benefit. The same story is told in Boston by former colleagues of a young oncology researcher, Dr. Brian Druker, who began working on this problem at Harvard's Dana-Farber Cancer Institute. They describe how hard it had been for Druker to obtain the materials and support he needed from industry sources to get his work off the ground. If successful, such a targeted approach could lead toward the holy grail of oncology research: blocking cancer cells preferentially without destroying normal ones, yielding a treatment that would cause many fewer side effects than conventional chemotherapy. Despite the excitement this novel molecular approach elicited among researchers, support from pharmaceutical companies was initially scanty. In 1993, Druker left Harvard and moved to the Oregon Health Sciences University to continue his attempts to treat cancer by blocking these signaling proteins. During the years in which his laboratory developed and performed the initial studies on the compound later sold as Gleevec, Dr. Druker's research was reported to have been supported 50 percent by the National Cancer Institute, 30 percent by the Leukemia and Lymphoma Society, 10 percent by his university, and 10 percent by Novartis, the company that later marketed the drug.

Convinced that blocking an enzyme called tyrosine kinase could make use of this new approach to treat leukemia, Druker asked Novartis (then Ciba-Geigy) to send him compounds they had developed that had this property, so that he could see which might work against CML cells in his lab. He discovered that one, called STI-571, had the effect he expected. According to colleagues at Dana-Farber, he tried to persuade the manufacturer to allow him to test it in patients "even though the drug company initially lacked interest. . . . Despite the promise of STI-571 in the laboratory, Novartis wasn't eager to produce enough for clinical trials unless there was evidence it might work in cancers besides CML." Read: unless it had greater market potential. Novartis had so little interest in committing resources to the drug's development that cancer researchers had to resort to the bizarre tactic of sending a petition to the company's CEO, signed by scientists in the Leukemia and Lymphoma Society of America, imploring him to make more drug available for clinical studies. Eventually, the company complied; the rest (and only the rest) is history.

The account of these events on the company's website is somewhat different: "Novartis saw the potentially significant patient benefits of Gleevec in early testing and took every step to ensure that Gleevec was made available to as many patients as possible and as quickly as possible." The company patented the drug and now sells it at an annual price of $24,000 per patient.

That cost isn't unusual for cancer drugs, and such pricing has created another fault line in the American medical care system. As with other drugs, the price is determined in the United States primarily by what the traffic will bear. For a very small number of products, such as newer monoclonal antibody treatments or other products of genetic engineering, production costs can be substantial, owing to the complex biotechnology required to manufacture such compounds. But for most other drugs, including most chemotherapy agents, once production has been established the incremental cost of making the next thousand doses is modest; these expenses account for only a fraction of the price charged for a given drug. This is why generic drugs cost so much less for the same chemical: much of the price of a patented drug covers the cost of marketing sizzle rather than paying for the underlying drug steak. (The relative amount that the sizzle factor contributes to the cost of medications is illustrated by the life cycle of omeprazole, the "purple pill" for stomach complaints. When it was first marketed as Prilosec, it cost about six dollars for each capsule. After years of litigation that vastly prolonged the process, by the time the drug became available generically and then over the counter, the per-pill cost for the same medicine sank to about thirty cents on the internet.)

This distinction between what it costs to manufacture a drug and how it is priced has produced especially odd spreads in the world of cancer care. While Medicare traditionally paid for very few pharmaceuticals, it reimbursed cancer doctors generously for intravenous chemotherapy treatments provided to patients. The rate of payment to the doctor was linked to the drug's average wholesale price, or AWP. But beginning in 2002, Medicare began to acknowledge a strange truth long known to nearly everyone else involved in pharmaceutical commerce: the AWP price was often made up out of thin air. It's like the surprising fact that many of us learned in high school about the Holy Roman Empire: it was neither holy nor Roman nor truly an empire. AWP has similar properties: it isn't average, it isn't wholesale, and it isn't really the price. For years people in the business (but apparently no one in Medicare) joked that AWP really stood for "Ain't What's Paid."

Traditionally, oncologists would administer chemotherapy to patients in their offices and bill Medicare a cost linked to the drug's listed AWP, often with a substantial markup added. But doctors actually paid far below AWP to buy the drug, and got to keep the rest. The General Accounting Office calculated that in just one year, Medicare spent a billion dollars extra because the prices it paid for these intravenous drugs for cancer (as well as a few other conditions, like arthritis) exceeded those paid by anyone else who bought them. The divergence between the reimbursed AWP-based amount and the actual cost of the drug to the doctor eventually became so extreme that the spread accounted for up to a third to a half of the annual income of many oncologists. Their professional association argued that this difference was needed to cover the related costs of giving the infusion, as well as other poorly reimbursed aspects of cancer care, like spending time talking to patients and their families. Medicare disagreed, and billions of dollars later finally announced its intention to relate payments more closely to the physician's actual costs.

This practice was not just another example of how medicine has been reduced to the manipulative push and pull of commerce even in the face of life-threatening disease. There is a more insidious aspect to the problem. Consider the situation of an oncologist facing a cancer patient in whom the usual first-line approaches of chemotherapy and/or radiation and/or surgery have failed to stop a tumor's growth. Sometimes there is an obvious next step with good evidence of efficacy, but often there isn't. One option would be to shift clinical gears and focus on preventing pain and maintaining the patient's independence and comfort as long as possible, rather than attempting an extremely unlikely cure. But there is almost always another kind of chemotherapy to try. There may not be any solid evidence from clinical trials that doing so will extend life, and this choice will certainly cause substantial side effects. But the patient may be willing to try anything, and the doctor genuinely wants to help. In such gray-zone decisions, economics may loom larger than either patient or physician would want in driving the decision to try another round of chemo.

The taint extends to the area of new drug development as well. A young oncology colleague told me with astonishment of an industry-sponsored focus group he had attended. A forward-looking pharmaceutical company was trying to gauge the potential market for several new cancer drugs it was developing. A representative described the early clinical trials of an oral version of an established chemotherapy product that had previously been available only in intravenous form. He noted with pride that the pill version seemed to work as well as the IV preparation, with just about the same rate of efficacy and side effects, and could cost less. He asked the cancer doctors how they might use such a new drug in their practices.

"Is it any better than the IV version?" asked one experienced oncologist.

"No," said the company rep, "but it seems to be every bit as good."

"Then I wouldn't use it," replied the doctor.

"Why not?"

"Because that's how I earn a living. The IV chemo payments from Medicare help pay for my nurse, my whole practice. Unless the pill form worked better, I'd have no reason to switch."

Oncology has been a growth business for the pharmaceutical industry in many respects, some of which influence clinical research as well. To market a new chemotherapy product, its manufacturer must present the FDA with evidence that it is effective in human trials. Thousands of patients must be enrolled annually in such studies, and companies generally pay physicians on a per-patient basis to enlist the requisite number of subjects. Many oncologists and cancer centers derive substantial support from enrolling their patients in these trials. In routine practice, the issue of the physician's economic incentive comes up again; in the academic setting, it can create a different kind of tension. Another young oncologist training at one of the nation's premier cancer centers was anguished as he told me of the pressures such research was causing in the institution. Here is the gist of what he said:

> We're all eager to enroll patients for studies of exciting new treatments. But more and more we're also asked to sign up patients for company-funded trials just so they can get approval for a drug that no one expects will be anything special. Most of those products are likely to work about as well as what we already have, since they're just clones of existing forms of chemo. But the center relies on the income it gets to run these studies. "It helps us fund our other research," they tell us. "It's how we pay for the nurses and the social workers and all the free care we give." That's probably true. But there's also a lot of pressure to participate in these studies for my own academic advancement, so I can be a co-author of the paper when it comes out. Where does that leave me when I have a cancer patient I've been taking care of for a long time, and I'm told to enroll them in one of these trials? They trust me so much after what we've been through together they'd jump off a bridge if I told them to. When I ask for their informed consent to enroll in one of these studies they just say, "Whatever you think, doc." Am I really doing this for them? Or so that I can have my name on some research paper? Or so that the drug company can market a ho-hum product? Or so we can pay for the expensive chemo that's really needed by some other patient who doesn't have insurance? It's getting so I don't know why I'm doing this anymore.

Figuring out how to contain this pervasive marketization of therapeutics could make treating metastatic cancer look simple in comparison.

THE TIES THAT ENTANGLE

Early in my career, at many elite institutions "drug company money" was seen, sometimes unfairly, as a lesser kind of research funding, inferior to peer-reviewed grant support from the National Institutes of Health. Things have changed. Manufacturers have become more willing to support basic biomedical research, as long as restrictive licensing and intellectual property provisions are put in place. At the same time, a more unpredictable federal budget threatens a financial squeeze that could put many researchers under financial pressure. Academic physicians traditionally had considerable flexibility in underwriting some of their activities with revenues from other sources. Public training subsidies to teaching hospitals helped pay the salaries of young doctors who also participated in laboratory work and taught medical students; clinical payments from patients with insurance helped cover the free care given to those who had none; and patient-care revenues contributed to the support of young researchers until their first grants came through. But at the same time that Medicare tightened the reins on its payments to doctors and academic medical centers, other insurers such as HMOs were doing the same. All the sources for cross-subsidizing research and junior faculty support became constrained at the same time.

Growing federal deficits now threaten an end to the rapid growth of NIH funding, which had seemed to offer so much promise to medical researchers at the turn of the twenty-first century. Concurrent tax cuts left little room for increases in any discretionary federal spending once entitlement programs like Social Security and Medicare were paid for. Add in growth in the military budget, and the prospects for further increases in publicly funded medical research became even dimmer.

Ever alert to opportunity, pharmaceutical manufacturers increased their research and training grants to the nation's medical schools and academic hospitals. The industry was flush with cash from record sales and profits, and was becoming more interested in the potentially marketable discoveries being made in university laboratories. For about the same cost as an all-out marketing blitz for a new product, a company could buy the rights to all the discoveries that came from a university-based lab it supported.

With the future of federal funding increasingly unsure, such industry support has become more attractive each year—even payment for marketing-driven clinical trials that have minimal novelty or scientific importance. Company dollars also stream in for support of medical school continuing education programs. One observer worried about the effect all this was having on universities' independence:

As a result [of reliance on industry-supported drug studies], the university's commercial interests are in conflict with its responsibility to reach honest, objective results, however harmful they may be to the sponsor's bottom line. The risks created by such conflicts are not fanciful; investigators have shown that clinical trials supported by industry are much more likely to arrive at conclusions favorable to their sponsors than independently funded work on the same drugs. . . .

The clearest example has occurred in medical schools where large pharmaceutical firms and medical supply companies have become very wealthy at a time when traditional sources of funding for medical education have tended to dry up. These trends have created a vacuum major corporations are all too willing to fill. . . .

Universities may not yet be willing to trade all of their academic values for money, but they have proceeded much further down that road than they are generally willing to acknowledge. . . . In the all-important domains of education and research, academic leaders still have the power to develop appropriate policies. A possible exception is continuing medical education, where the dependence on corporate support has reached such a point that it will be difficult for medical schools to free themselves of industry influence.

Skeptics might dismiss such dire warnings if they came from the pen of Ralph Nader or Noam Chomsky. But the words are those of Derek Bok, president of Harvard University from 1971 to 1991.

Shortly before the start of Bok's tenure, when I was just beginning my training, I was in a group of students who staged a brief sit-in in the dean's office at Harvard Medical School to protest (among other things) the fact that he had agreed to serve on the board of directors of Squibb Pharmaceuticals. It seemed to us that given his responsibility for our training in pharmacology, and for the clinical research that went on at the medical school and its teaching hospitals, this represented a potential conflict of interest, or at least the appearance of one. I remember the afternoon clearly, because of the irony of having to choose between going to the demonstration and attending an important lecture, "The Inflammatory Response."

Three decades later, few are surprised to learn that medical school chairs and teaching hospital CEOs sit on the boards of directors of the pharmaceutical firms with which their institutions do business; the practice no longer raises much controversy.

Potential conflicts of interest are often most pervasive at the nation's elite research-intensive institutions. The men and women who conduct cutting-edge medical research are deeply committed, sometimes driven people; they know that their work, if successful, could substantially reduce illness and suffering, maybe in millions of people, perhaps for generations. The progress of that work is all-important; the accounting details of who's footing the bill often don't seem as vital as the need to keep the research adequately funded. The academic community is deeply worried that governmental support for biomedical science is subject to the passing moods of Congress and the administration, and more recently to growing deficits. If the drug industry has deeper research pockets than government and comes with an open checkbook, it should not be surprising that its help is welcomed enthusiastically. Eventual ripple effects on the cost of medications, or on the identity of the university, usually go unnoticed at the laboratory bench.

The more that medical schools and their teaching hospitals become dependent on support from industry to fund their research and educational activities, the easier it is for their faculties to become convinced that what's good for those companies is good for their institutions—and for American health care as a whole. Add the prospect of personal gain if a study leads to a marketable product, and it's understandable that medical school scientists have accepted industry support so avidly.

Another kind of influence is at work here as well, at the personal level. Consider the situation of a university researcher who receives years of grants or contracts from a drug maker to help develop a new drug and then to conduct a clinical trial to test it. It's difficult to maintain the humility needed to conclude that the new treatment is only trivially better than other products already on the market, or isn't worth its price, or offers no advantage at all. This cognitive dissonance is intensified if the professor is also paid generously by the manufacturer to travel around the country reporting on the results of those studies to medical audiences.

Academic medical centers face one final set of conflicts if their faculty members set out to critically evaluate the worth of new medical technologies, whether they are drugs, costly invasive procedures, or diagnostic tests. Providing those interventions is what these places do for a living. It's what gives them an advantage over one another, and especially over lower-tech hospitals that the present business model depicts as the competition. Colleagues who ask impertinent questions about the possible overuse of these technologies, or their cost-effectiveness, threaten the tenuous fiscal integrity of the very institutions that employ them.

The architect Louis Sullivan taught us over a century ago that form follows function, but the lesson we need to learn in the present context is that *function follows funding.* For good reason, industry showers our academic medical centers with grants and contracts to study costly new treatments, and often provides us with those medications at cost, so our trainees can get used to prescribing them. The result is a tilt toward drugs that are new and scientifically fashionable, even if they are not a good value or are little better than what we used before. This in turn helps to mold the standard of care in these trend-setting facilities. Teaching hospitals are at risk of becoming an excessively user-friendly back-end entryway into the health care delivery system, through which very expensive new products are injected into routine practice. Even if each individual contract is a plausible agreement made between consenting adults, we have to worry about the effects this can have overall on the institutions that shape our trainees and set the tone for medical care as a whole.

There is one final concern to raise about the public-to-private shift in support for medical studies. Traditionally in American science, an individual researcher would come up with a good idea for a study, and then submit an investigator-initiated grant application to NIH or another federal funding source. The proposal would be judged by other academic scientists through a rigorous and highly decentralized peer-review system, made possible by the voluntary efforts of researchers at universities throughout the country. Funding depended primarily on whether a proposal was seen as scientifically important, regardless of its commercial potential. That process led to the most impressive flowering of biomedical discovery in human history. The checks may have been issued by the U.S. Treasury, but the nation's scientific community itself decided which grants to award.

We now face the growing privatization of medical research, indirectly funded (ironically enough) by oversized payments to drug manufacturers from governmental and private sources. This development may be welcomed by those who also seek the further privatization of education, welfare, prisons, defense, police, and other aspects of life, but it's not clear that it makes for the best science policy. With growing constraints on NIH budgets, as industry-friendly legislation and regulation enhance the flow of dollars to drug makers, we increase our dependence on these corporations for breakthrough medical discoveries. But market-driven incentives will primarily yield market-oriented products. Further commercial control over the process may give us more treatments for lucrative conditions like heartburn and allergy that will sell well, but it may not represent the smartest way to strengthen the nation's biomedical research infrastructure.

During his presidency, Dwight Eisenhower was an unwavering proponent of a strong national defense. But it was Eisenhower who coined the term "military-industrial complex" to warn that an excessively powerful defense industry could gain undue influence over the formation of national policy. Decades later, others modified the term to warn about the effects of a growing "medical-industrial complex." Like Ike, we can support the principle of a strong domestic industrial infrastructure at the same time that we work to ensure that its strength not be used to distort national priorities to meet corporate interests at the expense of the public interest.

14: WHAT THE TRAFFIC WILL BEAR

In trying to pay the nation's growing medication bill, Americans face a perfect storm of demographic, scientific, economic, and policy trends. People over sixty-five form an expanding segment of the population; our collective drug expenditure would rise on this basis alone even if everything else remained constant, since older people require more medications than the young. But of course everything else doesn't remain constant. Prices of drugs—both patented and generic—edge higher each year, considerably outstripping inflation. Medical research leads to the introduction of new products; a few are important breakthroughs and nearly all cost more, even if they aren't. Spurred by billions spent on promotion to both doctors and patients, market share is prodded toward the highest-priced drugs to treat a given problem even when they may not be worth their higher costs.

We currently spend more than $200 billion a year on medications in the United States. This accounts for only a small portion of a total health care budget that will soon reach $2 trillion, but its impact on the system as a whole is substantial. Spending on prescription drugs has become the fastest-growing component of all American health care costs, rising 13–19 percent per year and doubling between 1995 and 2002. This doubling occurred during the same period that spending for hospital care went up by only a fifth, and for doctors and other clinical services by only a third.

Drug cost increases may have initially been invisible to many doctors and the citizenry as a whole, but their impact eventually comes back to bite the patient, taxpayer, and employer. People fortunate enough to have generous prescription drug coverage (and their numbers are shrinking fast) used to think of their medications as being available "for free," or for a very modest copayment. State Medicaid programs traditionally covered virtually all prescription drug expenses for the very poor, though these budgets are now under unprecedented fiscal pressure. Several states, like Pennsylvania and New Jersey, established their own programs to pay for the drug expenses of less-poor elderly as well.

In recent years, the burden of high drug costs fell heaviest on the working poor who held jobs that didn't provide health insurance, and on the nation's elderly. The pressure on these groups was intensified by a cruel economic hit reserved just for them. Medicaid, the Veterans Administration, HMOs, and other insurers have massive purchasing power that enables them to demand price breaks from drug manufacturers, but individual uncovered patients don't. Ironically, those with no coverage are among the only Americans who still have to pay full price for their drugs.

As costs increased, even people with drug coverage found insurers raising the patient's share of each prescription, the copayment, from negligible to substantial. This helped contain insurers' costs, but left many patients to try to decide which of their prescriptions they could manage to fill. The anecdotal experience of many doctors has been borne out by several papers in the medical literature showing that patients in this vulnerable uncovered zone often did not take their prescribed medications because they just couldn't afford to. The consequences include the undertreatment of symptomatic illness, or a devastating event such as heart attack, stroke, or hip fracture that generates both misery and enormous cost.

When shifting the burden of payment to patients didn't contain expenditures sufficiently, many employers and HMOs put stringent limits on their drug benefits, or ended them altogether. The most extreme reaction was simply to terminate health care coverage—a course that small employers were often forced to take as their share of drug-inflated medical insurance became unaffordable. Ending coverage has also been an attractive business strategy for many investor-owned HMOs. In the 1980s, these companies entered what seemed to be a lucrative market by promising generous prescription coverage to older Americans frustrated that Medicare offered no help with their outpatient drug bills. But this loss-leader marketing strategy turned out to be self-defeating. The arrangement often proved unprofitable, particularly because of those rising drug costs. As a result many HMOs withdrew from the Medicare market, effectively "firing" millions of elderly enrollees by terminating their coverage. Most of those patients lost their drug insurance when they were bounced back into conventional Medicare.

Passage of prescription drug coverage under Medicare in late 2003 initially offered hope that the burden of unaffordable drug bills would be lifted for elderly Americans. But major lapses quickly became apparent. Negotiated largely behind closed doors with heavy input from the pharmaceutical and insurance industries, and passed with little time for debate (just one day's worth in the Senate), the bill raised as many problems as it proposed to solve. Whereas many nations enact laws to empower their governments to negotiate lower drug prices from manufacturers, this law did the opposite—it expressly forbade the government from seeking better drug prices for Medicare enrollees. (No such privilege is extended to hospitals or physicians, whose payments are set by the Medicare program.) It contained a dizzying collection of deductibles and copayments, crowned by what policy analysts termed a "doughnut hole" region in which coverage abruptly ceases for patients with high but not catastrophic levels of drug expenses. Another surprising prohibition: the new law made it illegal for older patients to purchase supplemental insurance to cover the numerous gaps the new law mandated.

Perhaps the greatest lapse of the Medicare drug entitlement lay in what it failed to do: it almost totally ignored the need to improve the appropriateness and cost-effectiveness of what doctors prescribe. In fact, skeptics worried that it would have exactly the opposite effect: by forcing the federal government to underwrite the costs of all marketed drugs, regardless of their clinical or economic value, it seemed destined to channel more and more dollars into the costliest (and hence most aggressively marketed) products. Within weeks of its passage, the White House had revised its projected cost upward by over a hundred billion dollars. Medicare enrollees might pay less at the drugstore, but far more would be paid (less visibly) in taxes and premiums, or through deficit spending.

Thus the new entitlement would likely do little to contain overall drug costs; to the contrary, it seemed designed to increase them. But for the private sector, the rate of increase in drug expenditures is unsustainable. For some large companies, paying the drug bills of employees and retirees now consumes fully a quarter of their entire outlay for health care. Few industries can tolerate such large annual increases in the expense of a major line item without feeling strong fiscal stress and reacting to that stress. When it comes to their drug benefit programs, American corporations are living out an allegory told in management courses as "The Tale of the Two Frogs." Frog One is tossed into a pot of boiling water on a stove; feeling the pain of the heat, he immediately jumps out and survives. Frog Two is tossed into a pot of cool water, and swims around happily as the burner is turned on. The increase in heat is gradual, and the frog doesn't notice how hot it has gotten until he has been boiled to death. Many of those responsible for drug expenditures in industry, HMOs, or government programs have begun to realize that they've spent the last decade behaving like Frog Two, and are desperately trying to escape the pot before it's too late.

If nearly all the other industrialized nations can ensure that their citizens are able to pay for the medications they need, why can't the United States?

SAME PRODUCTS, DIFFERENT PRICES

It is now widely known that a given prescription can cost an American patient up to twice what the same drug made by the same company will cost a patient in Canada, England, or most of continental Europe. The Organisation for Economic Co-operation and Development is a multinational consortium that tracks data on economic activity in about thirty nations. A recent OECD report compared drug expenditures in fourteen advanced industrial countries. The average amount spent per capita on medications in the United States was 65 percent higher than the average per capita drug expenditure in the rest of these nations, all of which have highly developed economies. At the time of the OECD study the U.S. figure was the second highest in the world, just a bit behind the pharmacophilic French. The survey data didn't include medications used in hospitals; if those had been counted, total U.S. drug expenses would have risen to number one. All of Western Europe, Australia, and Japan had per-person drug expenses substantially lower than ours. It is not because our population is older; many of those countries have higher proportions of elderly than we do.

We Americans are often perversely proud of how much we spend on things, perhaps assuming that if we pay a lot for a product or service it must be of high quality. (As Barbara Tuchman noted, this helps explain the popularity of powdered pearls as a treatment for the Black Plague.) But a systematic survey of patients in five English-speaking countries doesn't confirm the idea that spending more has made Americans more content about their prescription drugs. The U.S. citizens took more medications than respondents in Australia, Canada, the United Kingdom, and New Zealand, but they also reported the highest rates of side effects, of skipping doses to make a prescription last longer, and of not being able to fill a prescription at all because of its cost. (This last problem was reported by one in three American patients; an earlier survey found that the rate was one in two for the half of Americans with incomes below the national average, if they lacked health insurance.)

Our high-end drug expenses must be considered in the context of the rest of the U.S. health care system, which is also the costliest in the world. Here, too, the OECD comparisons are embarrassing. The group measured total medical care expenditures in nineteen advanced industrial nations in 2000—most of Western Europe, Japan, Australia, and Canada. In those nations the total average per capita price tag for all medical care, converted to U.S. dollars, was just $1,696 per year. In the United States it was $4,165—about two and a half times the average. (The per capita figure for 2004 is over $6,000, according to the Department of Health and Human Services.) Put differently, America spends about 15 percent of its entire gross domestic product on medical care, compared to only about 7–9 percent of GDP spent by nearly every other advanced country. In our $11 trillion economy, a few percent of GDP amounts to hundreds of billions of dollars. This is not a new trend; as far back as the 1980s, General Motors calculated that it was spending more per car on health care for its workers than it did on steel. For another industrial behemoth, General Electric, by 2003 health insurance had become the single largest category of expenditure across the entire company. These numbers have considerable implications for our competitiveness in a global economy, a concern we'll return to later.

Our outspending the rest of the world on drugs and other medical care might be worth doing if it produced better health outcomes for Americans, but it doesn't. OECD data show that the United States ranks nineteenth out of thirty countries in life expectancy at birth, fourteenth of twenty-nine in life expectancy at age sixty-five, and twenty-fourth out of thirty in infant mortality. For that measure, although different countries define infant deaths differently, of all the nations tracked by OECD only South Korea, Slovakia, Hungary, Poland, Mexico, and Turkey recorded worse numbers than we did. Nor are we more content with the care we get. In the five-country survey, 44 percent of American patients reported being dissatisfied with the nation's health care system, with 48 percent identifying its high cost as a major problem—over twice the rate observed in any of the other countries studied. A larger study of nationally representative samples of over seven thousand people across the same five countries found that 79 percent of U.S. respondents thought the health care system needed to undergo fundamental change or be rebuilt completely.

Americans who can afford it can indeed get some of the best medical care in the world. But these figures (and a great deal of other outcome data just like them) demonstrate that the average American pays much more for drugs and health care that aren't much better in quality or results than what the typical Western European, Canadian, or Japanese gets. And then there are the nation's over 40 million uninsured, most of them the working poor and their families, who have to rely on emergency rooms or charity clinics to get any care or medicines at all. These facts cast doubt on the supposed efficiency and quality of our marketplace approach to medical care.

It's unfair to compare the rate of rise in American drug costs to increases in other commodities like food and housing. A loaf of bread or a single-family house bought in 2004 may well be no better than the same commodity bought in 1974 (and in the case of the bread, it may even be worse). But today's medications are much better products than the drugs of thirty years ago, a fact often neglected in these calculations. It's therefore helpful to consider a different comparison.

The other great scientific success story of recent decades has been the information technology revolution. As with drugs, the latest tech products are dramatically better than what was available years ago. An Intel chip made in 1971 could handle about 100,000 instructions per second; a single microprocessor today can handle 3 billion instructions per second. The contrast is even more striking when we calculate the cost of information processing during these periods. At the start of the 1970s, one transistor cost about a dollar. Today, that same processing power costs one fifty-millionth of a dollar. Exponentially greater effectiveness accompanied by falling prices has also characterized information hardware, from cell phones to computers—remember that first clunky pocket calculator you bought in the 1970s for a hundred bucks? The science and power of computing technology have gotten amazingly better (would that our drugs had improved so much!), yet their costs have dropped at the same time. Granted, there are important differences between chips and drugs. But the information technology comparison raises provocative questions about just how much of the rising cost of drugs can be accounted for solely by the better-product explanation.

GRANNY AS CROSS-BORDER DRUG TRAFFICKER

We've seen that while some governments influence drug prices by keeping them down, ours has used its regulatory authority to keep them high. A new staple of the morning paper and evening news is the photogenic spectacle of groups of elderly people in Maine, Texas, and other border states climbing onto buses to go fill their prescriptions in Canada or Mexico. This geriatric hajj called attention to the remarkable discrepancy in the price of the same medicine for American patients versus our neighbors to the north and south. Outside the United States, the prices of prescription drugs are regulated by national governments (as in Canada), or kept low because that's all the market can pay (as in Mexico). These are often the very same products, made by the same major drug companies in the same factories that supply American drugstores.

This new kind of drug trafficking hasn't been limited to retirees. Since the mid-1990s, and even more frantically in the new century, state governments have seen their Medicaid expenses grow much faster than the rest of their budgets, with medications driving a substantial portion of that increase. These officials have begun coming together to consider joint purchasing arrangements to take advantage of cross-national price differentials. And individual Americans are logging onto the internet to fill their prescriptions at pharmacy sites based in Canada exactly as they would for mail-order pharmacy services based in the United States. They have read the headlines about the benefits of the new global economy and are acting accordingly.

In response to this growing trend and to demands that something be done to make drugs more affordable, several years ago Congress passed legislation called the Medicine Equity and Drug Safety Act of 2000, which had been quietly inserted into an agricultural appropriations bill. The law would have made it legal for Americans to buy drugs from sources outside the United States, such as in Canada, as long as those drugs were manufactured in the United States. That seemed innocuous enough, as did the requirement that before the new law could take effect, the U.S. secretary of health and human services would have to certify that use of such products would be safe and would save money for Americans, pretty plausible assumptions. But in the last weeks of the Clinton administration, HHS secretary Donna Shalala ruled that she could not certify either of these conditions, and the law was never implemented.

The pharmaceutical industry, although it benefits from many aspects of globalization, including the right to buy its supplies wherever on earth it can get the best deal, has not been as eager for American consumers or health care purchasers to be able to do the same thing. It raised fears about "foreign drugs" by casting xenophobic doubts on their safety and quality. In 2002, Congress again debated a bill that would make it legal for Americans to fill their prescriptions in Canada. Virtually all of these drugs were to be products manufactured by U.S. companies or their Canadian subsidiaries. Facing the threat of Americans importing drugs directly from those sources at lower prices, the drug industry mounted a response that might have come right out of *Dr. Strangelove*. It warned that "foreign handling" of these prescriptions would result in "loss of potency" and "adulteration." It ran an advertisement depicting two identical-looking pills over the caption "QUICK. PICK THE CAPSULE THAT HASN'T BEEN TAMPERED WITH." (Implication: it's the one that didn't pass through un-American hands.) The industry ad cited the support not just of the FDA and the HHS, but also of the U.S. Customs Service and the federal Drug Enforcement Agency, arms of government that usually worry about protecting us from very different kinds of drugs. The ad warned that allowing Americans to fill prescriptions in Canada "could open America's medicine cabinets to an influx of dangerous drugs," and closed with an exhortation to "KEEP BLACK MARKET DRUGS OUT OF AMERICA." In a further response to what might be called the Maple Peril, several large drug companies threatened to stop supplying their products to any Canadian wholesaler or retailer that knowingly sold them to American customers.

Recognition for the best commingling of fearful themes must go to HHS secretary Tommy Thompson. In arguing against the bill, he warned that "opening our borders to reimported drugs potentially could increase the flow of counterfeit drugs, cheap foreign copies of FDA-approved drugs [what the rest of us call generics], expired and contaminated drugs, and drugs stored under inappropriate and unsafe conditions." Granted, the unavailability of refrigeration in remote areas is a problem for vaccine programs in the Third World, but . . . *Canada*? Thompson's argument in 2002 climaxed with a strange conclusion: "In light of the anthrax attacks of last fall, that's a risk we simply cannot take."

One might have expected the FDA to intervene on behalf of the public and establish a means of certifying which imported drugs pass U.S. standards, exactly as it presently does for products manufactured abroad by large multinational pharmaceutical companies. Instead, it responded to the Maple Peril by aligning itself firmly on the side of the drug industry, stating that imported drugs could pose a major threat to the health of the nation, and that it was powerless to do anything about it. In the face of all the legitimate concerns of doctors and patients about real drug side effects, the FDA's most visible public pronouncements about risk in recent years dealt instead with the supposed hazards of drugs from Canada—despite the near-total absence of any scientific evidence substantiating this risk.

PATENTLY DISTORTED

Patent law is another tool governments can employ to influence the price of drugs as well as the pace of discovery. The patent system was originally intended to encourage innovation by enabling inventors and research-intensive companies to profit from their discoveries throughout a period of legally protected exclusivity, during which no one else could manufacture or sell a product they had developed. Yet the way these laws have been interpreted and enforced in the last twenty years has paradoxically also done much to spur *non*innovative pharmaceutical research. By the early 2000s, regulatory flaccidity and legal precedent had created an odd situation in which once a drug patent expired, the innovator company could routinely sue the first generic manufacturer that tried to market its product, automatically delaying availability of the lower-cost version by thirty months or more.

Industry lawyers went on to devise Byzantine new distortions of the basic patent concept. Beyond the patent on the original discovery, the courts allowed patents to proliferate on sometimes trivial details of the way the drug is made, minuscule changes in its formulation within a tablet or capsule, even its appearance. Suits based on such patents could then be stacked up in layers one upon the other, with each used to justify its own lawsuit and potentially its own lengthy patent extension, further delaying competition for years. In the business, this came to be known as "evergreening" an aging product.

Another practice is the use of chemical shortcuts to replace real innovation in drug research; it is starkly illustrated by two blockbusters, the allergy pill Clarinex and the stomach-acid drug Nexium. Clarinex was simply the normal metabolic product of the same company's older allergy pill Claritin, whose patent was expiring: when you take Claritin, your liver immediately transforms it into the molecule newly patented as Clarinex, hardly a medical breakthrough. Similarly, the new "purple pill" Nexium was simply the L-isomer twin of the older stomach-acid suppressor Prilosec—the same molecule made by the same company, but just the "left-handed" configuration rather than a mix of the left- and right-handed versions, with no clearly demonstrated clinical advantage. As new chemical entities, each could be patented and promoted afresh to add lucrative years to the blockbuster careers of both parent compounds. (Why anyone would want to prescribe, no less pay for, such costly chimeras is another matter, which we'll take up later.) In other instances, Congress has simply given away patent life extensions for activities that could have been seen as a routine cost of doing business, such as the six additional months of added patent protection for each product tested in children.

Although the pharmaceutical industry extols the virtues of unfettered markets, several companies have developed creative strategies to disable those very markets. A shadier response to patent expiration is for the innovator company to quietly pay a potential generic competitor *not* to produce a cheaper version of its product once the patent expires. The size of that payoff may be larger than the slim profits the generics maker would have earned in the first few years of production, and will cost the innovator company less than it would have lost to generic competition. Everyone comes out ahead—except for the patient or whoever is paying the drug bills.

Some of these tactics became egregious enough to provoke the ire of the Bush administration Federal Trade Commission, which became concerned about drug companies that appeared to value the "free" in the free enterprise system more than the "enterprise." In Senate testimony on competition in the pharmaceutical industry, FTC chairman Timothy Muris reported that some companies "attempted to 'game' the system, securing greater profits for themselves without providing a corresponding benefit to consumers." His accusations were laced with terms like "monopoly" and "abuses." In separate testimony before the House, Muris described an FTC report that analyzed what happens when a drug's patent expires. In 72 percent of the cases studied, he noted, the brand-name manufacturer initiated a patent infringement lawsuit against the first company that tried to market a generic version of its product. Of these cases, 70 percent were settled outside of court. Looking back over all such cases in which the courts did rule, the FTC found that the generic manufacturer eventually prevailed 73 percent of the time. Yet each such automatic lawsuit led to its own thirty-month delay in the marketing of a generic product. Legislation was proposed in 2003 to curb some but not all of these excesses.

The FTC used some of its strongest language in antitrust charges against Bristol-Myers Squibb, accusing the company of a decade-long pattern of illegally blocking the availability of generic versions of its drugs. According to the agency, the company "avoided competition by abusing federal regulations," deceived the Patent and Trademark Office by submitting fraudulent and misleading claims, and offered another company a $72 million bribe not to market a generic version of one of its products. The FTC was especially critical of the company's behavior in derailing generic competition for two widely used cancer chemotherapy drugs, Platinol and its profitable NIH-supported Taxol. A third manipulated product was the antianxiety drug BuSpar. I recalled a sales pitch I had been given for BuSpar when it was first marketed; the company sales rep urged me to try the tranquilizer in patients who were dependent on alcohol or narcotics, noting that it was free of abuse potential. He apparently was referring to its abuse by patients, not by patent attorneys.

In announcing a settlement with BMS, FTC chairman Muris brought the matter down to ground level. He charged that "Bristol's illegal conduct protected nearly $2 billion in yearly sales from the three monopolies, forcing cancer patients and others to overpay by hundreds of millions of dollars for important and often life-saving medications." That refers only to those who could pay; we cannot know how many cancer patients had to forgo treatment because they couldn't afford the higher-than-legal prices for the chemotherapy they required. To settle the FTC's antitrust charges, BMS agreed to curtail its practice of automatically filing new patent claims to block generic competition. Following litigation by several state attorneys general and other corporations, it also paid a $670 million settlement to resolve additional antitrust charges.

A RISKY BUSINESS?

Just as the effectiveness and safety of a drug depend on how it's handled in a particular clinical context, the price of a drug is also not a fixed property of the molecule. It doesn't really reflect the cost of manufacturing the drug, which is far smaller. It does not even closely track the cost of developing that drug. Rather, a medicine's price is a social and political construct shaped by the interactions of manufacturers, payers, and governments, as well as other less powerful players. A major explanation offered by the pharmaceutical industry for its high prices is that discovering new drugs is a vulnerable and expensive undertaking. Most new products are destined to fail somewhere along the lengthy pathway from lab to marketplace because they turn out not to work, or to have unacceptable side effects. As in any business, we are reminded, high risk must be accompanied by high reward or capital will flee elsewhere.

But if an economic argument is being made, the numbers need to bear up under scrutiny. If riskiness is determined by the predictability of return on investment, until recently the economic data made the pharmaceutical industry look about as risky as U.S. Treasury notes. For most of the past decade, the pharmaceutical sector has been the single most profitable industry group in the nation, year in and year out. Profit as a percentage of revenue has been more lucrative each year for the drug industry than for any other: 17 percent recently, compared to a median of about 3 percent for all Fortune 500 companies. It is true that many promising drugs fail before generating a profit. But for the large pharmaceutical companies, their stable of successful products has thus far been substantial and reliable enough to generate very handsome returns to investors every year. (Their recent downturn in profitability doesn't appear to result from greater inherent riskiness of the industry, but rather from the companies' problems in maintaining innovation, several high-profile side effect debacles, and growing resistance to very high prices.)

Another reason the companies have been so singularly profitable is their capacity to induce demand on the part of physicians and patients. Marketing a drug effectively can increase the number of people who want to use it and the amount that can be charged for it, well beyond its actual clinical benefit or economic value. This results from the very poor diffusion of expertise and decision-making clout in the health care system. The laws of supply and demand don't work well when those who control the supply also have a disproportionate influence over the demand. This conclusion is not ideologically driven: it is based on observing the astonishing mismatch between the way expensive drugs are used and the way their pharmacology suggests they ought to be used.

PAYING FOR LIFE

Consider the following segment from the evening news a few years from now:

[Wide shot of a crowd of about a hundred people marching slowly in a circle in front of a tall office building; many look chronically ill. Several carry signs that read "DON'T MAKE US DIE!" and "PATIENTS BEFORE PROFITS."]

FIRST REPORTER: We're standing in front of the U.S. headquarters of Croesus Pharmaceuticals. The Swiss-based drug giant is at the center of a firestorm of controversy over its pricing of Gonifimab, the new biotech blockbuster that is the first drug capable of actually curing several different forms of cancer. Let's talk to one of the demonstrators. *[Approaches one of the picketers, a gaunt middle-aged woman with pale skin and a few wisps of hair.]* Ma'am, what brings you out here today?

DEMONSTRATOR: I have colon cancer, the same kind of tumor that they showed Gonifimab could cure. I don't have the $60,000 a year it costs to buy the drug, and the disease is killing me.

REPORTER: Isn't there some way you could get help in paying for it?

DEMONSTRATOR: My company laid me off when I got sick, so I don't have health insurance anymore. I've been working two other jobs to put food on the table, but they don't provide any medical coverage. I'd have to quit work to qualify for Medicaid, but with all their deficits they can't pay for everyone who wants the drug. So they set up a lottery. It's only open to people under sixty, and I'm sixty-one.

REPORTER: What about Medicare?

DEMONSTRATOR: I won't be eligible until I'm sixty-five, and there's talk they're going to raise that to sixty-seven because of all the economic troubles. My doctor says I'll be dead long before that. He's trying to get me into a hospice for terminal care. It's just not fair.

REPORTER *[looking upward]:* Eighty stories above us, my colleague is talking to a representative of the company at the center of this controversy. Over to you, Susan.

SECOND REPORTER *[in a large office suite overlooking the city]:* I'm here with Dr. Rob Klepton, CEO of the U.S. division of Croesus Pharmaceuticals.

KLEPTON: That's "Mr.," Susan. I'm not a doctor.

REPORTER: Mr. Klepton, you have this major breakthrough product on the market, but many people with cancer can't pay for it and are dying as a result. What is the company doing about it?

KLEPTON: Of course, any death is lamentable, but medical research is expensive. We need to charge what we do to recoup our research costs in developing Gonifimab, and to enable us to discover the powerful new medicines of tomorrow.

REPORTER: But isn't it true that you didn't actually develop the drug, but licensed it from a small Japanese biotechnology company? And wasn't their work based heavily on discoveries made in Boston by university researchers funded by government grants?

KLEPTON: Susan, the business of drug development is very complicated and costly, and we can't get into all the details here. What matters is that we own the patent on the drug, and the courts have upheld our ability to protect that intellectual property. But the company has set up a program to help all Americans who may have trouble paying for the treatment.

REPORTER: Yes, we've looked into that program. It does lower the annual price to just $30,000 a year, and we've spoken to twenty patients who applied for it. Half were told that they didn't qualify, and the other half were put on a waiting list that is now eighteen months long. Don't you have a responsibility to make this drug more affordable?

KLEPTON: I feel great sympathy for all those people with cancer who can't afford to have it cured. But here at Croesus we have many responsibilities, Susan. I'm also responsible to our shareholders, who didn't invest their hard-earned cash with us so that we could give away our products, or price them at less than their market value. What company would do that? I'm also responsible to the next generations, so that we can take those record profits Gonifimab has made possible and plow them back into discovering the miraculous cures that will benefit future patients.

REPORTER: And so the debate continues. Back to you, Bill.

The example is only barely fictional. Each year sees the introduction of new products for cancer and other dread diseases, born of the accelerating revolution in biotechnology. They have Martian-sounding trade names like Bexxar, Ontak, Zevalin, and Raptiva, and some cost from $15,000 to $30,000 for a year or even a single cycle of treatment. The Gonifimab scenario is just around the next corner.

This is not an easy time to ask provocative questions about the limits of free markets. Despite the fond hopes of the left for a century and a half, state-controlled economies created systems that turned out to be fiscally, intellectually, and morally bankrupt. Even the kinder, gentler manifestations of European socialism have raised questions about whether too much governmental involvement in economic affairs can hamper growth and overall prosperity. Nations that have embraced free enterprise, from the United States to China, have increased their wealth substantially. At the beginning of the twenty-first century, many find it pathetically retro to warn of the dangers of unlimited corporate freedom.

But just as the last century proved the ineptitude of planned economies and excessive government intervention, we now risk demonstrating the opposite: the downsides of unfettered corporate license, and the risks of inadequate public oversight of markets. For many sectors of the economy, such as computers, clothing, food, and automobiles, the marketplace works reasonably well with only modest regulation. For others, like housing, energy, and telecommunications, history teaches us that more governmental oversight is essential. And for one key component of society, the delivery of health care, we are finding that a laissez-faire marketplace approach hasn't worked well at all.

In medicine, a fair fight between seller and buyer is implausible because a well-functioning market requires several conditions that just don't apply: the buyer must be able to understand the product well enough to decide on its quality, as well as the reasonableness of its price. He or she must be able to shop around and compare choices before making a purchasing decision. And society has to be comfortable with the prospect that some people may not be able to afford to buy the goods or services that others can, and may have to do without them. None of these assumptions can be counted on when it comes to health care. The ability of the typical patient to decide what medications he or she needs is inherently different from the decision to buy a sedan versus a minivan. It's hard even for experts to determine whether a particular drug is worth its sticker price. And although we can live with the fact that some Americans don't have cars or computers or cable, we are repelled (or should be) at the idea that our poorer citizens could become sick and die if they can't afford a lifesaving drug.

These problems explain why government's involvement in pharmaceuticals must be quite different from its participation in industries whose products are more easily evaluated, or don't impact so heavily on our basic human values. In health care, unbridled corporate zeal is like a powerful medicine of its own: as Paracelsus reminded us, whether it acts as a tonic or a poison will greatly depend on the dose. Profit may be the oxygen of commerce, but too much oxygen can sometimes be toxic. On the other hand, a completely government-dominated drug industry could suffocate patients, doctors, and researchers alike. The most productive political dialogue in the coming years will be the debate on which aspects of American life are best left to the market and which will need to be protected from it, and how. Nowhere will this conversation be more important than in the area of medicine in general, and medicines in particular.

Our imaginary vignette could have been even worse. Much important work that was once under the auspices of the federal Human Genome Project is now performed in spin-off corporations. Religious conservatives' antagonism to fetal stem cell research has shut off federal support in this area, driving nearly all of that promising activity out of the public sector, much of it into investor-owned laboratories. With the increasing privatization of so many aspects of medical research, the new cancer cure could well be discovered within the walls of one or more companies, and end up wholly owned by a single commercial entity. In our what-the-traffic-will-bear system, that company could in principle charge anything it wanted.

The phrase "Is nothing sacred?" comes to mind here. If we move too far down that road, there aren't enough antidepressants, sleeping pills, or anxiety drugs in the world to enable most of us to live comfortably with the likely outcome.

The nation resolved the question of whether the government should get involved in medical care decades ago, with the passage of the first Pure Food and Drug Act in 1906 and of Medicare and Medicaid in 1965. The issue for the coming decades isn't *whether,* but *to what extent,* and *in what manner.* The Gonifimab scenario is already here for some potentially fatal conditions, just not the most common ones. The more we develop amazing drugs that can cure incurable diseases, the more we will be forced to confront some of our most basic values. When free enterprise and the freedom to live clash, which freedom will we limit?

WHAT WE FEEL about the reasonableness of industry's research ultimatum will hinge on what we believe about the origins and motivations underlying important drug discoveries. I've lived in the belly of academe my entire adult life (and at only one university since 1969) and probably have a skewed understanding of such things. But in that time I've worked with many remarkably smart and productive people who didn't go into this line of work for the money. Some of them wanted to be scientists since puberty; others fell in love with research in college or during their doctoral training or at the bedside. In universities all over the country, people come to work at dawn, check on their tissue cultures on weekends, and fall asleep over their lab notebooks after midnight because they want to discover something useful. The best of them love the process itself; their relationship to their research is almost libidinal. Of course there are considerations of ego, and more and more the shadow of future financial gain looms over the ivory tower, but that is not the main thing driving most of these scientists. Despite the overwhelming sway that profit-driven models presently hold over policy discourse, we need to recall that useful human behavior can spring from other sources as well.

THE FUTURE OF U.S. DRUG PRICES

The pharmaceutical industry is quick to point out that since prescription drug costs still represent only about 10 or 12 percent of the total health care pie, even deep slices into this modest amount wouldn't do much to contain the nation's escalating health care bill. What, they ask, might be a plausible reduction to hope for in drug costs, even at the extreme? A quarter of the total? A third? Applied to the 12 percent figure, this would amount to just a 3 or 4 percent reduction in medical costs, but would leave untouched nearly 90 percent of the health care budget, where the biggest expenditures live. Or worse, they point out, excessive reductions in payments for the drugs that keep people out of the hospital and free of the need for other kinds of costly care could bring about an increase in use of those other services, and end up being counterproductive. This concern would prevail even if one totally discounted the research ultimatum argument.

The warning has some merit. Drug cost-cutting policies that are ill-conceived and badly implemented can do substantial damage to individual patients as well as to the health care system as a whole; a favorite reference used by the industry to defend that view is our group's study of the effects of the notorious New Hampshire Medicaid cutbacks. But since that study was published, additional evidence has been collected showing that containing the more pharmacologically inept forms of costly drug use can keep expenditures in check without any clinical downsides. More and more drug payers, even in government, are starting to identify the one or two drugs in a class that are available at the best price, and encouraging doctors and patients (through varying copayment amounts) to move use in their direction. Done well, this can be scientifically appropriate, clinically practical, and an economic godsend to those trying to keep drug benefit programs fiscally viable.

Stated differently, the research ultimatum comes down to the implausible argument that economically irrational prescribing is necessary so that a modest fraction of those proceeds can be redirected to help fund the discovery of new drugs. Surely we can think of a more efficient way to keep the engine of innovation humming without taking such a large fiscal toll on patients, governments, and all those who pay for prescription drugs. Now that the debate on U.S. pharmaceutical prices has taken center stage, such change is in the air. The fact that drugs constitute only a small part of our nation's total medical bill won't provide much refuge in a health care system increasingly driven to save every possible nickel. In one important way, savings on drugs are more attractive than reducing length of hospital stay, or number of procedures done, or tests ordered. Each of those other expenditures have fixed costs that cannot be easily lowered: unless the cuts are draconian (and not many of those are still possible), hospital beds must still be staffed, operating rooms maintained, laboratories kept active. But medication purchases are almost completely variable costs, with hardly any fixed costs attached for the payer. Savings on drugs go right to the bottom line; a dollar less of utilization is pretty much a dollar saved.

Drug companies have also begun to become more vulnerable politically. As health insurers shift more and more prescription costs to the consumer, they strip away the insulation that used to protect patients from the shocks of pharmaceutical prices. Consumers' resulting anger won't be directed at the local physicians who care for them or the hospitals in their communities, but to a small number of remote corporations that will find themselves with increasingly large public relations problems. This reversal of fortune has been postponed and attenuated by influence in Washington, but as political pressures rise over drug costs and accessibility, politicians are likely to take a tougher stance on the industry as a whole.

For all these reasons, pharmaceutical companies are likely to face continuing erosion of their pricing power and profits. Even though the proportion of revenues they spend on research is not as large as those self-congratulatory television commercials imply, it is still true that billions of dollars are committed by the best companies to important biomedical investigation; they hire excellent scientists, from basic organic chemists to clinical specialists, to try to discover important new products and bring them to market. Even if too much of the industry's prodigious cash flow is diverted away from research and spent on marketing and promotion, or on the development and protection of trivial "me too" products, we will still need to preserve that core of scientifically useful work as new policies make drugs more affordable. In a way, we will need to protect the companies from themselves—or more precisely, from domination by their marketing departments. As we will see when we take up the policy implications of all this in Part Five, this is quite possible. Medical research, like medical patients, does not require a high-fat diet to prosper. In fact, in both cases precisely the opposite is true.

THE ENORMOUS EDIFICE of the American pharmaceutical enterprise currently rests on two pillars. The first is the solid marble of science that supports the cutting-edge development needed for the next generations of drug discovery. The second is the clay pillar of oversold products that are no better than their competitors, but cost staggeringly more. We have seen two grotesque examples of what can happen when finance and therapeutics meet: the brain-dead solution of New Hampshire state officials in limiting the number of prescriptions poor people can fill, and the Alice in Wonderland calculus of drug pricing. There must be a more reasonable way to determine what a particular drug is *really worth* economically. Even if the prices of all our current medications were slashed, the population will continue to age, and research in molecular pharmacology and genomics will provide us with emerging products that will be increasingly expensive to discover and produce. Health care dollars will never be limitless, and we will still have to decide how best to deploy our constrained drug budgets, whether the "we" represents national governments, insurance companies, HMOs, individual doctors, or patients.

Faced with finite resources, shouldn't there be a more sensible way to measure a drug's true economic value? For a drug with a given efficacy and safety profile, *what should we be willing to pay for it?* As we saw with benefit and risk, the answer will require us to move beyond the boundaries of science and deep into other domains of inquiry. In doing so, we will come across some much better ways to approach this question, and some terrible ones, too.

15: NAVIGATING THE
THIRD DIMENSION

The development of new drugs with unprecedented power forces us to confront tough clinical, moral, and political choices. Innovative treatments for cancer, AIDS, and rare debilitating diseases are more effective than anything we could prescribe a few years ago—and more expensive. Things get even more complicated when we consider the growing burden of chronic illness and the benefits that drugs can provide in these conditions, sometimes at enormous cost. Some of these medications may make an unbearable illness easier to bear, or prevent hospitalizations; others reduce the risk of a bad event that might occur at some point in the future; still others can help profoundly disabled patients stay alive only to lead lengthy lives of disorientation or discomfort. How can we as physicians, patients, societies, know what ought to be paid for such treatments?

A century ago, most commonly used medicines were both cheap and useless, posing no great problems of distributive justice. But since then sharp increases in drug effectiveness and costs have forced health care systems in both the developing and industrialized worlds to try to figure out how to deploy finite budgets to pay for what patients need most. When Medicare was first introduced in 1966, few even thought it necessary for the program to cover prescription drugs. After all, many of today's pharmacologic mainstays weren't even on the radar screen then: there was no consensus about whether to treat mild to moderate high blood pressure; controversy raged over whether cholesterol levels should even be measured, no less managed; and depression was an embarrassing condition that was diagnosed only when extreme, and treated with a limited number of inexpensive products if drugs were used at all. So there was no uproar in the mid-sixties when the nation enacted a sweeping plan of national health insurance for the elderly that did not cover outpatient medications.

Within the span of my own professional lifetime, all that has changed. Randomized controlled trials completed in the late 1960s proved that anti-hypertensive drugs could prevent strokes in patients with even modestly elevated blood pressure. The "cholesterol controversy" was resolved by the completion of randomized trials showing that use of lipid-lowering medications reduces the risk of heart attacks and other cardiovascular disease. This was demonstrated first in patients with very high cholesterol levels and underlying heart disease, then in patients without underlying disease, then even in some patients with "normal" cholesterol levels. Whole new classes of breakthrough drugs came into use long after the initial Medicare regulations were engraved into legislative stone: beta-blockers and ACE-inhibitors to treat blood pressure and heart disease; histamine blockers and proton pump inhibitors like Zantac and Prilosec for ulcer-related problems; SSRIs like Prozac, first to treat depression and then for an ever-widening swath of psychological discomfort. Entirely new categories of drugs were developed to manage infection, pain, arthritis, cancer. Their clinical and public health benefits were enormous, but the new drugs also brought with them a growing hemorrhage of red ink.

For decades, Medicare simply ignored most outpatient drugs, and much of the rest of American medicine got by with a simple answer to the purchasing question: If the FDA has determined that every drug on the market works better than placebo, then just pay for them all, whatever the cost. With rising drug expenditures, the limits of this way of thinking became apparent. As the health economist Victor Fuchs noted, "In health care we can have anything, but we can't have everything." Even if we were to push American spending on all medical care from its current 15 percent of gross domestic product up to 20 percent of GDP (a change that is neither plausible nor desirable), there would still be a point at which we couldn't afford to pay for every imaginable treatment regardless of its cost; choices would have to be made.

Those responsible for managing health care budgets face a stark set of options. Simply paying for anything a doctor might prescribe makes budgets uncontrollable, or coverage unaffordable, or both. One easy solution would be to ration prescription drug use by wealth, with the rich buying all the medicines they want and the poor having to do without. Even though this is the consequence of much recent social policy, it is not an approach that Americans like to think of ourselves as implementing on purpose. There had to be a better way. . . .

COMPARING COSTS AND OUTCOMES

This topic brings us into a head-on confrontation with the third and final dimension of the benefit-risk-cost triad that underlies every drug use decision: *Is this medication worth its expense?* It doesn't help for us to declare that human health is too precious to place a dollar value on, or that the government should just lower drug prices, or that all medication costs, however high they are, should simply be paid for by somebody. Even in countries with strict drug price controls, even when lower-cost generics are used whenever possible, these choices still force themselves upon us. Those of us who have to make real-life drug decisions every day need better answers—solutions that can actually be implemented before the arrival of the Messiah. Earlier, we asked how efficacy and risk can be stacked up against each other to determine whether a drug's benefit is worth its potential for harm. It's now time to add the next level of complexity: For a drug with a particular set of benefits and risks, *what is it worth?*

> *You are responsible for developing policy on drug use and reimbursement for a large nonprofit HMO. National guidelines recommend much wider preventive use of cholesterol-lowering drugs to reduce the risk of heart disease; this could cost up to $1,000 per person per year. Other competing demands on your pharmacy budget include expansion of the childhood vaccination program and paying for a new blockbuster cancer drug at an annual cost of $24,000 per patient. Your drug expenditures have been rising at a rate of 17 percent annually, and senior management has determined that further increases of this size are simply unaffordable. The chief financial officer reaffirms that your drug budget for the coming year cannot possibly accommodate all of these additions simultaneously.*

How much should you be willing to pay for a given increment in benefit or decrement in risk? Grappling with this question draws us into a strange realm that lies at the interface of economics, pharmacology, ethics, clinical practice, and philosophy. To return to our case example: If widespread use of cholesterol-lowering drugs in the elderly saves lives, this would be an easy problem if it cost only $100 per life saved. But these drugs can be costly; what if a widespread program of such prescribing ended up costing $1,000,000 per life saved? Is any dollar amount too high to save a human life? If there is no limit, who's to pay? And what other expenditures will your health care system have to forgo if it runs out of money?

It would really help to have some standard way of measuring the amount of good a particular drug generates, so we could compare it with other worthy interventions. Can we possibly juxtapose the benefits of drugs that make you feel better (like an asthma medicine, a tranquilizer, or a drug for acne) with the value of medications that save lives? And in measuring those benefits, is the value of prolonging the life of an eighty-four-year-old to be counted differently from prolonging the life of a child, or a middle-aged worker? Should benefits that occur many years in the future somehow be discounted, as would be done in business? At what annual rate? These questions are not merely interesting case studies in applied philosophy; they are the bread and butter of real-world analyses with which many of us are struggling as we try to provide the best medical care that is affordable within increasingly constrained health care budgets.

The holy grail here would be a tool that enables us to know which medications are worth their cost and which are not. As with benefits and risks, any sensible approach must begin with an attempt to measure things systematically, so we could relate those measurements to each other in some logical and consistent way. Despite the enormous amount the United States spends on prescription drugs, huge sums are spilled about irrationally. Large segments of the population can't afford to buy the medications they need, and some patients with good coverage have a hard time paying their share of the drug bill. But at the same time, millions of others spend far more than necessary on their medications, sometimes even to the detriment of their health. If the randomized clinical trial is the polestar that guides decisions on efficacy, we could sure use a comparable tool that provides a reliable measure of the economic value of drugs.

Like any other good or service, some medications are great buys that produce substantial medical benefit for a modest cost; others are bad deals that consume many dollars while providing little or no health benefit in return. But just how do we quantify the benefits of medical interventions? Several approaches have been tried; each brings with it its own set of values, assumptions, insights, and problems.

SOME BAD SOLUTIONS

The economic analysis of medical interventions has a checkered reputation because of some terrible incarnations earlier in its evolution—some of which are still with us today. We'll look at some of these ugly avatars first, the better to discard them and move on to more promising approaches.

THE HUMAN-CAPITAL APPROACH

One early attempt to measure the benefits that come from medications and other health care interventions was based on the notion of "human capital," and flowed directly from industrial cost-benefit analyses. A decision on whether to repair a machine or retool a factory would start by calculating the future productivity expected from the equipment, given its age and condition. It might be worth fixing a broken-down but functioning machine if it had enough good years left in it to pay back the repair costs within a reasonable time frame. But an older piece of equipment with a shorter period of usefulness remaining, or requiring a bigger repair, would justifiably be thrown on the scrap heap. We've all confronted this kind of choice with our cars or refrigerators or computers, though usually not with our grandmothers.

An extensive and occasionally loathsome literature has tried to relate this economic approach to the maintenance and repair of human beings. In this method, the average national salary at various ages is used to calculate a person's economic worth, as measured by his or her future lifetime earnings. To mirror the marketplace more accurately, the earning power of men and women is often measured separately. Many early analyses used workplace salaries and didn't put any value on the productivity of women in the home; their human-capital value in such assessments came out as zero or close to it. Other studies attempted to assign an economic value to what homemakers do by crediting such work at the minimum wage for eight hours a day—a concept that will seem both whimsical and infuriating to anyone who has ever had to manage a family or a household.

Beyond the issue of whether parenting and maintaining a home should be valued so cheaply, this approach also does strange things to the "value" of older people. We saw earlier that economics aside, quality-adjusting each year of life based on disability can substantially reduce the calculated worth of each year lived by a person with several chronic illnesses. Things get even worse with the human-capital approach. If a person's economic value equals the income he or she produces, then the worth of an elderly person who stops working at age sixty-five plummets. One study made use of these adjustments to compute the value of a human life at various ages, with the value of a person dropping precipitously from young adulthood to the retirement years. Women did slightly better than men in the later years because it was assumed that they would continue doing housework until death, whereas the economic value of a man immediately fell to nothing upon his retirement.

Data like these have actually been used in cost-benefit calculations to predict which medications yield the most productivity dollars gained per dollar spent. Thus, a drug that would save the life of an eighty-five-year-old man (yielding a benefit of under a thousand dollars) would compare poorly with one that would save a thirty-two-year-old (yielding a benefit of hundreds of thousands of dollars). Granted, this perspective can more fairly take into account all the good that a drug does when it restores productivity in a working-age person (the antidepressants are an oft-cited example of this), but the inevitable downside, if we are to be consistent, is an opposite effect in valuing treatments for others. Such human-capital analyses lead inexorably to the conclusion that it isn't cost-effective to spend much on medicines or other health care interventions for the elderly. The absurdity and moral bankruptcy of this approach was highlighted some time ago with the release of a report prepared for the governor of New York on the economics of cleaning up toxic waste sites in various parts of the state. The report's author, an aficionado of human-capital methods, calculated the average economic worth of various citizens in different parts of the state, depending on the mix of ages, gender, and occupations—presumably to measure the cost to society that would result from the slow poisoning of each stratum of citizenry. A copy of the report was obtained by *New York* magazine, which duly published images of each category of New Yorker on its cover along with a price tag for each: it was worth several hundred thousand dollars to prevent the death of a stockbroker from Scarsdale, but only a few hundred to save a little old lady in Brooklyn. The governor's office quickly disavowed both the approach and the report.

Could these economists make things any worse for the elderly patient? Definitely. Some of them also measure future resource consumption as part of the cost-benefit equation in order to calculate a person's *net* human-capital worth. Viewed in this way, the meager productivity of an elderly person is further reduced or even brought into the minus column by taking into account the cost to society of the Social Security payments or publicly funded health care services they consume. In *Measuring the Monetary Value of Lifesaving Programs,* one author noted:

> One implication of this "net livelihood" procedure is that society is made better off by the death of those whose expected net present value is negative. This is true of retired people and those who are near retirement, some of whom receive disability and public assistance payments.

This logic is perfectly consistent with the concept that a lethal intravenous dose of morphine upon retirement would be the drug treatment with the most favorable benefit-cost ratio for older patients. This is the same methodology that produced the notorious studies showing that smoking is economically useful for society because it causes many of its victims to die quickly in late middle age from heart attacks or lung cancer, one of the faster-acting killers among malignancies. In doing so, it prevents them from growing old enough to develop Alzheimer's disease, have strokes, require nursing home care, or cash Social Security checks. From the human-capital perspective, it's far better to have people keep smoking and pass away sooner. Amazingly, this is just where the numbers do lead if one chooses to go down that path. Tobacco turns out to have a better benefit-cost ratio than insulin. As Woody Allen noted with equal insight, "Death is a great way to cut down on expenses."

Of course this is ridiculous. What is missing from this approach is any understanding of compassion, rights, one's debt to one's parents and fore-bears, or any sense of altruism or equity. Also absent is the vision that, as the medical economist Rashi Fein pointed out, "we live in a society, not just in an economy." If any further objection to the human-capital approach were needed, it would be its inability to take any account of pain and suffer-ing. One is either alive (and with luck, economically productive) or dead. Living with pain or chronic illness is of no consequence as long as one is working. For all these reasons, many health economists have moved away from the human-capital approach as a means of guiding allocation of resources for medications.

But before we leave behind this approach as if it were some kind of ethi-cally reprehensible roadkill, let me propose another clinical vignette that may suggest another way to look at the problem.

You are in charge of a local AIDS clinic in a poor country in sub-Saharan Africa. Western medications have been far too costly even to consider for your patients, since one year of a drug would cost hundreds of times the average per capita income of any one of them. For years, Western pharmaceutical companies successfully fought off attempts to produce more affordable generic versions of their AIDS treatments, cit-ing the need to defend their patent rights. When it became clear that this was doing little for their bottom line but had become an international public relations catastrophe, some began to make their drugs available to you at lower prices. This brought the annual cost down to only twenty-fold the available budget per person, but foreign aid from several Scandi-navian countries will enable you to cover the cost for a limited number of people.

This morning, you are seeing two such patients. The first is a twenty-four-year-old widow who contracted AIDS after being raped by her late husband's brother. She is one of the few people in the village who has completed secondary education, and is now the head teacher in the local school. She is also the sole source of support for her five children and her sister's four children. The second patient is a seventy-four-year-old man who acquired the virus from a prostitute. He has no family and has not worked for years because of a chronic problem with alcoholism.

Clinically, both patients are likely to experience a rapid downhill course over the coming year without treatment. Both are equally likely to show dramatic improvement if given the drug. Which one do you choose?

Few of us would pick the old man, or be comfortable letting a coin flip determine the decision. If we were in that doctor's shoes, virtually all of us would choose to treat the young teacher, and rightly so. But haven't we just embraced a drug coverage decision that was driven by some kind of human-capital approach? And hadn't we just concluded that this was an abhorrent method to decide who should get treatment and who should not? In many settings, yes. The paradox centers on the issue of scarcity.

This kind of triage-by-productivity may be a reasonable choice in a desperately poor Third World country where the amount of money available for medications is appallingly tiny and the need almost incomprehensibly large, so that only a fraction of patients can receive the drugs they need. Similar issues would come up at the national level in such countries in deciding how to commit resources to AIDS screening versus prevention versus treatment. This is the vision that underlies the United Nations Global Burden of Disease program, in which priority is given to preventing or treating the illnesses that deprive a nation of the most years of productive activity by its citizens—that is, conditions that preferentially strike the young and employable. That program considers illnesses and the value of treating them in terms of the number of years of work a given intervention could restore—a form of human-capital analysis. This may well be the best approach for a desperately poor country crippled with an intractable epidemic. But that does not make it an acceptable guide to policy in the richest nation on earth, where such scarcity does not (or need not) prevail.

WILLINGNESS TO PAY

Because of the ugly problems inherent in the human-capital approach, some economists proposed a different way to translate the benefits of medications into dollar terms. Known as "willingness to pay," the method was designed to have the quantitative precision of social science and the inherent egalitarianism of the marketplace. (These claims alone would appear to warrant its dismissal from any serious consideration.) The benefit of a medication is calculated by asking people how many dollars they would be willing to spend to achieve a particular outcome, like a 20 percent reduction in the chance of having a fatal heart attack. The technique is as simple as it is crude: healthy citizens are presented with a series of medical problems and asked to place a dollar value on what they would pay for a drug that could cure or prevent each one. In this way, it is argued, the pain and suffering of illness can be quantified, something that can't be done in the simpler dead-or-alive calculations of the human-capital approach.

The rationale is analogous to economists' attempts in other settings to infer the true worth of a given outcome by looking at the behavior of consumers and workers, or other so-called revealed preferences. For example, the wage differential paid to workers with hazardous jobs or the sums people spend on seat belts or smoke detectors are said to measure the dollar value they intuitively place on their own lives. Proponents claim that this approach permits democratization of health care policy, since it allows for the input of lay people in defining how desirable or undesirable particular clinical outcomes are, as expressed by their behavior in the marketplace. Skeptics think the idea is silly. I'm a skeptic.

In one example of this method, patients with arthritis were asked how much they would be willing to pay to be rid of their disability, as measured in terms of their total weekly family income. Over half of those questioned refused to answer. Those who did respond represented a subsample sharply skewed toward patients with college or graduate educations. The mean annual figures for relief of arthritis ranged from $120 for the poorest respondents to several thousand dollars for the wealthiest. To account for differences in economic status the amounts were then expressed as a fraction of family income. These also differed widely, with enormous variances at each income level.

That isn't surprising in light of the obvious noncomparability of spending decisions, including hypothetical ones, made by people of different economic status. We know that the rich make different allocations of their income (even proportionally) than the nonwealthy. This is even truer for people on limited and potentially shrinking retirement incomes compared with those who are still employed—especially if the older respondents are worried about paying for medical care in their later years. Studies that report the "unwillingness" of the elderly to pay much for drugs to avoid certain health outcomes may tell us more about how badly we look after our senior citizens than about the inherent worth of a particular treatment.

Data on willingness to pay have also produced wildly divergent figures on the marketplace value of a human life, ranging from under $40,000 to over $10 million. Some of this variance results from asking people stupid questions like how much they would pay to reduce their chance of dying from a given illness from 2 percent to 0.7 percent—a notion that is simply beyond the grasp of most of us, whether we are laypeople, physicians, or even economists. There isn't much comfort in the refinement proposed in one paper that we could "avoid the known irrationalities of general thought processes by having computerized models, not subjects, do the thinking."

It would be good to report that the irreproducibility and ethical problems of this method have caused it to fall out of favor outside isolated onanistic circles in academia and consulting firms, but sadly this is not the case. In 2003, the Bush administration was ready to embrace willingness-to-pay analysis in an odd replay of the New York pollution control fiasco of the 1980s. The Environmental Protection Agency sought to determine the economic value of reducing pollutants in diesel emissions that increase the risk of respiratory illness and death in susceptible patients. In its calculations, the agency cited the work of an economist who asked people of various ages what they would be willing to pay to reduce their risk of death from 1 in 200,000 to 1 in 300,000. We have already wondered whether the output of such questionnaires is good for anything but wrapping fish, but the study managed to obtain answers from 930 Canadians on the matter. Respondents over age seventy provided a dollar figure that was on average about 30 percent less than that given by younger people for this imponderable health advantage. A follow-up study on Americans didn't show the same differential, but the EPA went with the Canada estimates.

Plugged into the EPA's equations, the numbers would mean that it's less worthwhile economically to control air pollution in populations containing more older Americans compared with younger ones, because of the lower value the elderly place on life. The origin of these data was not prominently featured in the regulatory proposal that emerged, which projected the analysis over the entire population. It provided an apparent rationale for loosening pollution control regulations, on the grounds that they were not as fiscally justifiable as previously thought, in light of the price citizens put on the value of a human life. The new regulations were not greeted warmly by older Americans. As in the 1980s, once the public was alerted to the method behind the supposedly scientific calculations, the responsible officials backed away from their conclusions.

Like a virulent cognitive virus, the willingness-to-pay method has escaped the university laboratories in which it was first bred and gone on to infect cells of analysts all over the country, most importantly in the federal Office of Management and Budget.

A MORE HUMBLE APPROACH TO COST-EFFECTIVENESS ANALYSIS

It is beginning to look as if it might be impossible, on both moral and methodological grounds, to assign any reasonable numbers to the benefits that medications can produce. But that's unthinkable—it would mean we couldn't even begin to compare the economic value of drug A with that of drug B. Do we just have to pay whatever the manufacturer charges, with no way of differentiating a good investment of our limited health care dollars from a poor one? In fleeing wrongheaded solutions, we don't want to lurch into accepting the argument that no financial consideration should ever be undertaken for any medication that works—that they should all be paid for. Unfortunately, until recently that was the logic behind most prescription drug benefits in many private-sector and government programs, and it is the guiding principle behind the federal legislation to cover drugs under Medicare.

The problem with such a view is that it treats the category of prescription drugs as if it were some unitary construct, like oxygen or glucose. In most programs, the debate then moves on to dwell on smaller ideas, like the details of which patients are eligible for coverage, or what deductible amount the patient should pay before coverage begins, or what dollar share of each prescription should be borne out-of-pocket. As we saw, when the cover-everything strategy became unaffordable, many programs shifted more cost to the patient, limited coverage, or just eliminated it altogether.

The all-or-nothing view of paying for drugs has been the most important barrier to developing affordable prescription benefit programs in both the public and private sectors, and explains the great difficulty the nation has had in establishing a truly comprehensive drug coverage plan for all Americans. Without a better way to distinguish among products, open-ended entitlement programs can be tantamount to allowing the pharmaceutical industry to print money. It encourages marketing the highest-priced products even more fiercely to doctors and patients, causing program costs to balloon out of control. But we know that many drugs on the market got there simply by being a little better than placebo. Others are not as good as existing products, or grotesquely overpriced, or both.

In the search for a less objectionable method, many health economists have moved from cost-benefit analysis to cost-effectiveness analysis. The approach takes benefits out of the realm of dollars, and instead describes the good that a drug does in terms of its health outcomes. This approach can be used to develop a syllogism for drug coverage that is compatible with both clinical and fiscal reality:

1. Automatically paying for all marketed drugs is exorbitantly expensive, making drug coverage unaffordable.
2. Indiscriminate drug coverage sucks health care dollars into paying for medications of lower relative value, draining resources away from more efficient medical expenditures.
3. Limiting prescription drug reimbursement simplistically by rationing, "caps," or other across-the-board limitations is objectionable from an

ethical perspective, dangerous from a political perspective, and irrational from a medical perspective.

4. For a given condition, some drugs are much better than others in their effectiveness, safety, and/or value for money.

5. Therefore, if several medications are available to treat a given condition, we should figure out which ones provide the best effectiveness and safety per dollar spent, and preferentially pay for them.

Not rocket science, but still a conceptual leap that has been hard to make for many policy makers in government and in the private sector. But just how can we know which drugs give us our money's worth?

SEARCHING FOR A BETTER MEASURE

For economists, an ideal measure has two key properties: it can be put on a single one-dimensional line; and it has units that are equal and interchangeable—like dollars, for example. We might need to do some small corrections (as for inflation), but the unit is the unit is the unit. The cleanest kind of economic analysis is one that expresses everything in terms of such fungible units, so they can be swapped around like poker chips in valuing and executing transactions of all kinds. If things didn't work like this, if the worth of a dollar varied depending on the time of day, or the opinion of its owner, or what it was being used to buy, business would grind to a halt. It would be as if physicists learned that a meter varies in length according to how you measure it. (Of course, Einstein showed us that this is exactly what happens, and a similar paradigm shift is occurring thanks to behavioral economics. But we'll stick to the simple vision to start with.)

In classical economics, measurement of preferences also requires this kind of perfect fungibility. When early attempts to define the price of health and longevity led to unappealing moral and clinical weirdness, it became necessary to invent a system of discourse that would not require valuing life or health directly in dollar terms. One big step in this direction came from a surprising source: a seminal 1944 book by John von Neumann and Oskar Morgenstern called *Theory of Games and Economic Behavior*. It set forth the rules for "expected utility theory," a way of understanding how people prioritize their preferences and make choices designed to maximize their benefits, or utilities. They pointed out that preferences are best satisfied in a population when people can trade their poker chips of good and bad outcomes in exchange for other possible choices, or for money. Applying this perspective to medicine required the invention of a unit with the requisite von Neumann–Morgenstern properties of interchangeability, and the "quality-adjusted life-year" was born. In principle, this could allow a perfect parallel between business and medicine. In commerce, the best decisions are those that generate the most dollars (all other things being equal, which they never are); so in health care the best decisions would be the ones that generate the most QALYs. The concept was a breakthrough that had some similarities to the discovery of the internal combustion engine: it unleashed much useful power and a great deal of smog.

The most promising and the most problematic way of matching dollars with outcomes is a cousin of the decision-analysis tool we've already encountered, which assigns probabilities and weights to the good events that come from use of a drug as well as to the harm that it can do. Now we can try to use this same approach to compare both of these to the economic costs and benefits that flow from a drug's effects. But before we can do this we have to confront the appealing but untenable notion that human health and life are so precious that we should never think about cost in making any medical decisions. We'll have to exorcise that cuddly demon once and for all before we can get anywhere, so let's run the numbers on Futilon, a hypothetical drug.

A large randomized trial has shown that taking Futilon daily for twenty years will extend a patient's life span by one month on average, compared to placebo. The drug has no side effects, and produces no difference in health during this time—it just postpones death by a month if taken diligently over the preceding two decades. Leaving aside for now the sticky issue of discount rates, let's assume that the cost of Futilon is $2,000 a year, a price we've gotten accustomed to in medicine. (Its manufacturer has successfully fended off all generic competitors.) In a thousand people, paying for that extra month of life for all those patients would cost $40 million ($2,000 per year times 20 years times 1,000 people). For now, we'll ignore just who's paying that bill.

Do those numbers make Futilon a good value or a poor one? If you are the doctor in question and could direct where all the health expenditures in your practice go, would you really want to spend that $40 million to put all those patients on the new drug, or instead use it to pay for other needed medical care?

Now let's assume you're the patient: Would you demand that extra month of life if someone else (the government, your insurance company) were paying the $40 million? What if you had to pay for it with your own money? What if it were taken from the inheritance you'd leave your children? Or from the pool of dollars available to pay for all the medical care in your community?

I'm hoping that at this point even die-hard you-can't-put-a-price-on-human-life advocates will agree that as long as budgets for medical care are not infinite, it's worth trying to distinguish expenditures of very small value from more worthy ones. It's a little like the observation attributed to George Bernard Shaw when he asked a high-born lady whether she'd be willing to sleep with him in exchange for ten million pounds.

"I suppose I would," she replied.

"Would you do it for twenty pounds?" he asked.

"Of course not! What do you take me for, a prostitute?"

"We've already established that," Shaw responded. "Now we're just haggling over the price."

The high cost and tiny benefit of the barely mythical Futilon make it an easy case study to think about—but we should recall that many chronically administered drugs for hypertension or cholesterol reduction will on average add only about a month to the lifespan of many patient subgroups. What if another hypothetical drug, Plausinase, cost a mere $500 per year, and extended life by six months instead of just one? That sounds better, but how much better is it? Better enough to make Plausinase a good deal? The economic and moral challenges of such "Is it worth it?" questions may tempt some just to leave them in the hands of the doctor. That will be an idea to return to later, but for now it begs the question of how we doctors can know whether a given drug has a cost commensurate with its benefit and with its risks. The conscientious clinician would still need some way to make such a call, in case we once again are given full control over our prescribing decisions. The following real-world decision of several years ago illustrates how these decisions can be approached:

> You're a member of your hospital's Pharmacy and Therapeutics Committee, the board responsible for deciding which drugs are used by doctors at your institution. For several years the cardiologists and emergency room physicians there have been treating heart attack patients with the clot-busting drug streptokinase. Given intravenously within a few hours of the start of chest pain, this enzyme helps dissolve the clots that block these patients' coronary arteries; this can preserve heart muscle and improve the likelihood of survival.
>
> Today you're asked to make a decision about a new product that was developed through recombinant gene technology. Called tPA, it is a designer drug version of streptokinase and is supposed to work even better, opening the blocked artery faster and more thoroughly. One member of the committee is a cardiologist who is also a consultant to Genentech, the new drug's manufacturer. He argues forcefully that the hospital

should use tPA instead of the older product, because it makes so much sense physiologically.

A surgeon points out that many things in medicine that seem to make physiological sense don't work out as expected. How can we know, he asks, whether tPA's theoretical advantage actually pans out in practice, or whether its more powerful clot-busting power might even result in more bleeding complications, making it a worse choice?

The administrator who sits in on your meetings points out that the hospital receives a fixed payment of about $4,000 per heart attack patient from Medicare and most other insurers, whichever drugs are used. Streptokinase costs the hospital about $200 per patient; tPA would cost $2,000, or half the total reimbursement the hospital receives for all care delivered during the entire admission.

"Of course we want to do the best job we can," she says, "but what is the evidence that this new drug works any better than what we're using now?"

"We don't have any."

She persists. "Have there been any randomized trials published comparing these two drugs head to head?"

"No. The FDA approved the two drugs separately, years apart. Each one just showed that it was better than placebo."

Sensing where things are going, the cardiologist makes one last try. "Genentech is sponsoring a huge multinational study that is looking at just that question. The results should be published later this year."

The committee votes to defer the decision until the findings of that trial are available for review.

Six months later, the study is published in the New England Journal of Medicine. *It shows that the survival rate in heart attack patients randomized to tPA is about 1 percent better than those given placebo. The newer drug also results in a small increase in the likelihood of devastating stroke. The paper doesn't mention the tenfold price difference. The cardiologist requests that the question be resolved at the next monthly meeting of the P&T Committee. Before the discussion starts, the administrator asks for a moment to comment.*

"You're the doctors and I'm not," she begins. "As a nonprofit institution, our first commitment is to our patients—all our patients. We have no surplus to draw on for unexpected jumps in our expenses. What you decide today will determine which drug we use here. But please understand that whatever you determine, most of our payers still plan to give us just about $4,000 per admission. If you do decide that the $2,000 *drug is the one to use, I'm going to need you to tell me where we can cut back in other areas so we can afford to implement your plan. Is the new drug really so much better than the older one that you want to go that route?"*

In simpler times, hospitals used to receive cost-based reimbursement from most insurers: they were paid whatever they spent, plus a hefty proportional markup. This provided no motivation for containing costs—in fact, quite the opposite. In those days, a vigorous marketing campaign *(It's NEW! It's GENETIC!)* would have been enough to drive tPA to the top of the chest-pain charts. But by the 1990s the rules had changed, and hospitals received a flat fee from most governmental and private insurers for each heart attack treated, whatever their costs. The incentive to spend more and more had been transformed into an incentive to spend less and less. When tPA was first introduced, its early sales were not brisk. Genentech executives realized that unless they wanted to be stuck with an elegant expensive genetically engineered product that hardly anyone used, the company had to come up with a good comparative clinical trial to persuade doctors that its product was better than the cheaper alternative.

So Genentech went for the GUSTO—the acronym for the ambitious multinational controlled trial it mounted, called "Global Utilization of Streptokinase and tPA for Occluded coronary arteries." That trial can serve as a good case study to consider how costs, risks, and benefits can be related to one another. Genentech spent over $40 million to enlist doctors in Europe and the United States to randomly assign patients having heart attacks to receive either streptokinase or the newer tPA. While GUSTO was still enrolling patients, I received an inquiry from a small Swedish drug company called Kabi, which made streptokinase. I was asked if we could perform a formal decision analysis of the two competing products that would take into account their relative benefits, risks, and costs. In working out the terms of the research grant, I required as usual that the company allow us to use any data sources we chose and to perform the analysis however we saw fit; most importantly, they would have no control over our interpretation or publication of the results, whatever we found. Kabi agreed, perhaps secure in the expectation that no unbiased look at the data then available would ever conclude that tPA could be so much better as to justify its tenfold price premium. Dr. Susan Kalish, who was doing a research fellowship with me, headed up the project.

In the absence of head-to-head data from such a trial, a good theoretical case could be made on both sides of this life-and-death decision. Streptokinase had been around for years, was very well studied, and physicians had good experience with it. It had been clearly shown in very large, well-designed randomized trials to reduce death rates in heart attack patients. It was relatively cheap. The newer product, tPA, brought with it the cachet of recombinant DNA technology and the promise of better clot-reaming activity. In smaller studies, it too had been found to reduce death in heart attack patients when compared with placebo, at roughly the same rate as streptokinase. But experience with it was much more limited, particularly concerning its risk of causing stroke as an unwanted consequence of its blood-thinning activity.

Advocates for the new drug argued that theoretically, if it could dissolve clots more quickly, it might keep more heart muscle from dying, and so preserve more function and prevent more deaths than the older drug. But there was also that $1,800 per-patient price difference. A universal switch to tPA could represent a major burden for hospitals, as well as for the thousands of patients who lacked health insurance. The switch would add hundreds of millions of dollars to the cost of caring for heart attacks in exchange for a still-uncertain clinical benefit.

As we began our study, the GUSTO trial was still ongoing and no results were yet available. In the absence of data from head-to-head comparisons, we would have to resort to the next best alternative: trying to combine the results of all the published trials that had tested each drug against placebo. We could attempt to use that information to calculate the effect of each on mortality and adverse events, as well as on costs. But this approach is littered with methodological land mines. A streptokinase trial might have enrolled heart attack patients who were healthier or sicker than those in another trial that used tPA. We would have to try to make the studies comparable by looking at the death and stroke rates of the patients in the placebo group of each one, use that information to try to calibrate how sick the patients in that study were, and then adjust the outcomes in the active-drug arms accordingly—a complex and not very satisfying process. Its goal would be to simulate what would have been found in a single head-to-head trial that randomized its patients to one of the two active drugs.

Constructing a decision-analysis model is a little like practicing medicine: both force you to make choices in the face of uncertain or incomplete data. Doctors were treating heart attack patients by the thousands every day, and it would be important to have some evidence to guide those decisions until data from the multiyear GUSTO trial became available. Kalish and our team started wading through the trial data in the medical literature and building it into a computer model.

Then the results of the GUSTO study were made public.

Genentech's huge gamble on the trial had paid off. Of the thousands of heart attack patients who had been randomized to streptokinase, 7.3 percent were dead within thirty days; of the thousands randomized to tPA, only 6.3 percent had died. The fatality rates at one year continued to show a similar advantage for tPA. But stroke rates went modestly in the opposite direction: 0.8 percent of patients given streptokinase had strokes, versus 0.9 percent of the tPA patients. And when they occurred, the strokes in the tPA patients were slightly more likely to be severely disabling. There was a bit more bad news as well. For every thousand patients, three more in the tPA group went on to have a repeat heart attack compared to the streptokinase group, and seven more required a subsequent cardiac bypass operation. Had tPA rescued the sickest patients, who might have died if they had been in the streptokinase group? Perhaps tPA barely snatched them back from mortality at the price of requiring more invasive treatment later. Or, by contrast, it might have reduced the death rate but increased the absolute risk of other heart problems later on. We had to put this all together and then try to determine if the new drug was worth the sharply higher expense. This was no mere academic exercise; real everyday clinical decisions required the best possible answers to these life-and-death questions.

DEALING WITH A NEW REALITY

The day the GUSTO findings were published, doctors and hospitals all over the world were confronted with the difficult question facing the committee in our hypothetical vignette. Was a tenfold price increase worth that 1 percent reduction in mortality? Was this the trivial advantage of a Futilon, or the more compelling value of a Plausinase? What about those extra strokes? Would tPA still be a better choice if its mortality advantage were 0.5 percent and the accompanying stroke rate were twice as high? And if Genentech, emboldened by the favorable results of GUSTO, increased the price of tPA to $5,000 per dose—what then?

There are a limited number of ways to try to answer this question. The decision about which drug to use could be left up to each individual doctor, or to each hospital. But that begs the question as to how each doctor or hospital is supposed to figure out what to do. Others advocate letting the marketplace resolve the issue, perhaps by allowing the patient having the heart attack to decide which drug to get, and to pay for the difference. But how could anyone make such a decision in that context? And who could be comfortable with the knowledge that once again, the poor would end up having a higher death rate as a result? The analysis we eventually performed is instructive not just for what it says about the management of heart attack, but as a template for how this increasingly common benefit-risk-cost trade-off can be handled.

To see how this kind of assessment works, let's assume that we're giving a thrombolytic drug to two groups of a thousand heart attack patients each.

We can think of the streptokinase group as the base case, and use the GUSTO data to estimate the additional benefits and costs the tPA group would have above and beyond that. Let's say it cost the hospital in our vignette about $300 per patient to purchase streptokinase and about $2,200 for tPA, for a difference of $1,900 per patient treated. (Those were our hospital's acquisition costs for that year.) So every thousand people the hospital treated with tPA would cost it an additional $1.9 million. If the GUSTO outcomes apply, then for every thousand patients treated with tPA sixty would die; for every thousand treated with streptokinase, seventy.

If each heart attack survivor goes on to live for an average of about fifteen years more (a reasonable estimate if their mean age was sixty-five), those ten fewer deaths in the tPA group will result in 150 extra life-years gained in that group compared to the thousand patients given streptokinase. But how to factor in the extra nonfatal strokes and heart attacks and cardiac surgeries that the GUSTO data told us to expect from tPA? These complications don't just consume medical resources, they're human tragedies as well; how can we account for all that? As a very crude first assumption, let's say that people who have had a stroke value every year of life afterward as worth just eight tenths of a year in good health. We can equally crudely assume that people who have a stroke *and* a second heart attack value each subsequent year at only half a year of healthy life. If these "quality adjustment" factors are plausible (and they may not be), we can try to put a number to the expected disability of the surviving patients, based on the frequency of events that occurred in the clinical trial. We can also calculate the costs for the care of the extra strokes and cardiac interventions seen in the tPA group. All this could give the hospital in our vignette a better sense of what its patients would be getting for the additional $1.8 million it spent on the more costly drug. But it won't tell them whether to spend those extra dollars.

Our team used this method to create a computer model of the differing benefits and costs seen with each of the two drugs studied in the GUSTO trial. We found that when taking into account all the differences in benefit and risk, using tPA instead of streptokinase would extend the life of the *average* treated patient by about one month. Why so little? Because while it's true that for every thousand people treated with tPA there would be ten fewer deaths, the mortality outcome for the other 990 people would be the same whichever drug was used. That 1 percent mortality difference for the whole group of treated patients, when combined with the quality-of-life decrements among some of the survivors, would come out to just a one-month advantage averaged out over all patients entering the emergency room with a heart attack.

This may come as a surprise to those who thought the reduction of ten deaths per thousand patients made tPA an obvious choice, whatever the cost; if stroke were not involved, we might even have used the term "no-brainer" for this view. Some might be doubly surprised if they had previously decided that spending good money on Futilon just to gain one month of extra life seemed like an equally obvious waste of money. But the averaged-out perspective of this sort of analysis diverges sharply from the personal perspective of the individual doctor or patient. In the heart attack example, that one extra month didn't come from each tPA patient living just a little bit longer; it was an arithmetic convenience to describe the fact that a slightly smaller number of patients *died* during their hospital admissions. The difference occurred in terms of specific cardiac arrests, wakes, funerals, shivahs, affecting particular named individuals. Identifiable people became widows or widowers, destined to live with their loss for the rest of their lives. Whatever the average risk of death in a large group of people, if it happens to you it's 100 percent.

These numbers have the same strange property as those silhouette drawings of two heads facing one another—or is it a single goblet in the middle? Think about it hard enough, and you can get your mind to flip back and forth between the two perspectives, each of which is perfectly accurate in its own terms. The chief financial officer of a hospital system that handles a thousand heart attack cases a year may question whether it's worth diverting nearly two million dollars from other strapped programs to pay for a drug that will prolong the life of the average patient by only a month. But if I were a doctor working in that hospital's emergency room, I'd be very uneasy with the idea that sticking with the cheaper drug would mean that for every hundred heart attack patients I cared for (a number that's easier to relate to), one more patient of mine would die because of that choice.

If both drugs were free, that might be the end of the discussion: use the drug whose benefit-risk balance is even a little bit better. But drugs are not free. Someone will need to pick up the tab for that small benefit, whether it's the patient himself, or the governmental agency that pays for his health care, or his HMO or other insurer. And if no one does (a situation increasingly common in big-city hospitals that care for the uninsured), the institution itself will have to come up with the difference, usually by cutting back on other expenditures for patients.

That brings us back to the Futilon-Plausinase question. Does tPA provide a trivial gain for an unbearable expense, or is it *worth it*? We've abandoned the more businesslike perspective of cost-benefit analysis in which all outcomes are reduced to dollars, so we can't address our problem in conventional return-on-investment terms. But we can look at it in a different way: Compared to all the other things we do in medicine, all the other ways we could spend those very same scarce dollars, how good a deal is this?

For once, this is a question we can answer. The computer model we developed told us how many additional quality-adjusted life-years (QALYs) would be gained for each patient treated if a hospital always used tPA instead of streptokinase (that extra month comes out to about 0.08 years). It also calculated how many more dollars the institution would have to spend to achieve that: the greater expense of the drug and the cost of caring for its complications would consume about $2,500 more per patient. Dividing the latter by the former reveals how many additional dollars it would cost to achieve that incremental benefit: about $30,000 per additional QALY gained. (People who don't believe in QALYs can just run the numbers with every year of life valued as one; the results are similar.)

BUT IS IT WORTH THE PRICE?

Is $30,000 for a QALY a good deal? Faced with this question, most people feel the way I do when I have my car serviced and the mechanic says, "Dr. Avorn, you need to have the framistan replaced. I can get you a new one for $925." Aside from the dismay I feel at having been driving around a Volvo with a defective framistan, and the paranoia I feel over whether I *really* need to have the framistan replaced, I am left with the question: Is $925 a good price for a new framistan? How the hell should I know? Then the mechanic makes it even tougher: "You know, Doc, that's the price for a new Volvo framistan. If you want, I could probably get you a rebuilt framistan much cheaper, say for around five hundred bucks. It wouldn't be quite as good, you know, but almost. And it'll set you back only about half as much." Great. A whole new option to figure out. Feels like being back at the office.

In both instances, one craves a method that will take into account all the benefits of the new product as well as all its costs. Part of the appeal of cost-effectiveness analysis is that that is *all* it does. It generates a number we can bring to our beleaguered Pharmacy and Therapeutics Committee for them to factor into their debate. But we still need to determine whether a price tag of $30,000 per year of life gained means that it is "worth it" to use tPA. This is the point at which disputes can break out among ethicists, clinicians, insurance companies, doctors, and patients. It is the moment when a wise cost-effectiveness analyst will quietly leave the room, offering just one parting word of advice: "Look, I never said whether or not a life-year was worth a particular number of dollars. It's not my job to make those kinds of judgments. But you might want to stop beating on each other long enough to check out how that cost compares to what you're paying for other medical interventions that you're using routinely."

A virtue of this kind of cost-effectiveness benchmarking is that once we calculate the cost per extra QALY (or plain-vanilla life-year) that any new medication yields, we can look at it alongside the cost per extra year yielded by competing drugs, as well as by a variety of other medications and other treatments that we commonly use. The analyst can then say, "I don't know what the value of a year of human life is worth any more than the next person does. But I can tell you that new drug A for disease Z gives you more (or less) bang for the buck than drug B does. I can also tell you how it stacks up against a large number of other drugs for other diseases that we're already paying for."

Proponents of this field have examined a host of treatments the health care system regularly pays for—ones that are considered standard, of acceptable cost, and generally "worth doing" even before anyone ever thought about their cost-effectiveness. One commonly used example is kidney dialysis. For decades, our society has decided that this lifesaving treatment is clearly within the range of acceptable costs if a patient needs it. When researchers went back and calculated just how many dollars it costs to keep a patient on dialysis, the price tag kept coming in at around $50,000 per QALY gained. One recent assessment was conducted by Dr. Wolfgang Winkelmayer in my division, who noted how stable this estimate has been over many years, and across different countries. Other convenient benchmarks of cost-effectiveness price tags include the treatment of high blood pressure and the use of drugs to lower cholesterol in at-risk patients, both of which cost about $50,000 per QALY gained or less. Returning to our thrombolytic example, it turned out that despite the tenfold greater cost of tPA, according to the GUSTO findings those additional dollars bought that extra survival at a price well within the range of what we usually pay for other treatments. The new drug has now replaced streptokinase at most American hospitals.

So far so good. We can use exactly the same approach to provide guidance on which cholesterol-lowering drug our HMO should use, or which broad-spectrum antibiotic our hospital should stock. But in using cost-effectiveness analysis, we must consider two very important caveats. First is the distinction between "cost-effective" and "cost-saving." A relatively small number of medications are actually cost-saving, meaning that their expense is more than paid back by the clinical or economic good they do. Some examples of this are immunizations and aspirin used to lower the risk of heart attack in men at particularly high risk. By contrast, the vast majority of treatments are at best cost-effective: their price is reasonable in light of the good that they do, but they always require putting net additional dollars into the system.

This is a key difference, often lost on many prescribers and managers. It's analogous to going to the mall and finding a hundred-dollar bill on the floor, versus shopping the sales and getting a number of good bargains. In the former case, you're simply ahead a hundred bucks. In the latter case, you may have found a great $100 sweater for $60, a quality $400 suit marked down to $250, five $40 silk ties going for just $20 each, and a $25 dinner that costs just $15 as an early-bird special. Each may be a very good deal and a wise purchase, but you've still got to come up with the $425 to pay for all of them. It's exactly the same when we add cost-effective drugs to our medical shopping carts: even if each is a reasonable value (let's say $50,000 or less per QALY gained), they still add up to greater expenditures, not less. And we still need to find the money to pay for them.

Another concern about cost-effectiveness analysis is that it carries with it some heavy methodological and ethical baggage. Before embracing it wholeheartedly as a kind of clinical string theory that can tie together all the fiscal dimensions of drug decision making, we had better take a critical look at some of its loose ends.

SOME MESSY ASPECTS

One disadvantage of these calculations is that they are prone to facile applications. Readers with good memories, or those who are especially prurient, will recall the odd numbers that popped up when researchers tried to define the utility value of treating erectile dysfunction. That study was intended as a cost-effectiveness study of Viagra, although last time we encountered it we withdrew our attention before reaching its economic climax. As we saw, to come to an economic measure of the drug's worth the authors took the Beaver Dam data, some surveys of a few men, and a review of the puny existing literature to measure the disutility of impotence, measured as a reduction in quality-adjusted life-years. The researchers then plugged those findings into a computer model along with numbers on the cost, efficacy, and side effects of Viagra. A surprising finding arose: the drug was reported to cost only about $11,300 per QALY gained. Using the crude benchmark of $50,000 per QALY as the approximate threshold for a good buy, the analysis made Viagra look like an excellent deal. If we accept these results, any objection to the drug's cost, even at ten bucks a pill, goes limp. The difficulty arises in believing the inputs. The authors were astute enough to realize that cost-effectiveness analysis can rarely yield a single rigid number for such a complex issue, especially in the face of all those slippery assumptions. So they came upon an *a posteriori* list of plausible ranges for all the digits inserted into the model, to see if their output was sensitive to any of its members. This analysis showed that the findings stood up handsomely over a wide range of assumptions. It was, as the statisticians say, robust. But whether or not it was real is another matter: in the end, the flimsiness of the basic data used makes it difficult to consider this a hard number.

Other problems can also occur when cost-effectiveness analysts try to cut-and-paste general utility theory to create an all-purpose tool for assigning value to a given medication. One paradoxical issue is how time is handled. Because most cost-effectiveness analysis has its roots in the world of commerce, it treats the time value of health expenditures and outcomes the same way a banker would deal with the time value of money. In business, it makes good economic sense that money you won't get for several years should be valued less than money you'll be paid immediately. If you invested those immediate dollars they could bear fruit right away in a commercial opportunity, or earn interest in the bank. Moreover, inflation will make $1,000 received ten years from now worth less than $1,000 today. So in economics it's logical to discount the value of future financial benefits or debts in calculating their net present value.

But how does this translate into thinking about health care outcomes? If we go down this road, both theory and mathematics require us to discount the value of future clinical events at the same rate used for discounting future dollar expenditures. As a result, the value of a year of good health added to my life in twenty years (e.g., by taking a preventive medication every day starting now) must be reduced by a fixed percentage per year to determine its net present value, exactly as if it were a financial windfall that would come my way in two decades. The logic also requires that future bad events also be discounted: the negative impact of a heart attack I'll suffer in twenty years would be attenuated sharply by calculating its net present value of badness. This substantially reduces the impact of most events that will befall people when they are old. But that's the life stage when most medical problems occur, as well as when the benefits of most preventive drugs kick in. Many of the dollars required for medications to achieve those future health benefits have to be spent starting today, well before what budgeteers call the out-years. This ends up devaluing the impact of benefits that accrue to people after they enter the geriatric age group.

Controversy rages about the correct discount rate to use in such studies; recommended numbers have ranged from 0 percent to 10 percent per year. Because of the many years of use required for the preventive therapies we prescribe, the discount rate chosen will have an enormous impact on how these calculations come out. Sometimes, the recommendations that flow from such analyses depend more on which discount rate is used than on any other variable considered; opposite recommendations may result from the same analysis, depending on the rate picked. Because that rate can feel awfully arbitrary, especially as it relates to clinical events, these supposedly objective analyses can be terribly fragile, to put it kindly.

OTHER PROBLEMS WITH UTILITY THEORY

If we think carefully about what we ought to pay for a drug, before you know it we're grappling with one of the most fundamental problems in philosophy: What is good? What should medical care provide to people? In the larger scheme of things, what are medicines for? Longevity, control of symptoms, freedom from pain, reduction in disability? Of course it's all of these, but in what order of priority? And what if one good (say, pain reduction in a patient dying of metastatic cancer) is at odds with another (prolongation of life)?

The one-dimensional map of life-years added doesn't always fit the shared goals that doctors and patients should have, especially at the end of life. Even if we quality-adjust those life-years, in these analyses prolongation of living (or of dying) is nearly always assumed to have value. This is the inverse of the human-capital model, in which any prolongation of life in a nonproductive person has no worth, or even a negative dollar value. But in trying to put the richly complex mission of medicine on a one-dimensional scale in which more is always better or always worse, economic models can risk distorting the most human aspects of illness and healing. In caring for a terminal cancer victim in constant pain, discussions with the patient may lead to the decision to use as much morphine as needed to alleviate that discomfort even if it means shortening life. That may well be the right decision, but for reasons that are way beyond the metric of cost-effectiveness analysis.

Used poorly, cost-effectiveness analysis of drugs or any other health care intervention can even run against the very grain of the medical enterprise. The problem has its roots in the beginnings of utility theory—back at least as far as the eighteenth-century English philosopher Jeremy Bentham. In his *Introduction to the Principles of Morals and Legislation* (1789), he laid down the bedrock set of assumptions on which all such analyses rest. Bentham argued that the basis for any action should be whether it promotes utility—the creation of pleasure or the prevention of pain. All governmental activity and individual behavior, he contended, should aim at increasing society's overall utility so as to provide, in his famous phrase, "the greatest happiness of the greatest number." Most contemporary cost-effectiveness analysis in medicine is a direct descendant of Bentham's "felicific calculus," and this can create some curious anomalies. Utilitarianism calls on society to spend its resources on interventions that yield the most life-years or QALYs per dollar spent, working down to those that yield fewer until all available resources are used up. That way, the finite pool of dollars available will be deployed in a way that yields the most benefits for the most people, maximizing the overall amount of utility that can be squeezed out of whatever budget there is to spend.

This sounds like a great idea, but like any simple rule it can produce some ethical catastrophes. Consider this bizarre hypothetical application: if the goal of generating the greatest medical good for the greatest number were all the moral guidance we needed to make resource allocation decisions, it would be perfectly fine to take a large group of healthy elderly people and harvest both kidneys from each to transplant into twice as many young renal failure patients. If no replacement were provided for their kidney function the oldsters would soon die, but not all that many years before they would have died anyway. In doing so, each person would have provided a nephrological twofer, yielding far more life-years for twice as many younger counterparts—more than doubling the available pleasure, to use Bentham's term. Of course this is unthinkable, but it helps to analyze why: in mindlessly counting up life-years saved, the plan fails to take account of any other overriding ethical principles. Similar problems can occur if we use utility theory uncritically to drive resource allocation decisions for medications.

More subtle variants of this paradox can put the requirements of utilitarianism on a direct collision course with my role as a doctor. Considering clinical problems from the perspective of the greatest good for the largest number of patients can be incompatible with the sense of one-to-one moral responsibility that a conscientious physician feels toward the individual patient who has come asking me for help. Treating the inherited disorder Gaucher's disease can consume tens of thousands of dollars per year, which doesn't yield a very pretty number per life-year gained. But would cost-effectiveness analysis have me manage all my patients with high blood pressure first (along with everyone else with a more favorable cost-per-QALY figure) before I wrote a single prescription for any patients with Gaucher's? Some advocates of this approach would say yes, a view at odds with much of what medicine is about.

It's no accident that the idea of transferring this concept to health care came primarily from policy analysts and mathematicians rather than doctors. The patient I'm taking care of expects me to do everything possible to treat the problem at hand, not to prioritize society's use of resources and withhold some care so as to leave more for other patients. It's a little like the situation of the little girl who falls down a well in a small town. The citizenry expects that no expense will be spared to help this one identified child, and understandably so. Yet those same citizens may the same month vote down a tax bill to fund programs in health or human services that would have had an enormous impact on the health and welfare of much larger numbers of the town's children in general.

These issues will become more common as we discover more costly drugs to help small numbers of patients. Increasingly, we will be forced to ask whether there is any limit to the bedside doctor's love-the-one-you're-with orientation. For if we physicians have total disdain for our role as stewards of medical resources, it will make medical care unaffordable for many, as has already happened. The direct result of that moral choice is a health care system that spends so much on medications for some patients that others are unable to afford drug coverage at all. Happily, we will see that a more thoughtful approach to the problem can reconcile both perspectives and spare us from the unappealing outcomes either extreme would produce.

WHOSE PERSPECTIVE TO USE?

The all-against-all marketplace vision of American health care acts like a powerful magnet in health economics, causing many physicians, managers, and academics to line up like iron filings in its force field. This can foster a silo mind-set, in which each component of health care is seen as its own cost center or revenue stream. Each is then considered separately from the unique and inward-looking perspective of a particular economic player. When this view is applied to patient care, it leads to assessments that can sound grotesque to a doctor and, I expect, to most patients as well: "We're starting to see a negative margin for our portfolio of mental health products," or "Our cancer product line showed good profitability in the last fiscal quarter." (The latter statement would make sense only on the lips of a tobacco company executive.)

For prescription drugs, the most common version of this approach analyzes the drug bill of a given hospital or HMO in sublime isolation from any clinical outcomes. In this view, higher drug expenses are bad, lower ones are good. But of course the cost of a medication has to be looked at along with how its effects reverberate throughout the rest of the health care system. This requires understanding its impact on nondrug domains, such as improving the patient's clinical status, shortening the length of hospital stay, or preventing the need for readmission. Ideally, we should be looking at these questions from the widest possible perspective, that of society as a whole, rather than from the narrower standpoint of a given health maintenance organization or hospital or insurer.

That broad perspective can give an answer that may differ from the view seen from a single component of the health system, especially in the short term. For example, it may well be in the best interest of society as a whole for older women with very thin bones to be treated with medications for osteoporosis to reduce their risk of fractures. But a health maintenance organization having trouble meeting its existing drug budget is not likely to warm to an ambitious program designed to increase its expenditures on these costly drugs. At present about 20 to 30 percent of HMO patients disenroll from their plans each year—what managed care people call the churn rate. But the advantages of osteoporosis drugs, like drugs for blood pressure, cholesterol, and glaucoma, don't emerge until years later. The fact that a cohort of patients will have fewer fractures or heart attacks or strokes years from now is little comfort to a managed care pharmacy director berated for exceeding his budget for the current quarter.

"Why should I commit a huge amount to these drugs now," an HMO drug benefit manager once asked me, "when by the time these people are ready to have their hip fractures, a lot of them will be covered by Medicare or in some other HMO?" It's a savvy business insight, although it makes for crappy health care. There was a time when I thought this kind of current-fiscal-year thinking would never be seen in a government-sponsored health care system that covered an entire province or nation, since those systems could naturally take a larger, population-oriented view. Not necessarily. Even societally based health care systems can find themselves putting budgetary concerns over wider public health goals: several European systems of universal health care have levels of use of drugs to manage osteoporosis or high cholesterol that are lower than that in many American HMOs.

Our research group came upon a vivid illustration of this conflict between clinical and managerial goals in a study we conducted about a difficult treatment decision in hemophilia. Patients with this disease cannot make a protein needed to coagulate the blood; when they bleed, they must be given those blood factors intravenously to control the hemorrhage. Even worse, a subset of them go on to create antibodies to that clotting factor that deactivate it as quickly as it can be given. As a result, they can bleed uncontrollably for days at a time and require truly massive volumes of factor to stop the hemorrhage; at our hospital, one patient with this problem consumed over a million dollars of clotting factor in a single year.

These patients can be cared for in two ways. They can be treated episode by episode, using high doses of factor at the time of each hemorrhage, pouring it in faster than the patient's antibodies can chew it up. Alternatively, we can try to overwhelm the antibodies, by giving a still greater amount of factor along with immunosuppressive drugs in an attempt to defeat the antibody once and for all. This generally works well, but the gargantuan amount of clotting factor required for the initial treatment makes its expense astronomical, often amounting to hundreds of thousands of dollars. A study we performed, led by Dr. Alan Colowick, then training in hematology at the Brigham, calculated the costs and outcomes of each approach. Here again, there had not yet been any head-to-head comparison of the two approaches, just individual trials of each method separately. By reviewing these and a host of other papers on the costs and outcomes of care for these challenging patients, our group constructed a computer model that "virtually" pitted the two strategies against each other. It showed that although the proactive immune tolerance strategy has a much higher up-front cost, it works better in eradicating the dangerous antibody, and so increases patients' life expectancy. The interesting twist was this: this method also turns out to cost less over a patient's lifetime, because less clotting factor is needed year after year once the initial treatment is given. Despite this, many health care systems are still reluctant to initiate this therapy because of the massive front-end expense they would have to incur. Immune tolerance treatment may have the best outcome for the patient and cost society less in the long run, but its initial economic burden still makes it unattractive to many of the players in our atomized health care system.

There are many such examples in which the best therapeutic decision for the patient, even the best decision for society as a whole, looks unappealing to the piece of the health care system that has to pay for it now. This will continue to be a problem as long as health care decisions are driven more by the short-term fiscal needs of specific payers than by the big-picture clinical needs of patients. Cost-effectiveness analysis can demonstrate how changing the perspective of the analysis (from the payer's short-term view to a long-term societal view) can radically influence the results of the calculations.

A MODEST CONCLUSION

As long as it is employed humbly, cost-effectiveness analysis can help us understand the trade-offs we inevitably face between drug expenditures and outcomes. But when the analyses become too grandiose, tossing around numbers with little quantitative basis or pitting all treatments for all diseases against each other, the method risks losing both intellectual and moral legitimacy.

These analyses can be powerful policy medicines if used appropriately, but like drugs they can also have unintended consequences that may be dangerous, particularly if undetected. As a doctor, I find the method most valuable for comparing different ways to get the patient to a given endpoint: curing the pneumonia, dissolving the blood clot, eradicating the cancer, controlling the diabetes, and so forth. It forces us to look at all the inputs and outcomes of treatment, not just the price of the drug, and obliges us to think hard about which sector of the health care system is spending how much to achieve what results. If we used such analysis only for this circumscribed purpose, it could take us far in identifying the most efficient ways to achieve some common clinical goals—without having to address the unanswerable question of whether it's more "efficient" to treat diabetes, cancer, or AIDS.

All of us who venture into the arcane world of cost-effectiveness analysis must constantly remind ourselves that it is by definition an oversimplification of complex problems. As Einstein pointed out, not everything that counts can be counted. The probability data we need to use may simply not exist if they were never collected in clinical trials or large epidemiologic studies. Or the neat calculus of utility theory may not match the real world occupied by sick people and those who care for them. Can we really assign accurate numbers to define how bad Mr. Smith's emphysema is compared to Ms. Jones' kidney failure? And the analyses do not address vital questions such as whether more public benefit would result from a billion more dollars spent on medications versus foreign invasions versus tax cuts for the wealthy. Those cost-effectiveness comparisons are enormously important, but lie in a larger realm.

In our smaller universe of prescribing choices, many comparisons of cost versus outcome are doable, and worth doing. For any drug, well-made generic versions work exactly as well as the brand-name version of that molecule, usually at a fraction of the price. Similarly, the ALLHAT study showed that for most hypertensive patients, thiazides work better and cost less than higher-priced blood pressure regimens of other types. These entry-level cost-effectiveness analyses could be done by a first-year medical student on the back of an envelope, yet wide application of their conclusions would save billions of dollars on the annual U.S. medical bill, and enable the nation to afford all the drugs our citizenry needs. Other calculations take more work, but have equally important lessons: lowering cholesterol in high-risk patients provides wonderful results at a reasonable cost; vaccines are a fantastically good way to spend health care resources; wise use of anticoagulants yields major clinical benefits for a modest investment. Yet in everyday practice, even these obvious lessons are often honored more in the breach.

BUDGETS AND BEDSIDES

The future of medicine will require physicians to keep one eye on how wisely we deploy the health care resources that society has (for now, at least) put under our control. But our gaze must also remain fixed on the individual human being sitting or lying in front of us. Insurance companies or HMOs may see medical care in terms of covered lives or groups of insureds, but as a doctor my responsibility is also to see it in terms of sick people, one at a time.

Common sense can point us to a reconciliation of these conflicting viewpoints. We can use—indeed, we need to use—a stripped-down, humble version of cost-effectiveness analysis to help answer important questions about the comparative value of the drugs we prescribe for particular conditions. It's much less clear that this tool will provide the overarching answers to complex clinical and social priorities that many of its proponents envision, and that's okay. Rather than push the technique beyond its appropriate limits, I'd prefer to go with the good sense of a well-trained and compassionate physician. This may require anguished choices that are more painful than looking up a drug on a table and deciding if its use is "worth it" in a given patient. Goethe reminded us that for some matters feeling uncertain is uncomfortable, but feeling certain is ridiculous.

WHERE DOES ALL THIS leave us with respect to the cost-effectiveness analysis of drugs? Humbled and encouraged. Humbled by realizing that this technique is built on some sweeping assumptions that may conflict with the values underlying the human and social enterprise of medicine. Humbled as well by the frailty of measurements that rely heavily on judgments about illness that are probably beyond the capacity of the human mind to measure, and whose application to individual patients may miss the mark entirely. But used with circumspection, these tools can provide a helpful starting point for many clinical and policy deliberations. They can help us distinguish medicinal silk purses from sow's ears, not to mention eye of newt. That may not be satisfying to analysts who make their living by extrapolating such findings to four decimal places, but it's still an important contribution. The approach can also help justify the use of drugs with a legitimately high sticker price, if we can show that they actually have a far more modest economic impact when the good they do is also factored into the equation.

At a time when the nation thinks it is unable to afford even basic drug coverage for millions of people while we waste billions of dollars on overhyped drugs of limited worth, basic cost-effectiveness analysis can point us toward a first-approximation way to identify which drugs represent truly good value, and which are indefensibly overpriced pharmacological baubles.

Now for some good news. No denial of care will be needed to shrink our nation's bloated drug budget down to an affordable size. *We are already spending enough on drugs in the United States to meet the pharmaceutical needs of every man, woman, and child in the country.* There need not be an irreconcilable clash between my role as the compassionate physician trying to do the best for the patient in front of me, versus the pragmatic utilitarian shepherding the nation's scarce drug resources to yield the greatest good for the greatest number. All the billions we need could be saved just by reducing the sums we waste on products that are not at all better than their cheaper alternatives—just more expensive. Nor should we uncritically accept the assumption of scarcity that underlies so much of the drive to define the cost-effectiveness of specific drugs. There is so much waste and inefficiency in the way we employ medications that we can have a revenue-neutral solution to our drug access problem without recourse to rationing.

Rather than resort to that "r" word, we need to look more critically at the lifeboat mentality that characterizes so much discussion of the economics of medication coverage. In that metaphor, a society confronting limited medical resources is likened to the passengers on an overcrowded and sinking lifeboat, who have to choose whom to throw overboard so that the rest can survive. But the sinking-lifeboat metaphor is only partly correct. True, there are increasing numbers of Americans floating about in the pharmaceutical equivalent of small leaky vessels, wondering who among them will be tossed into the sea. But a wider view reveals that the lifeboats are encircled by a fleet of cabin cruisers and destroyers, their decks filled with well-dressed experts offering suggestions and commentaries on how such life-and-death decisions should be made. Instead of focusing on the content of those recommendations, energy would be better spent on redeploying the fleet to rescue some of the victims.

TO RETURN to the real world of medical practice, it's time to admit that even the best cost-effectiveness analysis doesn't influence prescribing very much, any more than does erudite pharmacology or practical epidemiology. Like those who study efficacy or side effects, those who study the cost-effectiveness of competing drug therapies mostly talk to and write for each other. Our findings appear in medical journals, but that is only a small factor shaping the everyday decisions doctors and patients make about medication use. The biggest bullhorns of information transfer are outside our hands. Understanding how prescription drugs are used today in the United States requires more than a grasp of the science and economics involved; we need to see how information about that knowledge is or isn't transmitted to the doctors and patients who are the frontline drug decision makers. That is one of the biggest reasons so many Americans can't afford the drugs they need; we'll take it up in the next part.

PART FOUR: INFORMATION

16: SIGNALS, NOISE,
AND THE BIG VOID

The high cost of individual drugs explains a great deal about why the nation's rising drug expenditures have seemed to defy the laws of economics and even, it seems, of gravity. An equally important cause is how physicians make decisions about what we prescribe. Those judgments in turn depend on what information about medications flows or doesn't flow to us and to our patients. Let's return to our comparison with the skyrocketing effectiveness and dropping prices of computers. Anyone with a subscription to *PC Magazine* can make a reasoned decision about whether the new Pentium chip is worth an upgrade, or whether Compaq's latest laptop is better than IBM's. But drug-use decisions are far more complicated, and they are controlled by a relatively small cadre of specialists: we doctors, for the most part.

Why aren't we doing as well as the computer folks? A major reason is that doctors don't always have access to the kind of neutral "tech support" we need, especially in the United States. But we are awash in inputs of all sorts designed to inform us about the drugs we prescribe. Medication decisions, while more reality-based than a century ago, are still heavily influenced by the triumph of hype and hope over data, of the politics of self-interest over coherent science-based policy. Many physicians and patients are seduced by the latest medication fashions, gorge on expensive clinical junk food and empty pharmacologic calories, haven't a clue as to what it's all going to cost, and don't feel like it's their problem.

One of the most active areas of basic biological research is a field known as signal transduction. It turns out that an enormous amount of what an intelligence operative might call "chatter" is going on continuously inside the body's cells, and between them as well. These biochemical messages keep cells informed about what's occurring around them, which new developments might affect their function, whether there is an imminent hazard to guard against, or when there's a tasty molecular morsel floating by that can be ingested and put to some higher use. Some signals activate a specific activity or tune it down; some help cells know what others are up to and whether they should produce more or less of a given substance themselves.

Several diseases seem to have their origins in the failure of signal transduction. If cells are unaware of what other cells are doing, or don't respond appropriately to that awareness, they can't function properly. If a group of them continues to reproduce despite signals from neighboring cells that doing so is robbing them of nourishment and even eating into their own boundaries, we call that cancer. The malignant tissue may go on growing for years, and can eventually destroy the biological system in which it developed.

Several levels of organization up, we have a big signal transduction problem in medicine, especially when it comes to drugs. The individual action units, whether doctors or patients, often don't receive the vital messages they need for dealing with opportunities, hazards, and resources in their immediate environments. Some signals don't turn on the right actions, so that needed prescriptions are never written. Other, misplaced signals abound—messages that say a given product is desirable when it isn't. Many of the functional units in the health care system are bathed in a hyperconcentrated brew of rogue signals that jerk us around, overstimulating this action, suppressing that behavior. To use a media analogy, it sometimes seems as if all the transmissions from Public Broadcasting System stations were being jammed by nonstop MTV, broadcast at maximum volume.

DRINKING FROM A FIRE HOSE

Churchill once observed that the problem with the Balkans is that the area produces more history than it can consume. A similar point can be made about medicine: each year, literally each day, ongoing research produces more findings than we doctors can possibly assimilate. New biomedical facts accumulate at an exponential rate, their quantity doubling at regular intervals. Medline, the National Library of Medicine bibliographic service, contains some ten million abstracts, to which it is presently adding over seven thousand new ones every *week*.

For a physician, trying to keep up with drug-related advances can feel like drinking from a fire hose, except that there are multiple fire hoses, each one spewing hundreds of gallons of new facts at us from a different angle. The *New England Journal of Medicine,* the *Journal of the American Medical*

Association, Lancet, and the *Annals of Internal Medicine* are some of the biggest nozzles for an internist like me, but vital papers about drugs appear unpredictably in dozens of other publications as well, and each specialty has its own sources. Then there are the professional meeting info-fests and continuing education courses, whose open data bars offer everything from the tonic of good clinical trial findings to sparkling promotional concoctions, as well as intoxicating sponsored brews that tastily answer all the wrong questions. The flow goes on and on.

The difficulty of taking all this in is evoked by the wonderful scene in Disney's *Fantasia* in which Mickey Mouse, as the sorcerer's apprentice, casts a spell on a broom to make it carry buckets of water for him, and then can't get it to stop. Each time he whacks it in half with an ax it becomes two brooms carrying water, then four, then eight, then sixteen, flooding the sorcerer's den: arcane knowledge run amok. It's no coincidence that one of the first publications on technology assessment in health care was named *The Sorcerer's Apprentice.*

There's a perverse paradox here: those of us who see the fewest patients have the most time to keep up with the latest advances. My friends who spend twelve- and fourteen-hour days in clinical practice could make much more use of this information than I do, but they don't have as much time to acquire it. Each year, they're obliged to see more patients per hour, perform more procedures, and deal with more administrative busywork. The journals pile up, their vital discoveries undiscovered. The efficiency of the marketplace strikes again: data, data, everywhere, but no time to stop and think. The resultant blockages in the flow of information constitute one of the most important—and underappreciated—reasons our health care system cannot deploy medications or other resources more appropriately and affordably.

THE EDUCATIONAL VOID

The overload problem begins in medical school. Those years could be an ideal time to inoculate physicians-to-be with the cognitive sensitization they'll need once they're in practice: teaching them how to systematically compare a treatment's benefits, risks, and costs, how to understand the complex interplay of drug use, expenditures, and outcomes in the health care system. But in most schools these topics are either omitted from the curriculum altogether or touched on glancingly and then forgotten amid the necessary din of biochemistry, neuroanatomy, and genetics. Today's graduates know more than I ever will about DNA transcription, but many of them lack the savvy about real-world drug use that was once common among third- and fourth-year students.

In many medical schools, clinical pharmacology has lost its curriculum time to more modern fields such as molecular biology. The hours of pharmacology teaching that remain are increasingly given over to topics like the biochemical basis of drug action—vitally important, but one more remove from teaching students how to choose and use medicines in intact patients. This shift was reflected years ago in an organizational change at my own institution: Harvard Medical School no longer has a Department of Pharmacology; that function was folded into the Department of Biological Chemistry and Molecular Pharmacology. Similarly, many post-residency fellowships in clinical pharmacology have difficulty recruiting enough talented trainees, while others, such as the program at Harvard, have shut down altogether.

Events at the cellular and molecular levels are enormously important; they underlie the effects of every drug we give. But using medications well also requires expertise at levels higher in the organizational system. Curriculum committees often despair at the prospect of giving first- and second-year students the details of currently available antibiotics, cardiovascular medications, or cancer drugs. After all, they reason, many of these drugs will be obsolete by the time the students are finished with their training six or even ten years after the start of medical school. According to this inherent obsolescence perspective, it makes more sense to teach students about the basic molecular mechanisms of drug effects. The idea is that knowledge about how to prescribe actual drugs to sick people can then be "picked up along the way" as the students begin their internships and residencies, and later on in practice.

This presumption of drug obsolescence isn't always correct; some of the most effective drug groups of today have been around for decades. Ironically, the basic concepts of how drugs work at the cellular level are also prone to obsolescence, as new and better models supplant older ones. The molecular mechanism of the moment, like the specific drug of the moment, may well be passé by the time our students are writing their own prescriptions. As one of my medical school professors put it years ago with atypical humility, "As research advances, about half of what we will teach you over the next four years will turn out to be wrong. The problem is, we don't presently know which half." But one area of knowledge that will never become outdated is the capacity to evaluate evidence rigorously, the sense of healthy skepticism, and the tools of inquiry that these habits of mind require. When it comes to pharmacology, the nation needs to do a much better job of teaching those timeless skills to our medical students.

THE SCIENTIFIC VOID

Once in practice, the physician must live daily with the "water, water, everywhere" paradox of drug information. The informational fluid in which we're awash is a mixed blessing. There's the pure distillate of well-filtered scientific findings, but there's even more saltwater promotional material surrounding us. When it comes to data on medications, doctors and patients need more fresh water to survive in our little informational vessels.

Even the finest aqueducts can't move along the flow of information if the spigot at the source is turned down to a trickle. To see the beginnings of the problem, we can start in Rockville, Maryland—home of the FDA. We saw in Part One that the agency generally does not require a manufacturer to demonstrate that a drug works any better than available alternatives—just that it's better than placebo. In fact many new drugs are *not* better than already available alternatives. But if a manufacturer isn't required to perform comparative trials they are much less likely to occur, and the data needed to feed our distilled-information thirst are never produced. With a few notable exceptions, the slack has not been taken up by others in the private sector (such as HMOs or other large insurers/payers), governmental programs (Medicare, Medicaid, or those two huge drug purchasers, the Department of Veterans Affairs and the Defense Department), or the National Institutes of Health, and certainly not by the FDA itself.

The two landmark NIH-funded studies published in 2002 that we've considered before illustrate what can be accomplished when common drug questions are addressed with well-funded systematic investigation. The trial of hormone replacement therapy found that some of the most widely prescribed drug products in America did not decrease the risk of heart disease, but did cause breast cancer, stroke, blood clots, and other bad outcomes. The ALLHAT study showed that using newer, more expensive blood pressure medications resulted in more strokes and heart disease than the old-standby thiazides, and drove up drug costs as well. What was remarkable about these studies was not that they were done, but that they were performed decades later than they should have been, and that there are not dozens more like them to address the myriad other medication-use questions that remain unstudied.

Thirst is a powerful drive. Survival guides offer the unappealing advice that if you're ever stranded at sea, it helps to drink your own urine for the first few days because it will be less toxic than the sea water around you. Starved for purified data, many doctors do the self-referential information equivalent: they feed their decisions with their own recent clinical experience. This may be better than relying solely on promotional material in the same way that drinking urine is better than relying on salt water, but "In my experience . . ." is usually a less reliable guide for choosing a drug than "The clinical trial data show . . ." That's how our hypothetical Dr. Vasily failed to prevent Stan's stroke in the Prologue; millions of such evidence-starved decisions are made daily.

TRYING TO FILL THE VOIDS:
THE NEED FOR SYSTEMATIC DRUG ASSESSMENT

When you're dying, you'll try anything. That's how Noelle Merino felt when her doctor told her the breast cancer had returned. But there was one final possibility: a new treatment that used extraordinarily high doses of chemotherapy. This is toxic to the bone marrow and can destroy a patient's capacity to make blood cells, so the drugs are followed with a transplant of healthy bone marrow, where such cells are made. More drugs are then given to prevent rejection of the transplanted marrow. The regimen would be lengthy, painful, and expensive. Although data were still being gathered about the approach, Noelle's doctor felt it represented her last hope. Her insurance company disagreed; the administrator on the phone informed her that her policy would not cover the new treatment.

"You're signing my death sentence!" she screamed at the disembodied voice. "I can't afford to pay for this myself!"

"I'm sorry, but that's the way the policy is written."

Unknown to Ms. Merino, change was in the air. Thousands of women across the country had confronted the same situation she now faced: their doctors had recommended high-dose chemotherapy plus bone marrow transplantation to treat their breast cancer, and their insurance companies had declared the therapy experimental and refused to pay for it. Local news channels told their anguished stories; letters were written, lawsuits threatened. Patients' rights groups and the companies that made the drugs joined forces to apply pressure. State and federal legislators held hearings to condemn the insurance companies, accusing them of valuing their profits over saving lives.

Within weeks of Noelle's confrontation with her insurer, she received a welcome phone call. Her doctor told her that the lobbying and several successful lawsuits against recalcitrant HMOs had worked; her state had just passed a new law requiring all insurers to pay for the high-dose chemo plus bone marrow therapy. Like women all over the nation, she was admitted to the hospital and began the long and grueling treatment. Thousands of patients who had previously been denied a therapy they hoped would save their lives could now get the care their doctors recommended, and their insurers would be legally obliged to pay for it.

The regimen was as rough as her oncologist had predicted. First came the wrenching vomiting, the painful erosions in her throat and esophagus, and multiple bouts with fungus infections. Then Noelle developed graft-versus-host disease, a grisly condition in which white blood cells formed by the newly infused marrow perceive the patient to be a foreign protein and attempt to destroy it. The condition caused her to slough large areas of skin, requiring her transfer to the burn unit for care. A fungal abscess started growing in her brain; her kidneys were damaged by one of the antibiotics required to treat it. After a ten-week hospitalization, Ms. Merino died.

"We fought this tumor as hard as we could," her doctor told Noelle's husband shortly after her funeral. "At least we know we gave her every chance possible."

That year and in the years that followed, litigation and legislation gave women like Noelle access to high-dose chemotherapy and bone marrow transplantation as their one last chance to try to beat their tumors. Not all had as excruciating a course as hers, but it was a painful and arduous treatment for each of them. Some improved; some died. But for all women with health insurance, the new law made sure that their coverage would pay for the costly care, which averaged about $80,000 per case.

Six years after passage of the law in Noelle's state that guaranteed cancer patients access to the innovative treatment, several medical journals published the results of randomized clinical trials designed to systematically test whether it worked. The studies found that despite the pain and complications that the treatment invariably produced, patients who received it did not fare any better than identical patients randomized to receive older, less invasive forms of care. The legislation and lawsuits had forced public- and private-sector payers to cover a costly, excruciating treatment that didn't work. Forty thousand patients and over a billion dollars later, the legislation was repealed. The treatment is rarely used for breast cancer anymore.

Signal transduction in health care delivery can succeed or fail at several different points. Specific studies can be funded or not, and their findings can be heeded or not. Information transfer can proceed well or poorly at the societal level. It is surprisingly hard for a prescribing doctor—or even for the formulary committee of a large health care organization—to find reliable information that compares the benefits, risks, and costs of comparable drugs. One would expect that a matter so important would have numerous organizations, both in the private sector and in government, churning out analyses and information on a daily basis to inform these decisions—especially since their consequences can literally be a matter of life or death, as well as involve huge sums of money. But this is not the case. Our health care system remains ill-equipped to generate the vital benefit-risk-cost information we need about medications, and we often ignore it even when it exists.

A DEPRESSING HISTORY

Several times since World War II, attempts were made to establish federally sponsored programs to measure the effectiveness of health care interventions, including drugs, and disseminate those findings. A quick review of this history is sobering, if not downright depressing. One of the earliest initiatives was the National Center for Health Care Technology Assessment, established in the 1980s to support rigorous studies of this kind. Concern arose in the industries (such as medical devices and pharmaceuticals) whose technologies were to be assessed, and the program was quietly shut down not long after it started.

Few believed that the same fate could befall the respected Congressional Office of Technology Assessment. For decades, the OTA provided nonpartisan scientific advice to Congress on legislative questions that had dense technical content, and its work was widely respected on both sides of the aisle. OTA had a small staff by Washington standards, only about 130 people—but half of them had doctoral degrees, generally in the sciences. They worked with independent scientists to assemble facts and identify policy options for Congress on complicated topics from nuclear power to genetic research. I learned this firsthand by participating in an OTA study of medical research and the pharmaceutical industry in 1992 and 1993. The project's format was typical: bipartisan sponsorship, freedom for the outside experts to present our views regardless of the political consequences, and an adept core staff of technocrats who managed to summarize our deliberations in language even a congressman could understand.

Our report's format reflected its process: like all OTA documents, it did not make recommendations, but instead listed the available legislative options and their likely consequences. This was exactly the kind of information you'd want if you were a conscientious legislator trying to make policy in an area whose technical aspects were over your head. In a city in which everything is politicized, OTA's reports were legendary for their fairness and balance; it was not unusual for senators or representatives on both sides of a given issue to cite an OTA report as backing their position.

But in the process the agency also made enemies, particularly in the corporate sector.

In 1995, as part of the Republican revolution to shrink government activity on all fronts, Congress voted to terminate the OTA—even though at $22 million its annual cost was barely visible in the federal budget. It was also a Republican, Representative Amo Houghton of New York, who led the fight to save OTA: "We are cutting off one of the most important arms of Congress when we cut off unbiased knowledge about science and technology." In fact, eliminating OTA probably did increase the efficiency of government; it is much quicker just to have a lobbyist for the involved industry explain the issues and recommended policy alternatives, bypassing all that troublesome data and time-consuming debate.

With the abrupt shutdown of OTA, its staffers and consultants worked extra hours to finish the requested reports that were still in progress, but couldn't get to them all. One of the studies they were working on before the budget ax fell in 1995 was to assess "how to protect against weapons of mass destruction that fall into the hands of third parties like terrorists or small nations." The report was never completed. But the federal budget was protected: that year and every year since, Congress' decision to eliminate the OTA saved eight cents in taxes for every man, woman, and child living in the United States.

One of the boldest attempts to grapple with the benefit-risk-cost triangle in medicine was the Clinical Guidelines initiative of the federal Agency for Health Care Policy and Research. This runt cousin of the National Institutes of Health is chronically underfunded but has supported some vitally important research on medical care delivery and its consequences. Under a previous name, this was the agency that had helped my own research on drug use to get off the ground. With its new name, it became universally referred to as AHCPAR (pronounced *AK*-par); its mission was to unite health care research with policy. (I thought it would have been more logical for "research" to precede "policy" in its name, but an experienced Washington hand explained that given the tendency to sound out acronyms, the agency would then be referred to as AH CRAP. This was the same fellow who explained to me why the NIH didn't name the Human Genome Project the National Institute for Genetics Research.)

The guidelines project was to represent the flowering of evidence-based medicine, clinical epidemiology, health services research, and cost-effectiveness analysis. These were all relatively young disciplines ready for prime time; the new program was designed to bring them together in awesome synergy. The enterprise would tackle a series of common clinical problems ranging from cataracts to prostate disease to chronic back pain, assemble all the studies that had ever been done on these topics, and have them reviewed critically by experts in these areas. It would then produce a synthesis of all this information in a compact, user-friendly guide to the best therapies, one version written for clinicians and another for their patients.

The opposition did not take long to see the problem. Ophthalmologists became concerned that the new cataract guidelines could, if followed, cut down sharply on their most common and lucrative procedure. The pharmaceutical industry worried that evidence-based prescribing guidelines might discourage use of high-margin patented drugs whose price tags were often much larger than their therapeutic credentials. In the end, the coup de grâce came from the nation's back surgeons. They were infuriated that the program's back pain guidelines, based on a careful review of all published studies of surgery versus less invasive treatments, concluded that these operations were unnecessary and potentially harmful for many patients. Several of the offended surgeons had repaired congressional backs (or thought they had), and they joined with other adversaries to mount an effective lobbying campaign to clip the agency's wings. With little fanfare the guidelines program was wound down, and AHCPAR's name was subsequently changed again, reemerging as AHRQ, the Agency for Healthcare Research and Quality. The linkage between research and policy had been formally renounced, and the nation took one giant step away from bringing science to bear on the systematic assessment of therapeutics.

The most recent attempt to establish a federal program to provide unbiased assessment of drugs was the CERTs project: Centers for Education and Research in Therapeutics. The initial vision called for a network of centers across the country that would conduct research on drugs' effectiveness and risk, and provide education on their optimal use for physicians, other health care professionals, and patients. Only a limited amount of funding was made available from governmental sources, and the effort became a "public-private partnership," with support coming from large drug manufacturers such as AstraZeneca, Aventis, Bristol-Myers Squibb, GlaxoSmithKline, Roche, Janssen, Lederle, Merck, Pfizer, Pharmacia, and Wyeth. The former head of Glaxo's drug epidemiology programs was appointed to chair the federal panel that determined how the public dollars would be spent, as well as to run the steering committee that guided the centers' work. He continued as a consultant to the company while running the government's CERTs selection and oversight committees.

Despite initial hopes that CERTs would provide comprehensive assessments of the safety, effectiveness, and value of comparable drugs, the centers' output thus far has focused more on specific studies of isolated topics in pharmacology, often paid for by the companies that manufacture those products. Little has been done as yet in the way of comparative assessment of competing drugs. The program's "Vision Statement" declared that "Americans should expect CERTs to be a permanent, trusted resource when they need answers to questions about therapies." The promise of this private-public partnership has not yet been realized.

FOR YEARS, many of us have argued that the nation needs systematic, publicly funded, rigorous research to measure the comparative benefits, risks, and costs of drugs. But who will be responsible for making that happen? The FDA has enough trouble fulfilling its "is it better than nothing" mandate for drugs, and finds this added responsibility unthinkable. The pharmaceutical industry, which could make the FDA's work a daily nightmare if the agency got into this area, has made it clear that it agrees. Both industry and the FDA have pointed out that the agency's enabling legislation authorizes it to approve drugs based on their efficacy alone, and makes no mention of the obligation or the mandate to compare drugs with one another, or to consider cost. Routinely requiring head-to-head studies might be defensible under a broad reading of that legislative authority, but would certainly trigger litigation by manufacturers. The NIH itself has had limited interest in these questions, preferring to spend its resources on exploring the molecular basis of disease.

THE REGULATORY VOID

If we shift our focus from inadequate policy to inadequate prescribing, we find that things are not under very good control here either. Patients and legislators seem to believe that most doctors have all the information we need to make prescribing decisions effectively, and that someone is out there making sure that we do. Quite the opposite is true: many of us don't choose drugs optimally because we were never taught how, or because the necessary comparisons have never been made. And even when the data are available, most of the time no one knows or cares whether our prescribing is compatible with the best evidence. Once a drug is approved for sale, there is alarmingly little oversight of its use, and no locus of responsibility for ensuring that it is being prescribed appropriately.

Once a doctor receives a medical license at the conclusion of training, most states never require any demonstration of competency in prescribing or any other clinical skill ever again. If I become a soft touch for junkies and start to issue narcotics prescriptions in great volume, and if I do it long enough and flagrantly enough, *and* if someone notices what I'm doing *and* turns me in, the federal Drug Enforcement Agency (not the FDA) might take away my right to prescribe controlled substances for a while. But this leaves untouched the vast majority of prescribing decisions that don't concern drugs of abuse, for which no such surveillance exists.

Once we are licensed, we are not required to keep up with emerging information about new drug products, or anything else in medicine for that matter. Despite this near-total lack of quality control, many physicians manage on their own to find time for the extra work required to stay up to date. Thousands attend excellent continuing-education lectures and multi-day courses offered by medical schools, teaching hospitals, and professional societies. These doctors make heroic efforts to keep up with the cascade of new research findings that relate to their clinical work, and spend hundreds of hours of their own time poring through medical journals. Thousands more study for and take voluntary recertification exams in their chosen fields. Unfortunately, about two thirds of continuing medical education is supported by the drug industry, but many programs are not. For example, I give a lecture on geriatric pharmacology for Harvard Medical School's annual continuing education course on the care of elderly patients. Each year, some two hundred physicians carve time out of their impossible schedules to come to Boston, often at their own expense, and sit through three long days of lectures and workshops to learn how to do their job better. Doctors sign up voluntarily for similar courses all over the country.

But the key word here is "voluntary." A large proportion of doctors don't keep up, or nourish their expertise primarily with company-sponsored freebies or mind-deadening pap at pro forma weekly rounds. In medicine—of all fields—there is no consistent quality control for staying competent; my fellow physicians have successfully blocked all attempts to make such a requirement a condition of our continuing licensure or payment.

Each state empowers a legally authorized board to determine who can practice medicine within its borders. But I have to do more to renew my Massachusetts driver's license than to renew my Massachusetts medical license. At least the state's Registry of Motor Vehicles periodically requires me to show up in person and demonstrate that I can still see. By contrast, the state Board of Registration in Medicine asks only that I sign a form every two years stating that I have been present for fifty hours of some form of continuing-education activities per year. The requirement is usually fulfilled when a physician reports having sat for an hour each week in a large darkened room in which a lecture occurred. The self-attestation is virtually never audited, and we certainly don't have to show that we actually learned anything during these sessions. A wide variety of activities can satisfy the requirement. It may involve actively studying in a rigorous and demanding continuing-education course, or taking a catnap at a local hospital's weekly Grand Rounds lecture (with both the speaker and the snacks provided by a generous drug company), or eating your way through a scientifically dubious industry-sponsored infomercial with dinner.

I once asked a member of our state's Board of Registration in Medicine why the state didn't require us to demonstrate some minimum level of pharmacological competency every five or so years before it would renew our medical licenses. A straightforward test could be given on the basics, just to make sure that some of the most important advances in therapeutics are known by every physician who continues taking care of patients. Politically infeasible, he replied. Granted, the board has in the past had trouble keeping up with even more basic expectations, such as disciplining physicians who rape their patients or commit major Medicare fraud. Subtler issues like competency are probably not within its grasp yet. The situation is similar in most states.

WHEN INFORMATION ISN'T APPLIED

What evidence is there that this causes problems? Examples abound showing that even when important facts about drugs are available, they aren't consistently translated into doctors' prescribing decisions. Despite clear evidence that overuse of antibiotics leads to the growth of resistant bacteria, not to mention wasted dollars, they are still widely prescribed for minor viral illnesses. Millions spent on consumer advertising made the first "purple pill" Prilosec (omeprazole) the most demanded prescription for bellyache or dyspepsia, even when a drug that costs much less than six dollars a dose would have worked as well for many patients. Calcium-channel blockers for high blood pressure do not have exceptional therapeutic credentials, but heavy marketing caused them to eclipse similar medications that were better and cheaper.

On the opposite end of the spectrum, perfectly good drugs are often underused—a problem that can't be blamed on insufficient trial data or promotion. Some of the most elegant and comprehensive clinical studies have shown over and over that cholesterol-lowering drugs reduce the risk of heart attack, stroke, and even cardiac death in high-risk patients. But years after these studies appeared, these drugs are severely underprescribed by doctors, despite intense marketing to us as well as directly to our patients. As we saw in earlier chapters, anticoagulants like Coumadin (warfarin) are still omitted in the care of patients with atrial fibrillation, despite copious evidence that they reduce the risk of stroke by two thirds. Medications like Fosamax (alendronate) reduce the risk of hip fracture by half in patients with severe osteoporosis, yet when Dr. Dan Solomon and I looked at the drugs taken by these patients, we found that only a small fraction of high-risk women were being treated. Worry over cost was not the problem in most of these instances, since the underuse occurred in populations with total or near-total drug coverage. Studies at the Brigham and elsewhere have proven that the humble aspirin, taken in very small doses, can markedly reduce the risk of heart attack. It's cheap, it's safe, it prevents a major medical catastrophe—yet its utilization still falls far short of the ideal.

A final example comes from another study led by Dr. Solomon in which we looked at use of the now-notorious Cox-2 drugs, products like celecoxib (Celebrex) and rofecoxib (Vioxx) that were designed to be safer than older anti-inflammatory drugs such as ibuprofen (Motrin), and about a dozen others. Even before their risk of heart disease was publicly known, it was clear that these expensive drugs weren't any more effective than older products, although they appeared to reduce the risk of gastrointestinal bleeding somewhat. Several of the risk factors for such bleeding are well understood: being older, using steroids or anticoagulants, having a history of ulcer disease, and so forth. Solomon wondered whether doctors were preferentially using these slightly safer but very expensive drugs on their higher-risk patients, and staying with the older, more affordable medications for patients at lower risk of drug-induced bleeding. So he extracted from our database a large sample of patients who had been prescribed either the older Motrin-like anti-inflammatory drugs, or their newer, costlier Cox-2 cousins.

Surprisingly, we found that a patient's bleeding risk was not a strong predictor of which drug was prescribed; many people vulnerable to drug-induced bleeding were still being given the older products, and most of the patients who took the new, costlier drugs had no apparent risk factors for bleeding. Was prescribing completely random? Not at all. When we looked at the prescribing patterns of each physician in our database, Solomon found that a doctor's practice habits were the strongest predictor of which patients got which drugs. Physicians who believed in the newer, more expensive medications gave them to most patients regardless of their risk profile, while doctors who weren't big fans of these products used them rarely, even in patients who needed them. The drugs were being both overused and underused at the same time. Dr. Phil Wang, a psychiatrist-epidemiologist in our division, has made similar observations about the use of antidepressants.

THE SOUP WE'RE IN

The lack of surveillance over what we prescribe is accompanied by weakening oversight concerning the promotional information that we and our patients see. The FDA's strict standards for accuracy in drug advertising were once the envy of doctors and governments throughout the world, but in recent years those standards have begun to erode. It is not just the excesses made possible by the removal of drugs calling themselves "supplements" from any real governmental oversight. Misleading promotion of prescription drugs is less egregious, but more and more claims that skirt the edge of verifiability now murmur seductively from the pages of medical journals and lay magazines. When a new administration assumed power in 2001, the FDA announced that it would reduce its enforcement actions related to problematic ads, and has been accused by Congress of failing to carry out its responsibility to stop misleading promotion.

If this trend continues, the situation could come to resemble that fast-growing spectator sport, professional wrestling, a bizarre example of postmodern American athleticism. Colorful, grotesquely musclebound combatants (themselves the beneficiaries of considerable medication use) prance around the ring breaking the rules while a small and pathetic referee protests vainly, jumping up and down and gesticulating impotently. No fans are surprised that the combatants don't heed the ref—that's just the way the game is played.

THE ECONOMIC VOID

Gaps in our knowledge about the comparative effectiveness of drugs are compounded by even bigger gaps in our grasp of their economics. In very round numbers, if the American medical system spends about $200 billion a year on drugs inside and outside hospitals, and if about 600,000 physicians account for most of the prescribing decisions, then each one of us on average is responsible for over $330,000 of medication expenditure annually (and several million dollars more for each of us in the other health care expenditures we order). You'd think that this financial stewardship would lead to a universal exposure to at least some medical economics in our training, but it doesn't.

The resulting fiscal innumeracy has particularly ornery effects on how we use drugs, and sets the stage for an additional set of problems related to the flow of economic information about them. We've seen that these products differ from most others because the purchasing decision is not made by the person who uses the product (the patient), but instead by a decision maker (the physician) who usually doesn't have any financial stake in that decision. Even more unusual for most marketplace transactions, many patients have traditionally gotten off the hook economically, protected from financial consequences by their insurance coverage or a government entitlement program. As a result, many participants in frontline drug purchasing decisions have until recently been about as cost-conscious as players in a late-night game of Monopoly after a few beers.

We have considered the roles of the pharmaceutical industry and politics in influencing the prices of prescription drugs. But there is an important information transfer story to be told here as well. The single largest cause of bloated drug bills is the mundane, relentless use of expensive products when far less costly ones would work every bit as well. This day-to-day financial hemorrhage is made possible by several kinds of information deficit on the part of doctors: not knowing what the prescribed drug costs, not knowing whether a given product is any better than less expensive choices, and not knowing whether the patient can afford to fill the prescription.

Several studies confirm that much prescribing looks like the work of people who have had economic lobotomies. This is not completely the fault of us doctors. It is not easy for practitioners to find out how expensive the drugs we prescribe are; prices vary widely for the same product, and are often not in open view. In our project to improve prescribing described in a later chapter, some of the doctors we visited told us that apart from all the relevant clinical information we presented, simply letting them know what various drugs actually cost was one of the most useful parts of the educational program; no one had ever shown them those numbers before.

THE GRAND ILLUSION

Plausibly enough, most doctors believe that after we give a patient a prescription, it is brought to a pharmacy, filled, and then taken pretty much as directed. This often does not occur. The problem is known variously as noncompliance, poor adherence, or impersistence. Whatever it's called, it is too rarely acknowledged, and it dramatically reduces the real-world effectiveness of prescribed treatments. One important cause is financial; in some studies a third to a half of American patients report failing to fill a prescription because of its cost. With rising drug prices, this problem will only worsen; increasing copayments and deductibles will intensify it for those who have prescription drug coverage as well. But one aspect of the problem is independent of economics. Our research group was able to study this by looking at patterns of prescription filling in several government-sponsored programs in which the patient bears little or none of a drug's cost.

Some large databases in pharmacoepidemiology are built from information about what a doctor prescribes. A good example is the United Kingdom's General Practitioner Research Database, an enormous collection of information maintained by the British government; it is built from data collected as physicians write prescriptions on their office computers. But that tells us only what medications the doctor *wanted* the patient to take, and a substantial fraction of those prescriptions never make it as far as the pharmacy. An advantage of the paid-claims information that we work with in our studies is that it is built from the bills that drugstores send to a government program for reimbursement, *after* a patient (in Medicaid, for example) has come in and filled a prescription. No filling, no bill; no bill, no data. This has provided us with a powerful way to know what medications a patient has actually obtained, and in what quantities, and how often. There is often a sharp contrast with how the doctor expected these drugs to be used.

We've looked in particular detail at drugs used to control hypertension and cholesterol—medications that do not produce any symptomatic benefit (sometimes quite the opposite) and must be taken for a lifetime to manage risk states. In studies conducted with Drs. Mark Monane, Jacques LeLorier, Eric Knight, and Josh Benner, we found a striking pattern that was consistent across patient populations, disease states, and even countries. Up to a fifth of patients filled only their first prescription, and then no more; within five years of starting on a supposedly lifelong regimen, only half or fewer were still filling any prescriptions at all in that drug class. These were all people who had generous government-provided drug coverage, so cost was not an issue. The problem didn't occur just among the indigent and chronically ill patients in our Medicaid database; we found a similar pattern in the beneficiaries of a state-run program for middle-class elderly in New Jersey, as well as in the entire over-sixty-five population of the province of Quebec.

Some interesting trends provided clues to deeper issues. In our U.S. populations, poorer patients with full drug coverage complied less well than middle-class patients; blacks complied less well than whites, even after we controlled for poverty; and the oldest patients were less likely to take their medications regularly than were the "young old" patients aged sixty-five to seventy-five.

Something is happening, or not happening, in the doctor-patient encounter that is causing a large fraction of our patients to disregard our well-intentioned recommendations, and the disconnect is greatest for our patients who are poor, nonwhite, and oldest. Since all our data came from populations with comprehensive drug coverage, the findings are a sobering reminder that merely providing payment for drugs will not ensure that they are taken as intended. A great deal more research is needed into this often-overlooked problem, drawing on the combined expertise of clinicians, epidemiologists, anthropologists, and psychologists.

INFORMATION FOR PATIENTS

However well or poorly we physicians handle information about drugs, a separate flood of communication washes over our patients once they leave the office. Each year consumers have access to more medicine-related information, a growing stream with its own torrents and whirlpools, crystal-clear eddies and toxic outflows. In olden times, before the internet and consumer advertising, the doctor's consulting room and the drugstore were the main places where such information was transferred to the patient. In the late 1980s, many of us took heart when Congress passed a bill requiring pharmacists to talk to patients about the drugs they sell them: what they do, how they should be taken, which side effects to watch out for. This education was to be offered for each medication dispensed unless the patient expressly refused it.

The plan held great promise: pharmacists' substantial knowledge about medicines is vastly underutilized in the American health care system. But faced with the imperatives of a high-volume marketplace, many chain pharmacies quickly sank to a solution familiar to anyone who has filled a prescription: a loose-leaf notebook is proffered along with the pill bottle by the person behind the counter (often a technician rather than a fully trained pharmacist) and the customer is shown where to sign. Most people think this is a kind of receipt for the drug, but next time you're asked to sign, read the small print above. It says that by your signature, you are declining counseling about the drug you are getting. When this shortcut around the new law was first devised, the pill bearer usually said something like, "You can talk to a pharmacist about your medicine if you want to; if not, just sign here." Within a few months, in many chains the phrase turned into "Sign here to get your prescription." In some stores even that has been replaced by a grunt, a gesture, and a pen on a string.

With the transformation of the corner drugstore from a mom-and-pop operation into a branch of a national company, the local druggist has suffered the same fate as the local GP, but to an even greater degree; considerations of turnover and output now impose enormous pressure on pharmacists to get the pills into the bottle, affix an adhesive label, ring up the charges, and move on to the next customer. The dispensing fee is the same whether or not any meaningful conversation occurs, producing an economic disincentive for patient education. It also provides no incentive for the pharmacist to call a doctor to discuss a prescription that may be problematic or duplicative. If a diligent pharmacist perseveres despite this, it will take a while to reach the doctor by phone; if the conversation results in eliminating the unnecessary prescription, the druggist is rewarded by losing the dispensing fee as well as the markup on the retail sale. It is remarkable how many pharmacists still try to preserve their professional role despite these erosive pressures.

The FDA has made its own attempts to improve the communication of drug information to patients; these have been consistently well intentioned and frequently frustrated. Beginning in the 1970s, the agency tried to require manufacturers to provide patients with a brief lay-language summary of the uses and side effects of each of their products, to be made available whenever a prescription was filled. A regulation was written in 1980 mandating an ambitious program of such patient-oriented educational materials. The pharmaceutical industry resisted the plan because of concerns that explanation of possible side effects could be bad for sales. Many pharmacy companies didn't want the responsibility of stocking hundreds of leaflets and making sure the right one was included with each new prescription. Some physicians were wary that giving patients too much information might cause them to second-guess the doctor's prescribing decision.

Soon after Ronald Reagan assumed the presidency, the Department of Health and Human Services aborted the program. Its termination was followed by assurances that the free market could generate this information comprehensively and voluntarily, with no need for meddlesome government involvement. There were some stirrings in this direction. For several years I worked with AARP in producing its own elder-friendly patient information leaflets on drugs, which filled an important niche for the nation's older medication users. Several drugstores began to produce their own informational materials or license them from third parties; some of these were quite good, but many were poor. For the average patient, the quality and even the availability of such information remained unpredictable.

By 1996, new congressional legislation further limited the FDA's capacity to exert quality control over private-sector activities in this area. The agency's own efforts were sharply curtailed, and it was left with the capacity to require "Medication Guides" only for a few drugs that "pose a serious and significant public health concern," including birth control pills. To date, such guides have been completed for only a small number of products.

In early 2000, Dr. Sidney Wolfe's Health Research Group compiled a report showing that many of the private-sector leaflets routinely dispensed by pharmacies omitted mention of major risks and precautions for several commonly used drugs. In response, the FDA commissioned its own survey, in which patient information leaflets were sampled from pharmacies around the country and evaluated by groups of experts and consumers. The experts found unacceptably low levels of accuracy concerning risks and general information; the consumer panels found major problems with the leaflets' comprehensibility and even their readability. Despite this, extensive lobbying has blocked Congress as well as successive administrations of both parties from restoring the FDA's authority to produce drug information for patients, or even to implement quality and accuracy standards for materials produced by others. This may illustrate the effectiveness of the free market in action, although here it appears to be the market for politicians rather than for products.

GOING STRAIGHT TO THE CUSTOMER

Patients may not have routine access to scientifically vetted information about their drugs when they fill their prescriptions, but they get plenty of input from advertising. Before the mid-1990s, many drug manufacturers were wary of entering the expensive world of consumer advertising, since promoting their products to doctors had traditionally been all that was needed to increase sales. But when HMOs sought to contain costs by restricting use of expensive drugs, the ground rules changed. The drug companies hoped that direct-to-consumer promotion could give them an unprecedented way to market their products to patients, bypassing both the physician and the managed care formulary committees. In 1997, the FDA agreed to remove most prohibitions on such advertising.

A former FDA commissioner once asked whether such promotion was "misleading in a way that constitutes a public health hazard." In the disarmingly binary thinking that sometimes characterizes regulators, the agency declared that it was not. But a more interesting and important question is what effect this advertising has on the way medications are used in the United States. In nearly all other countries, such promotion is still not permitted; are we better off because we allow it?

It's appealing to think that consumer ads might help patients detect diagnoses that have been unnoticed or undertreated by their physicians. After all, our health care system performs badly in the management of elevated cholesterol, hypertension, and diabetes, among many conditions. Other diagnoses suffer the dual liability of underdetection and undertreatment, including depression, incontinence, and osteoporosis. Advocates of pharmaceutical promotion raise an interesting point when they suggest that advertising to patients could increase awareness of these conditions and thus improve decisions on both sides of the prescription pad, a process that could in theory bring about an eventual public health benefit.

It is likely that some patients didn't know they were clinically depressed until they saw an ad for Zoloft, or weren't aware that there was a useful treatment for impotence until Bob Dole told them so in a Viagra commercial. And it's also probably true that numerous patients found the courage to tell their doctors that they constantly wet themselves, and wanted treatment for it, only after they were exposed to promotion of a drug for incontinence. But from a public health point of view, is this the best way to spend $4 billion on health communications to the public? Even if more patients with high cholesterol or depression came into treatment because of ads for the costly drugs Lipitor or Prozac, how many more could have been treated using equally effective but much cheaper generic products in the same classes? And if the older thiazide drugs are both better and cheaper than many newer ones for the management of hypertension, what was the net public health benefit of all those costly ads for calcium-channel blockers, and the promotion-driven use of the expensive products that they generated?

To fully assess the health impact of direct-to-consumer health communications, we would need to ask what the incremental benefit would have been had we spent some of those billions instead on messages about diet, exercise, or alcohol, drug, and tobacco abuse—or the importance of compliance with a prescribed drug regimen, regardless of which company manufactures the product. Perhaps some drug ads can make patients more informed consumers in some situations, and patient education and empowerment are in general good things. Yet some of the most lavish spending has been for overpriced products for heartburn and hay fever that were virtually identical to the expiring-patent products that preceded them. The real benefits of these drugs were high margins for their manufacturers, not improved outcomes for patients.

Direct-to-consumer ads can also have adverse effects on the doctor-patient relationship by turning the prescription into a kind of zero-sum negotiation between conflicting parties. The patient brandishes the latest glossy ad from *Newsweek* and demands the promoted product, while the doctor defends the original prescription—or just caves in altogether. The evidence indicates that for doctors faced with impossibly short visit times and reluctant to displease patients, the latter occurs more often. We needn't pine for the old days when the prescription was a sacrosanct gift bestowed by an omnipotent physician upon a grateful and unquestioning patient. But we are not benefited either if the transaction becomes an adversarial encounter, with doctor and patient circling each other warily in the consultation room, each trying to prevail over the other.

If we really want to increase the public's awareness of depression or incontinence or heart disease prevention, we could do so directly; those same talented people at the advertising agencies would be quite willing to put together promotions that are not product-specific if someone paid them to do so. If statins and antihypertensive drugs are underutilized (as they are), systems approaches to physician and patient noncompliance could work at least as well as, or better than, ads for specific products. Some might object that this is implausible—that pharmaceutical companies are willing to spend money to advertise their own products, but the nation itself lacks the resources to pay for public-interest medical messages. This is not true. In the end, the advertising bill is already being paid by the public.

Patients, employers, insurance companies, and numerous government health care plans are ultimately providing the $4 billion spent on promotion to consumers, and more. It is not just the cost of all that airtime, the magazine pages, and the advertising firms that put the whole enticing package together. That is covered through the higher drug prices needed to pay for such expensive advertising. It is also the cost of using a more expensive patented product when nearly identical generics are available, and the cost of wasted physician time spent convincing a patient that her heartburn will respond as well to a generic drug as it would to the latest "purple pill." And it is the emotional cost to the cancer patient who learns that his fatigue and weakness are due to the malignancy itself, and will not disappear with a $1,500 dose of Procrit as the television commercials imply.

The United States has made its choice about drug ads for patients, and it is unlikely that the genie can ever be put back in the bottle; defensible free-speech arguments and less defensible lobbying activities will guarantee that. We will probably see an increase in such advertising in the United States for the foreseeable future, even though most other nations seem able to run quite effective medical care systems without it. But somehow, the dollars aren't there for pro bono messages to educate the citizenry about medications. We lack the will to mount noncommercial programs on the same topics, and the health care system perceives that it cannot afford to do so. After all, it has trouble meeting its own rising costs for the current fiscal year—increases that ironically are caused in large part by rapidly swelling expenditures on these same heavily advertised drugs.

At issue is not the fact of pharmaceutical promotion, but the way it has come to have such a heavy influence on the drug choices made by doctors and patients. More ominous is a larger issue: these ads and commercials are helping to transform the medical care system from a professional enterprise focused on the health of people to just another marketplace, like those for fast food, cars, and pop music. The name of the game is buying as big a media splash as possible, catching the eye of the consumer, winning market share. The proliferation of this noise is simply another aspect of the commodification of medicine. It is born of our confused conviction that corporate self-promotion on all fronts is the most effective way to advance the health of the public. In this model, there is little room for health-oriented communications that don't advance a particular sales agenda.

Ironically, despite all the drug information lavished on patients by those who seek marketplace solutions to medical decisions, one kind of communication is strangely lacking—information for the consumer about what these products cost. Considering how central price information is in all other aspects of commerce, it's odd that its near-total absence from most brand-name drug ads has not been a topic of concern for most medical free-marketeers. They seem willing to endow drug decisions with only selected pieces of the free-enterprise model—heavy on information about benefits, light on risks, and nothing at all on cost.

But Americans are resourceful, and many have begun to use the internet to put the market to work in their own interest by searching out the best prices for a given drug. As we have seen, that search often leads outside our borders. But when patients seek to act on *that* kind of consumer information, the drug industry and federal government warn in strident terms against doing so. When consumers persisted in trying to be price-sensitive and buy American-made drugs from Canadian pharmacies, the first reaction of the FDA and drug makers were threats to block the transactions and to shut down that open commerce.

WE'VE SEEN THAT after the FDA releases a drug for use, the molecule enters a world of laissez-faire chaos where normal scientific and economic standards suddenly loom small. Once the final wording on the package-insert label is negotiated, it is usually no one's job to make sure that prescribers know how the drug stacks up against the alternatives, or that we and our patients use it properly. But nature abhors vacuums of the informational as well as the physical kind. In the absence of a coherent societal agenda, others are more than happy to fill this cognitive space—with a free lunch thrown in as well. That vast sucking sound you hear is the pressure of commercial hype rushing in to fill the conceptual void.

17: INFORMATIONAL KUDZU

Vaginitis, of all things, provided me with an early lesson in how adept the pharmaceutical industry is at filling this vacuum. As a new junior faculty, I arrived at work one morning to find one of the secretaries admiring a coffee mug. It had been dropped off by a drug company sales rep, and had two thick blue horizontal stripes on its sides. Between them was the logo for Monistat 7, an antifungal medication extensively used then to treat yeast infections. Now a modified version was being introduced—a solid vaginal suppository the patient could insert without the nuisance of applying a gel or a cream. But how would the active ingredient get from the suppository into the surrounding inflamed tissue? "Hey, watch this," the secretary exclaimed, pouring hot coffee into the mug. Before my eyes, as the mug warmed up, the blue stripes—applied with heat-sensitive dye—faded away to reveal a phrase printed underneath: MELTS AT BODY TEMPERATURE. As the coffee cooled, the blue stripes returned, obscuring the message. I served a colleague some tea in the mug; the message reappeared. A practical lesson in applied pharmacokinetics, delivered in a way I'll long remember.

Pharmaceutical marketing is the most important source of knowledge about new drugs for most physicians, and a major form of continuing conditioning as well. Companies have high motivation to bring their information to physicians, and often there isn't much nonindustry competition to elbow aside to get our attention. Medical journals publish papers reporting the results of clinical trials, and many run review articles that provide dense overviews of a given field of medicine. But we've seen that important findings about the benefits or risks of a new drug or an old one might appear in any one of dozens of journals. These reports are necessarily in the arid format required for rigorous scientific communication, often emphasizing the methodology of a study more than its implications for everyday practice. Visually, their appearance is just a little more engaging than a phone book, with pages of edge-to-edge type relieved only by the occasional table or graph, until recently exclusively in black and white. Keeping up with all this literature is an arduous task that few of us have the time or the stamina to perform comprehensively.

Contrast this with the communication we get from pharmaceutical companies. In most medical journals, the scientific reports are interleaved with at least as many pages of ads. The latter are bright, colorful, engaging, with large headlines, appealing pictures, easy-to-understand graphs, and unmistakable take-home messages exhorting us to prescribe that product. The same multipage ad campaign is likely to run in a number of journals at once, ensuring that it will be seen by physicians who read any one of several publications. In case the battle were not one-sided enough, the industry has two additional advantages. First, although I have to open the journal to read a paper and plow through its dense text to glean a practice-relevant message, the sales pitch for a drug comes to my doorstep in the form of an amiable sales representative. He or she will turn up whenever I want at the location of my choice, bearing trinkets and even lunch. Or the company will host a dinner at one of the better restaurants in town, interspersed with a well-tuned slide show touting its products. They might even pay doctors to attend.

The result is that most of us who practice medicine are surrounded by an almost suffocating plethora of information of very uneven quality, a sort of informational kudzu. (Non-Southerners may need to be reminded that kudzu is a prolific and fast-growing vine that was imported from Japan to the southeastern United States during the Great Depression to control soil erosion. It grows over nearly everything in its path, and can kill a tree by climbing up it and absorbing all the available light. Once established in an area, kudzu is very difficult to eradicate and is now considered a major agricultural problem; it is sometimes called "the vine that ate the South.")

What is the effect of all this ubiquitous and hardy promotional material—does it really influence how we physicians actually prescribe drugs? Of course it does, although it is surprising how many "influence deniers" are still out there. ("I take the gifts, I talk to the reps, I attend the dinners, but none of that has any effect on what I prescribe.") Common sense would lead to a very different conclusion, as does a growing scientific literature in this field. With the possible exception of the companies that sell beer, cola, and autos, pharmaceutical manufacturers are the most adept organizations on earth in designing, implementing, and evaluating marketing campaigns. These advertising programs are shaped with exquisite care over months, using focus groups and pilot tests to gauge and refine their impact throughout their costly development. Once deployed, their effectiveness is closely monitored. Pharmacies all over the United States are paid to provide market research companies with detailed information on exactly which physicians are prescribing which medications to what kinds of patients. The largest of these, IMS America, sells this information at a very high price to the pharmaceutical industry, whose member companies use it to evaluate their marketing efforts in a given region and focus them ever more precisely. Sales representatives' commissions or bonuses are determined on the basis of these sales data.

AD NAUSEAM

The first research study I ever published began as an idea in my early student days. There we sat in the amphitheaters of Harvard Medical School, hearing erudite lectures on the most subtle details of physiology and biochemistry. But on those rare occasions when we caught glimpses of actual practice by typical doctors, their use of drugs seemed much less science-based. Products that made little pharmacologic sense and had unimpressive clinical trial data were prescribed widely, and the elegant mechanisms and biochemical strategies we were learning about didn't seem to count for much. What caused that change? Was it related to all those ads and free meals and personal sales visits in which our fully trained forebears in the community were marinating?

To try to figure that out, with the help of two student colleagues I identified a random sample of primary-care physicians in the greater Boston area, and asked them what shaped their prescribing decisions: their own training and experience, advice from colleagues, patient demand, advertising, or the sales reps known as "detail men" (because they provided the details about the drugs they were promoting; there were few detail women in those days). This was the first half of the study; my sociology course in college had taught me that their answers would be heavily colored by socially acceptable responses. That part just laid the foundation for the next set of questions. Nonetheless, even those initial responses yielded some surprises: fully a fifth of physicians reported that detail men were an important source of influence on their prescribing, and only a few classified these sales reps as "minimally important."

The more significant part of the survey came next. I had identified several drugs that had one interesting property in common. Clinical trials had shown that they were either ineffective or no better than over-the-counter products, but each was widely used and the subject of vigorous marketing campaigns extolling its virtues. The real test of how physicians got their information about these products, I reasoned, would come when we asked them how well these drugs worked. The answers we received were disturbing, and cast doubt on whether the doctors' responses in their earlier part of the interview, however sincerely they were intended, were at all accurate.

One of my favorite examples from that study is a drug that is still used surprisingly often. It is Darvon, whose generic name is the much less pronounceable propoxyphene. Before the advent of the nonsteroidal anti-inflammatory drugs like Motrin (whose generic name is the much less pronounceable ibuprofen), Darvon was heavily promoted by its manufacturer as a strong analgesic, with the clear implication that it was more effective than aspirin or Tylenol (whose generic name is the much less pronounceable acetaminophen). A distant chemical cousin of narcotics like morphine and heroin, Darvon was advertised as having narcoticlike pain-relieving capacity, but without the side effects of addiction, respiratory depression, and disorientation. There was only one problem: the clinical trials did not bear out these assertions. When Darvon was given in double-blind studies to patients in pain, it didn't work any better than aspirin or Tylenol.

The problem was worse than that: a little like OxyContin decades later, this opiate derivative turned out to have many of the same downsides of its more notorious relatives. It was prone to abuse and could cause confusion, especially in the elderly. Paradoxically, its image of safety was also a hazard. In its heyday, Darvon was one of the commonest causes of both unintentional and intentional overdoses that resulted in trips to the emergency room or the morgue. No better than aspirin or Tylenol, potentially addictive, high overdose risk—yet it was one of the best-selling drugs in America.

Another group of medications I chose for the survey also had a great image in its ads but little or no evidence to back that up. This was the category of "cerebral and peripheral vasodilators." Unrelated to the modern vasodilators used today for the management of high blood pressure and some kinds of heart disease, these earlier drugs were shams. They were promoted by their manufacturers as being able to open narrowed arteries all over the body, thus restoring life-giving circulation to the brain, the leg muscles, the fingers, and even the uterus. At the apex of their popularity, these drugs' FDA-approved labeling listed uses including the treatment of senility, inadequate blood flow to the fingers or legs, frostbite, and threatened miscarriage.

A NEW DISEASE

Given my interest in drugs taken by the elderly, I was particularly struck by the ads that recommended these products for senility. One evocative multipage spread featured a picture of an agitated gray-haired man who looked as if he was about to commit mayhem. An adjacent headline read, "RECOGNIZE THE 'OBNOXIC' PATIENT?" There is no such word in medicine as "obnoxic"; it was invented by the company by combining the words "obnoxious" and "hypoxic," which describes a state of oxygen deficiency. The goal was to convey the idea that this poor guy didn't have enough blood supplying oxygen to his brain, rendering it hypoxic. That in turn created his confusion and foul temper, rendering him obnoxious.

What could be done for this fellow? Logically enough, the ad encouraged us to open up the blood vessels supplying his brain so they could provide it with the oxygen it craved, rendering him more docile and less threatening. We could do this by prescribing Cyclospasmol, a then-popular "cerebral vasodilator." A few pages later in the ad sequence, our patient has gotten his Cyclospasmol and he's doing just fine. A drawing superimposed over his now-smiling face shows a rich network of blood vessels flowing abundantly throughout his head; the next photo shows him cuddling with a cute little girl under the headline "JUST A LITTLE HELP HERE" (in his now well-circulating brain) "MEANS A LOT HERE" (the grandchild-cuddling photo). Warmly engaging, definitely appealing—totally bogus.

In fact, sluggish blood flow to the brain had already been discarded by neurologists as the cause of most mental impairment in the elderly. And if this man did have any circulatory problems, they were likely caused by the irreversible changes of atherosclerosis, which litters the insides of arteries with fatty deposits, hard calcifications, and inflammatory gunk, none of which would be touched by a tiny dose of Cyclospasmol. No adequate controlled trial had ever shown that this drug produced any benefit in patients like this. Another clue should have been that these same products were advertised as opening up arteries in the legs and fingers, and, in theory, throughout the body. If they had had any real pharmacological effect, they would have dilated blood vessels all over, causing patients' blood pressure to drop and making them fall down. Fortunately, because the drugs were generally inert, this rarely happened.

"PERHAPS IT WORKS"

How could such drugs have been sold? These were still the wild-and-woolly-headed days of the FDA's years-long DESI project, which took two decades to get such useless products off the market. During that time, these questionable medications continued to be promoted under the category "possibly effective." One of the most popular vasodilators was manufactured by Marion Laboratories in Kansas City, Missouri, an operation run aggressively by Ewing Marion Kaufman. A story in *Fortune* magazine titled "Ewing Kaufman Sold Himself Rich in Kansas City" described the entrepreneur's remarkable skill at purveying anything, implying that he could have sold rubber crutches to a cripple. That is comparable to what these drugs did, and did well enough that his company prospered handsomely.

Like the therapeutics of the Middle Ages, the vasodilator story was satisfying conceptually even if it was totally unsubstantiated by fact. But a good story was enough, and sales were brisk. The problem this caused wasn't just that physicians obliged elderly patients to spend their money on products that didn't work. Equally worrisome was that the heavy promotion of these drugs perpetuated an incorrect understanding of senility. Even then it was becoming clear that mental failure in the elderly was far more complex than just "hardening of the arteries in the brain." Whereas most textbooks of medicine and neurology by the late 1970s and early 1980s had moved beyond this outdated notion, the vasodilator ads kept it alive and well in the forefront of physicians' minds.

So the vasodilators also earned a place in our study as a group of drugs that looked great in the ads but fared poorly when actually tested. In the second part of the survey, after physicians had reported that their knowledge of drugs was shaped heavily by the scientific literature but hardly at all by promotional materials, we asked another set of questions. One was "Is inadequate blood flow to the brain the main cause of senile dementia?" Fully 71 percent of the physicians answered that it was. This was not a concept they would have found in contemporary journal articles or textbooks. But there it was, all over, in the vasodilator ads.

We also asked whether they thought Darvon was a stronger analgesic than aspirin. The doctors were told to ignore patient preference, side effects, and all factors other than pure pain-relieving ability. Six of the seven published randomized trials then available had shown that it was not, and the seventh suggested that the two drugs might be about equal. There were no published trials that showed Darvon was better. But only 20 percent of our respondents got this question right. Nearly a third reported that they thought Darvon was as good a pain reliever as aspirin, and the largest group—49 percent—believed that Darvon was stronger, even though there were no published studies that had come to this conclusion. The doctors may have felt that the information they got through sales channels didn't affect what they understood about drugs, but their answers revealed a very different situation. The findings of this study sowed the seeds for a new way of thinking about the problem of poor prescribing, described in detail in the next chapter.

BIOPSIES OF THE SYSTEM

How widespread is this problem today? The most egregiously useless drugs are gone, but the underlying issues remain. As a university-based researcher I can't afford the market data that the drug companies purchase, but our research unit's drug utilization database works about as well. As described earlier, we periodically ask various state programs to send us the paid-claims data on all the prescriptions they paid for in a recent year. For programs like Medicaid in a large state this can yield a treasure trove of utilization data; we also receive information from states that run large drug benefit programs for elderly people who don't qualify for Medicaid. Extreme care is taken to remove any personal identifiers that could violate patients' privacy; all we need to know is what kind of patient was prescribed what drugs, and how. The FDA may not have a great interest in the details of how specific drugs are being used in practice, but we do; the database we constructed over the years has proven to be a powerful tool for collecting and analyzing just such information.

Since that first study, we have used these files often to find out how drug use is influenced by marketing rather than clinical trial data in other clinical areas. We first focused on the treatment of high blood pressure, and "biopsied" our prescription database over several years to see how well doctors' actual prescribing lined up with the clinical trial findings and recommendations published in medical journals. By the 1990s, several major studies had proven that treating this condition could reduce strokes and other terrible consequences. Most of those trials had used the thiazide diuretics, a venerable class of medications that had been around for decades and had a solid track record of effectiveness and safety. A second group of drugs whose credentials had been clearly demonstrated were the beta-blockers, another well-established medication that lowered blood pressure safely and had the added advantage of reducing the risk of death after a heart attack. In studies I performed with Drs. Mark Monane and Eric Knight, we found that these drugs were becoming less and less popular choices for doctors throughout the 1990s, even as more and more papers were being published demonstrating their effectiveness.

What was the problem? The older drugs were being edged aside by the newer calcium-channel blockers, or CCBs, heavily marketed and selling fantastically well. This created two problems. First, the CCBs were very expensive, with the brand-name products costing up to $900 or more per year, compared to less than $60 for a year of thiazides. Second, during the many years covered by our initial studies, essentially no large-scale clinical trials had been published proving that the CCBs could actually prevent the strokes, cardiovascular disease, and kidney damage that were the main reasons for treating high blood pressure in the first place. The products had been approved by the FDA because their manufacturers had shown in studies lasting a few months that CCBs lowered blood pressure better than placebo did, and that was enough.

Thiazides and beta-blockers had long ago gone off patent and were being produced by numerous generic manufacturers at very low cost. That's good for patients and others who pay the bills, but it doesn't fund the exorbitant marketing efforts that drive doctors' practice patterns. Little or no promotion was going on for these older generic products, but the CCBs were protected by patents that would last for many years. Large profits followed each time a patient was started on one of them, usually for life. This made it worthwhile for manufacturers to put thousands of sales reps in the field, pay for millions of dollars of multipage ad spreads in the medical journals, sponsor hundreds of "special educational seminars," and feed tens of thousands of meals at dinner symposia—all with the goal of convincing doctors that CCBs were the most up-to-date way to manage this common clinical condition. It worked. In droves, doctors abandoned the very drugs that had been the most carefully tested and shown to be both effective and safe. We academics kept giving our talks at continuing-education courses explaining that thiazides and beta-blockers were still the most rational first-line drugs for most new patients with uncomplicated hypertension, but the sales data showed that we were voices crying in a non-evidence-based wilderness.

Our research team next studied subgroups of blood pressure patients to see if the picture looked any more encouraging at a higher magnification. If clinical trials had proven that heart attack patients lived longer when prescribed beta-blockers, were hypertensive patients with this condition likelier to be prescribed those drugs? No, CCBs. The damage wasn't limited to the oldest drugs alone. Another class of blood pressure drugs, the ACE-inhibitors, had been shown to protect kidney function in many patients with diabetes as well as to reduce the risk of death in patients with heart failure. When we looked at the hypertensive patients who also had heart failure or diabetes, were most of them on ACE-inhibitors? No; CCBs were capturing much of that market as well.

THE ENGINE OF MOTIVATION

A car salesman trying to get me to buy a Mercedes would have to convince me that the thousands of additional dollars I'd spend on his product would buy an incremental benefit over what I'd get if I spent the money on something else. But when a doctor is spending other people's money, whether it's from a large insurance company, a government health program, or the patient, he's likely to worry less about what the drug will cost somebody else. If a new medicine has an appealing modern-sounding physiological mechanism, or a theoretical rationale for slightly better effectiveness, or offers the possible hope of fewer side effects, it's easy to brush away resistance to a higher price tag. And if the doctor doesn't hear the other side of the story or doesn't even know what the price tag is, it's hard to act otherwise. A volatile mix of chemistry, hopes, fear, and money, all swirling around in a vacuum of information about relative effectiveness, costs, and coverage, makes a foolproof recipe for problematic prescribing.

> *The young man seated next to me at dinner is flushed with enthusiasm and some very fine red wine. We are in the private dining room of a trendy New York restaurant, and he's describing how he had risen in the ranks at the pharmaceutical company he works for. "I remember this one regional sales meeting," he tells me. "They had us in a huge auditorium. All the sales reps in our area were there, along with the company's VP for marketing, a guy we hardly ever get to see. They were motivating us about a new product the company was bringing out. Some well-known KOLs were there too."*
>
> *KOLs? "You know," he explains, "key opinion leaders. Doctors like yourself, from major medical schools, big experts in their field. Several of them were involved in the early clinical studies of our product, and they gave talks explaining to us why it was such an important breakthrough. And then, after all the talks were finished, onto the stage drives this brand-new BMW convertible. They announced that whichever sales rep moved the most product would get to drive that Beemer for a full year." He looks at me with disarming seriousness, and now speaks softly and slowly. "I decided at that very minute . . . I was going to be the guy to drive that Beemer."*

Our dinner had followed an all-day working meeting at which a small number of scientists from around the country had been flown in to confer with physicians and senior managers at a large pharmaceutical company. The purpose of the session was to evaluate new findings from clinical and laboratory research and to discuss what they might mean for the care of patients with a particular disease, as well as for the company's product line. This wasn't one of those thinly veiled marketing sessions that had become so common, in which heavy prescribers would be paid $500 as "consultants" to sit through a long sales presentation over a good meal. This had been a day of genuine give-and-take in which our small group, including department chairmen from several major medical schools and hospital clinical departments, reviewed controlled trials that were about to begin or about to be wrapped up.

We combed through new evidence about the effectiveness and side effects of the company's product, as well as those of its competitors. I was there to discuss a study we were conducting about side effects in patients who took the company's drug. I declined the $2,000 honorarium provided for the day's work, requesting that instead it go to a nonprofit charitable fund. The meeting had been productive, with a lively exchange across disciplines. The dinner that followed was for a much larger group, including people from the company's marketing department who had not attended the scientific discussions. There were to be no presentations before, during, or after dinner—just excellent food, conviviality, and an open bar.

Because of my interest in what shapes physicians' prescribing practices, I was genuinely interested in the story of this young man, who had no scientific background to speak of. "So what did you do to try and win the Beemer?" I asked.

"I memorized everything they gave us about our company's drug," he said. "Its method of action, the clinical trial results, its advantages, its safety, the problems with the competitors' products, which patients the doctors should give it to, everything. Then I made sure to visit every single doctor in my district to give them each free samples, hand them the journal reprints we were supposed to distribute, review our product's advantages over older drugs, the usual." He went on to explain the important role of that pivotal decision maker in this form of continuing medical education: the "office girl."

"Once you get her on your side, you're home free," he explained. "But if she's a real bitch, or she decides she doesn't like you, *fuhgeddaboudit*." Do whatever it takes to co-opt the office girl, he explained: ballpoint pens, mouse pads, clocks, calculators, and other office tchotchkes are a bare minimum; occasional flowers and chocolates are often required as well. "If she's on your side, she can tell you what time to come by to get a few minutes when the doctor will be available, or she can sneak you in between patients if she wants to do you a favor." My dinner partner scored a real coup with one heavy-prescribing KOL when the office girl explained that the doctor had to go to a different location once a week for a meeting; the travel time there plus parking really cut into his working time. "So I found out when these meetings were, and every time he had to make that trip I just turned up at the front door with my engine running. He got a free lift with no hassles, and I got a few minutes with him as a captive audience to detail our products. It got so if I didn't turn up, he went out looking for me."

PAYING FOR THE BEEMER

I replied that the product he was promoting seemed to have a lot going for it, although it was rather expensive.

"It had better do well," he responded. "The company's counting on it for a big chunk of our revenue growth for this fiscal year, and I have all my options and 401(k) plan tied up in our share price." Not to mention his salary and annual bonus. A massive marketing machine had turned its costly and prodigious focus on putting this drug's name on the lips of every physician who might conceivably prescribe it, beating the drum at a deafening pitch for as many years as remained on its patent.

The rules of the game are simpler when viewed from this perspective. University medical centers, governmental health programs, nonprofit HMOs—each have multiple agendas: delivering health care, keeping the budget from going too far into the red, stretching toward some goal of equity, and for the academic medical centers, also performing research and training the next generation of medical professionals. But for any publicly traded company, the ultimate bottom line ultimately must be the bottom line. This is not a moral failing, or some unnatural kind of corporate greed: it's just a normal fact of business life, and one that we shouldn't try to explain away. If Merck or Pfizer or Glaxo fail to bring in impressive earnings each quarter, Wall Street analysts will lower their recommendations, individual and institutional investors will sell their shares to buy those of companies that provide better earnings, and the stock price and market capitalization will drop. Large and increasing sales can keep this from happening and drive the numbers in the opposite direction. It's not helpful to pretend that pharmaceutical companies are bound by a different set of economic rules that are somehow gentler or nobler than those that determine the fates of companies that sell oil, food, or hair care products.

This iron discipline is not mentioned in the image ads we see on television for individual companies or for the industry as a whole, nor is it a part of the presentations made to physicians. But like many forces of nature, its power increases exponentially the nearer one is to its source—in this case, the profit and loss data. Get very close to this fiscal gravitational pull, and those attractions can become strong enough to distort motivations and goals, bending both to fit the economic force field at its center. Does the world need another cholesterol-lowering drug just like all the others, or for hypertension to be managed with more and more calcium-channel blockers? It's not about need, or about public health, and certainly not about cost-effectiveness. It's about sales. This is not evil and should not be shocking. Nothing personal—it's just business. Forget this single key fact and it's impossible to think clearly about the realities of medication use in America.

IS THE DEVIL IN THE DETAILERS?

The situation my dinner companion faced is well described in a little how-to book for drug detailers called *Be Brief, Be Bright, Be Gone: Career Essentials for Pharmaceutical Representatives:*

> Your district manager . . . routinely checks reports on your performance, doctor by doctor, hospital by hospital. Your performance is also being compared with that of your colleagues in your district, your region, and your division. Making 100% of your sales quota for each of the products you are selling is great unless others average 115%. In that case, 100% may not be enough.

His diligence in moving product won him the BMW, which he drove with pride for the full year. This was a bright young man, clearly very hardworking, and it is probably safe to say that before his career is over he will have shaped the prescribing practices of more physicians than most medical school faculty members. Because the stakes are so high and the industry has been so profitable, its sales representatives are well rewarded for this kind of diligence: bonuses alone, based on the prescribing patterns of the physicians they cover, can add $30,000 to $50,000 per year to a generous base salary, as long as one moves enough product. (Thus their pay, like their influence, also exceeds that of many junior faculty at the nation's medical schools.) The stakes are so high because the physician's clinical decision to write a given prescription is the golden door through which all pharmaceutical sales must pass. Getting several minutes every few weeks alone with a heavy prescriber is worth all the ballpoint pens, dinners, chocolates, and football tickets that are needed—and then some.

How this is accomplished is concisely detailed in *Be Brief, Be Bright, Be Gone.* Early on one of its authors, an experienced sales rep, sets out the stakes with the hyperbole that often marks their presentations:

> During a divisional expansion in which I was involved, my company received approximately 60,000 résumés for five hundred open positions. You may have better luck applying to and getting into Harvard, Yale, or Stanford than landing a sales slot at a major pharmaceutical company. Consider this, too: Countless pharmaceutical products are considered to be "me too" products. For example, most major companies in the cardiovas-

cular marketplace sell blood pressure drugs that are extremely close in chemical composition, mechanism of action, side effects, dosing, and cost. So part of your job may be to convince doctors that your company's drug is better, when, in the eyes of your customer, there is little or no difference at all. As I said, it is not an easy job.

In choosing sales reps, do companies take their pick of the best science students from the most prestigious universities? No, that's not really the point. The handbook's author is quick to reassure potential entrants into the field that despite the competitiveness, a familiarity with drugs or science is not required. An MBA may help, but for most frontline reps what really matters is the ability to sell. Everything you need to know about the products you'll be promoting, and the diseases they're designed to treat, will be provided by the company in a concise training program. After just a few weeks, you'll be totally ready to go out and teach people like me how to take care of our patients.

Pharmaceutical sales reps learn early to home in on the KOLs in a given community. Not only are these people often heavy prescribers in their own right, they're also frequently the early adopters whose practice patterns and recommendations have a ripple effect throughout their area. For a small number of eminent medical school–based opinion leaders, the ripple effect can be national and even international. Larger enticements are available for these doctors, including participation on the company's speakers' bureaus, through which the manufacturer will arrange lectures at $500 to $5,000 per talk throughout the year. For national-level experts, the perks are far more lucrative: well-paying memberships on scientific advisory boards, generous support of a professor's academic training programs or research laboratories, or leadership of multimillion-dollar clinical trials.

NO ONE'S IN CHARGE

All this works so effectively (for the companies, at least) because so many physicians' prescribing decisions are left to the laissez-faire environment that governs much of health care. The idea, rarely articulated, is that there is no need for anyone to have oversight over what we know or what we prescribe, since with all those competing companies hawking their wares and touting the advantages of each, the practicing physician can just evaluate all the claims and counterclaims in order to decide which are the best drugs to use. The marketplace model has a logical corollary: no one has to worry about the impact of our prescribing on the public's health or the public till, either. Individual physicians, patients, and payers, each pursuing their own interests, will take care of all that as well.

The whole notion, charming in its naïveté, is similar in many ways to belief in Santa Claus or the Tooth Fairy. It was articulated well in a 2003 statement from the Bush administration on the role of markets in spreading knowledge: "Research indicates that markets are extremely efficient, effective and timely aggregators of dispersed and even hidden information." That statement was a defense of a Pentagon plan to set up a futures trading market to predict terrorist attacks and assassinations, but it reflects the same quasi-religious belief in the ideology of the marketplace. That particular faith-based initiative was canceled before it began, but fervent allegience to the gospel of commerce-as-panacea continues to thrive, both inside and outside Washington.

In tune with this spirit, the pharmaceutical industry has created an evocative portfolio of television commercials and magazine ads promoting its commitment to research. We have acknowledged that many of the companies do sponsor important scientific work, both within their walls and in outside laboratories. Yet we've also seen data that suggest the industry's commitment to sales and marketing is much greater. According to numbers published by the industry's own trade group in its *Industry Profile,* member companies reported employing 86,226 people in marketing, compared to only 51,588 in research and development.

That massive marketing personpower extends far beyond the sales reps. I was once asked to participate in a panel discussion of how pharmaceutical promotion influences doctors' prescribing. Another speaker was a man employed by a large public relations firm that worked mainly for drug companies. (It turned out that he was the person who designed the vaginitis mug; he was delighted that his work had left such a lasting impression.) During the question period, a medical student complained about the prominence of drug ads in medical journals. His response included the most chilling line of the evening. "The ads are really the least of it," he declared. "If you really want to get upset you should worry about all the other kinds of messages we send you that don't even look like ads."

He was right, of course. Such stealth promotion can take a wide variety of forms. One of the largest companies in this field, Grey Healthcare Group, offers drug makers a range of services that is particularly broad. Its website lists some of them: market conditioning, online thought-leader management services, advocacy development and mobilization, medical education, congress optimization, strategic publications planning, medical symposia and meetings, monographs, opinion-leader registries, medical cybercasting, slide kits, speaker training, and celebrity communications. Such a daunting arsenal of weapons of mass distraction can make powerful synergies possible. Patients may come to their doctors asking for a medication they heard about on television—not in a drug ad directed at consumers but in a talk show interview in which a famous guest mentions how much better her energy or arthritis is since she started taking a certain prescription drug. It took years of such appearances before it became widely known that these people were often hired spokespersons, paid to drop the name of a company's product into a carefully planned interview.

Equally unobtrusively, public relations firms spend considerable energy and money shaping the opinion environment in which we physicians live. Some companies specialize in setting up and paying for clinical trials solely to showcase the virtues of their client's product, sometimes by comparing it to another drug given at a dose that is unusually low (for efficacy studies) or high (for side-effects studies). The results are then reported in medical journal papers that may not reveal the details of the study's origins. Other firms arrange for sponsored continuing-education sessions at meetings of professional societies, featuring academic speakers carefully selected to deliver a predictable message touting a given medication. Hidden product placements can occur in teaching hospitals when a drug, championed by company-friendly experts within the institution, is provided by the manufacturer at an impossibly low price to get the residents and medical students into the habit of prescribing it.

Low prices aren't the only way a company tries to win its drug a coveted place on the formulary, or preferred-drug list, of a teaching hospital. It is often a staff physician close to a particular manufacturer (by virtue of research support, speaker fees, or a consultancy) who proposes such an addition. If that doctor is also the local expert in the condition the drug is meant to treat, the endorsement can mean a lot. In one bold variant of this approach, no fewer than three senior physicians all wrote impassioned letters recommending the addition of a particular costly new drug to a hospital formulary because of its wonderful properties (which had eluded the notice of the rest of the committee). The impact of the three letters was lessened considerably when it was noted that the letters were all identical. An enterprising sales rep had persuaded each of the three doctors to give him a sheet of stationery, onto which the rep had printed the same glowing endorsement, which each then signed.

The area of pharmaceutical company influence on physician decision making has become a small research field in its own right. The respected *British Medical Journal* devoted an entire edition to this topic; the issue's title, "No More Free Lunches," borrowed the name of an American website, www.nofreelunch.org, which tracks this problem. In an editorial the journal's editors declared that "doctors and drug companies [are] being entangled in an embrace of avarice and excess, an embrace that distorts medical information and patient care." Compared with the highly focused and effective influence of the manufacturers, the editors wrote, "medicine is a disorganised mess. Doctors have become dependent on the industry in a way that undermines their independence and ability to do their best by patients." Articles in the issue documented ways in which pharmaceutical sponsorship can distort the very design of clinical trials, as well as how they are reported and promoted to doctors. Physicians must also bear some of the blame for this situation, the editors argued, noting "it takes two to entangle."

KEEPING UP APPEARANCES

I have seen at close hand how compelling such enticements can be. Often the seduction is accomplished through an intermediary such as a "medical education company." These are enterprises that derive most of their income from programs sponsored by drug companies, often with predictable effects on their content. But the sponsorship is typically listed as a group with a bland name like "Continuing Education Associates" or "Postgraduate Medical Training Institute." These firms don't limit themselves to putting on courses for doctors. Like many of my colleagues, I have been approached by such groups to author an overview of a given topic for publication, sometimes with an offer that the content could be ghostwritten. The company can then pitch it under the name of the academic author to a series of journals until one of them takes it; or it may be preplaced for publication in a supplement to a reputable medical journal. Many medical journals allow outside groups to buy an entire supplement to one of their regular issues, for a price. It then is published along with the regular issue, appearing to the naive observer to have undergone the journal's usual peer-review process (it hasn't), though the content is often revealingly one-sided. The come-on usually begins plausibly enough. "Dr. Avorn, because of your expertise in this area, we'd like to invite you to write an overview of this clinical issue. To compensate you for your effort, we can provide an honorarium of $2,000. We realize how busy you are, so we'll prepare a draft to save your valuable time. You can then review and approve it, and we'll take care of the rest." I politely reply that I write my own material.

It's hard to overestimate the effect of all these pressures on the totality of medical communication. If I want to put together a study on the side effects of a commonly used drug, or the virtues of an off-patent generic product compared to those of a newer one, I have to struggle to find funding for the work, confront the usual tribulations of getting the research done and the piece written, then face the possibility that it will be seen by journal reviewers as a Luddite tract that casts doubt on the ever-upward spiral of medical progress. Contrast that to the response I got to a study I was beginning on the cost-effectiveness of cholesterol-lowering drugs in the elderly. No data were in yet, but the idea that more of these drugs should be used in older patients was a concept the manufacturer was keen to put before as wide an audience as possible. A medical communications company contacted me and offered to write my talk, prepare my slides, pay me a generous honorarium, fly me business class to the annual meeting of a professional society in Europe to present a lecture, and put me up for a few extra days to help with the jet lag.

I had quite a different reaction in connection with another study we were conducting, to investigate a potentially hazardous adverse effect. A medical communications company was working with that drug's manufacturer as well; its representative invited me to present my findings at a meeting in New York, again complete with honorarium, travel, and luxury accommodations. In the course of planning the presentation, I was asked what I'd be presenting. I mentioned that our study found that the company's drug increased the risk of a serious side effect substantially. A few days later I received a brief e-mail from the communications company indicating that my time would probably be better spent that day by staying in Boston.

KUDZU ON THE NET

The tightly controlled promotional binging and purging that characterizes the flow of drug information can also purvey useful information, but overall it does not work well for the public health, or for public and private budgets. Industry domination of the informational space is only one part of the problem. A larger issue is the general disarray in the marketplace of ideas and products that marks American medicine as a whole. The 2002 *JAMA* paper reporting the downsides of prolonged estrogen use triggered a wave of debate and disorientation among patients and doctors, centering on whether women taking hormone replacement therapy should stop it. In the year after the paper came out, with that debate in full swing, I was studying the clinical websites prepared by medical groups in England and Australia, described in the next chapter. For comparison, I was curious to see what a typical net-surfing American patient or doctor might find on the same perplexing issue here at home.

So I logged on to Google, the most commonly used internet search engine, and tapped in "estrogen." In nanoseconds I was presented with a wealth of informational resources. Most prominently posted were two sponsored links: www.shopping.com, which promised SAVINGS ON ESTROGENS! and www.yesnutritionworks.com, which offered new ways to treat premenstrual syndrome and a free consultation on nutritional supplements. Among the nonsponsored sites, the first ones listed were, in order: (1) www.teamestrogen.com, a company that markets women's bicycling apparel; (2) www.estrogenmusic.com, a site established by a musician named Karen Kusowski but then abandoned so she could focus on her new album; (3) www.jama.ama-assn.org, a link to the original text of the July 2002 *Journal of the American Medical Association* research paper on the Women's Health Initiative study (a good hit, but without context for most lay web surfers); (4) www.eeletter.com, an industrial newsletter about environmental chemicals that can interfere with hormone function (subscriptions available at $515 per year); (5) www.dmeb.net, the site of the Darth Maul Estrogen Brigade, a treasure trove of material written by female *Star Wars* fans; (6) www.jackie.nu/estrogen/, a site for online casino and video games; and (7) www.theestrogenfiles.net, which described itself as a "cyber sitcom," whatever that is.

I next tried an internet site that was exclusively medical, hoping for a more focused perspective. I used WebMD, the most widely used medical site on the net. Looking up "estrogen" linked me directly to WebMD's "Menopause Center." So far, so good. The most prominent listings there were:

- an ad for an upcoming television show on the birth control pill;
- an ad for a sponsored site that matches patients to clinical trials seeking subjects;
- the lead article, "Exercise Alone Trims Tummy, Health Risks";
- the second most prominent article: "Most Women Not Quitting HRT."

The site also directed me to other articles. The first one was "HRT Should Treat Menopause Symptoms," and the second, "Tofu May Prevent Breast Cancer." Further down there was a link to several short WebMD articles: "HRT May Reduce Diabetes Risk," "HRT Protects from Endometrial Cancer," and a third on the FDA's warning that HRT can increase the risk of breast cancer, stroke, blood clots, and cardiovascular disease. A patient or doctor who managed to get that far would find just a listing of those side effects, without much additional information. It took several more clicks to get to a link from WebMD to a Cleveland Clinic site that eventually led to a reasonable overview of HRT risk information.

The relevant facts about hormone replacement weren't completely missing on WebMD, but they were hard to find in the midst of a great deal of dreck. Better sources are available, but only if you can find them—and for some, if you can afford them. Some excellent subscription-only medical sites based in the United States can be accessed electronically (their URLs can be found in the Notes); a small selection follows. One good source is the Medical Letter, a nonprofit organization that publishes a biweekly review of new drugs for clinicians and has a refreshingly skeptical point of view.

Subscriptions are inexpensive, and its website offers several medication overviews at no charge. One of the most comprehensive medical websites is from UpToDate, a Boston-based group of physicians who do a remarkable job of maintaining a current encyclopedia of clinical knowledge on their website. But a subscription costs about $500 per year, and it reaches only a limited audience.

Another entrant into the information arena is a company with the cute name of ePocrates. It provides a comprehensive electronic listing of nearly all medications, doses, adverse effects, and interactions, but its main product offers little in the way of evaluation or comparison. Most interns I know carry it around with them on a Palm Pilot for reference, replacing the little dog-eared notebooks my peers and I used to call our "peripheral brains." The information can be constantly refreshed with updates from the company's site whenever you dock your device into its base for charging— at the same time that messages can be downloaded from the company's commercial partners, and data on the information you've searched for could be uploaded to the company (no free lunch again).

TOO MUCH OF TOO LITTLE

In his 1976 book *Medical Nemesis,* the social critic Ivan Illich used a term, "paradoxical counter-productivity," that could also be used to describe the present situation concerning prescription drugs. He noted that in our attempts to facilitate transportation in big cities, we build so many cars and roadways that more and more people end up stuck in rush-hour traffic and actually have a harder time getting to work. The same problem occurs when substantial sums of energy and R&D money are channeled into research to extend patents and expand markets, followed by lavish promotional campaigns to get people to use these no-better-than-what-we-have new products. It may look as if more new drugs are being developed and more physician and consumer education are going on, but the end result is that medication use becomes more irrational and unaffordable. Drugs like Clarinex and Nexium cost us twice: first through all the research and health care dollars they absorb, and then through all the informational space they occupy in the eyes, ears, and minds of doctors and patients.

Another metaphor from biology suggests itself here, akin to the signal transduction analogy of the last chapter. In 1982, Dr. Eugene Braunwald and his colleagues were studying an interesting clinical paradox. Patients with long-standing hypertension or other heart disease often develop congestive heart failure, a common and serious condition in which the exhausted organ loses its capacity to pump efficiently. At first, the body responds by producing adrenalinelike substances and other chemical messengers that flog the heart into performing better. But Braunwald and his collaborators found that even though this hyperstimulation is adaptive in the short run, over years it effectively numbs the heart muscle, further impairing its function. This chemical arousal overload was called "chronic stunning." It creates a vicious physiological cycle that leads to ever more severe heart failure, which in turn prompts the body to churn out even more of the stimulatory substances. Untreated, the process can eventually result in death. But if the excessive prodding is interrupted pharmacologically or surgically, much of that biochemical noise can be tuned down. Experiments and later clinical experience showed that if that can be accomplished, the dazed and confused heart muscle can regain its cellular senses and return to more normal function. Doctors, patients, and heart cells have this in common: barraging us with incessant and noisy stimulation may flog us into increased action in the short term, but if it continues relentlessly we become numbed by the chronic stunning and function poorly.

Other information-flow problems help explain why our rising drug expenditures are not being matched by commensurate increases in clinical benefit. Many parts of the problem cannot be laid at the doorstep of the pharmaceutical industry; often, larger systems issues are at fault. Despite the more than $20 billion spent annually to promote new drugs to doctors and patients, as a health care system we still aren't using drugs—old or new—optimally. Numerous studies document disturbing undertreatment of several common medical problems: blood pressure in poor control nationally, cholesterol levels off the charts, depression underdiagnosed and undertreated. All this has occurred despite massive efforts by the drug industry to increase use of its products for these conditions. At the same time, other drug classes are rampantly overused: tranquilizers and sleeping pills in the elderly, Prozac-type antidepressants in patients with no evidence that they need them, outmoded products that have become clinically obsolete, diet drugs in patients in whom the risk doesn't come close to matching any possible benefit.

IN THE PAY-AS-YOU-GO marketplace of American health care, drug information behaves like medical care itself. Excellence is there if you can find it, though sometimes at a steep price. There is also abundant mediocrity, and even some very bad product. The American info-landscape for medications is marked by towering peaks, dank swamps, and the cognitive equivalent of numerous strip malls. A typical searcher, whether doctor or patient, may have to wade through drivel about tummy tucks, tofu, and bicycling apparel to discover vital facts about drug-induced cancer or stroke.

There is so much that we physicians and our patients need to learn about how to deploy the powerful arsenal of drugs available to us: potent new products undreamed of just a few years ago, new ways of thinking about existing products, and occasional unanticipated hazards from both. Is this really the best way that the wealthiest and most technologically advanced nation on earth can manage such vital life-and-death information transfer? No . . . as the next chapter shows, we could be doing it much better, even within the context of the present nonsystem.

18: DEVISING AN ANTIDOTE

In England, the Elizabethan era was a time of commercial ferment as active as the pharmacological ferment of our own day. Currencies of wildly differing worth proliferated across Europe and within countries. One of Queen Elizabeth's main economic advisers was the financier Sir Thomas Gresham (1519–1579). He noticed something about the way people used money that has some parallels with the properties of medical information today. Often two kinds of coin would be in circulation that had the same face value but different intrinsic worth—one might be made of gold, the other of a base metal. Gresham discovered that over time people tended to use the coins of less intrinsic worth in their transactions rather than the more valuable ones. As a result, the former eventually displaced the latter in commerce. Reduced to a catchy phrase, as many great concepts are, the insight became known as Gresham's law: "Bad currency drives out good." Others later found that the same principle applied to counterfeit coins.

For most of human history, a kind of Gresham's law of therapeutic information loomed over medicine: easily manufactured but bogus nostrums were used more widely than truly effective treatments. Over the centuries, in the absence of reliable methods to determine their worth, well-hyped but inferior remedies were used far more widely than effective ones. Thousands of elixirs, tonics, cathartics, laxatives, and botanicals flourished in the clinical marketplace, harming far more patients than they helped. In Part One we examined the two mid-twentieth-century developments that raised us out of that chaos: the acceptance of the randomized clinical trial and the empowerment of governments to demand that drugs must be proven to work before they can be sold.

At the start of the twenty-first century, we are ready to move on to the next two fronts in the therapeutic information wars: establishing a higher scientific standard than "better than nothing," and disseminating such knowledge effectively to participants in the health care system. This will be necessary to overcome the clinical manifestations of Gresham's law. We need to make sure that evidence-based, unbiased clinical knowledge becomes the dominant currency of clinical thought and action, edging out baser forms of information that are driven more by tradition, superstition, or mainly commercial agendas. Diffusion of this idea will be the next logical step in modern societies' approach to health care, and especially to medicines. But how can we get there from here?

DE-MARKETING: USING THE INDUSTRY'S OWN MEDICINE

The FDA has now done a good job of clearing the underbrush of totally ineffective drug products, at least for the categories over which it has jurisdiction. But even good drugs can be misused, or underused, or overused, producing a mismatch between the best available science versus actual day-to-day prescribing. We medical school faculty may have a neutral and comprehensive view of the data, but we are not great communicators; in our efforts to educate practitioners we preach only to those who come to attend our lectures or courses. In doing so, we usually present old-fashioned didactic speeches from a podium, ignoring nearly all adult learning theory since 1960. We sometimes inflict on those audiences erudite but obscure discussions of physiological mechanisms that often have little to do with the prescribing decisions our listeners will have to make the next morning in their offices. We obsess over nuanced arguments, counterexamples, subtle caveats. That kind of hesitancy doesn't encumber the others who communicate with clinicians about the same subjects, the salespeople who have been hired to push drug product. It is the same problem Yeats observed almost a century ago in a very different context: *"The best lack all conviction, while the worst / Are full of passionate intensity."*

Growing up as I did in the sixties and living since then in the cloistered setting of academia have either informed or deformed my understanding of what drives human behavior. I believe that most doctors *want* to prescribe well, and when we don't it's usually because we lack the right information about a drug's effectiveness, safety, or cost. To this day, I have not met a physician who knowingly preferred a less effective drug when a more effective one was readily available, or a medication with bad side effects when a safer one could be prescribed. Poor prescribing is common, but most of that can be explained by our spotty training and the fact that after residency no one is really minding the store of our drug knowledge, except for those trying to get us to sell their wares.

In thinking about how this problem could be fixed, I wondered what would happen if the powerful and elegant strategies of communication and behavior change that the drug industry uses so well could instead be employed to promote more appropriate prescribing. This concern led me in an unexpected direction: I read up on the federal government's agricultural extension service. As American farming grew during the last century, small farmers throughout the country were having trouble keeping abreast of new discoveries about crops and animal husbandry. To address the problem, the government sent men out to travel from farm to farm, bringing word of these new methods to practitioners in the field, so to speak. The programs were eventually based in the land-grant universities, where they continue to function today.

I began to wonder whether a similar service could be provided to individual physicians in their own clinical fields. Like farmers of an earlier time, we are often isolated from important new findings as well as from one another. Perhaps doctors, too, could benefit from a proactive, noncommercial source of information about new developments. But how to deliver that information? Those of us on medical faculties might have an excellent window on new developments in pharmacology, but it wouldn't work for us to try to share that knowledge in the same old-fashioned way that we traditionally dispensed continuing education.

Instead, I wondered if we could co-opt the approaches the pharmaceutical industry had honed so well, and which it employs so effectively in changing prescribing practices. Maybe their powerful medicines of information-transfer and behavior-change strategies could be used to achieve more pro bono goals. Such a pharmacological extension service could deploy medication educators to visit physicians in their own offices just as drug company sales reps do. Like the manufacturers, we could choose these outreach workers based on their ability to communicate effectively and congenially. But unlike the companies, we would also require that every one of them have solid training in clinical pharmacology. Their messages would be evidence-based, relevant to the quality of patient care, tightly focused, cost-sensitive, and presented accessibly. Recommendations would be backed up by vivid print material laden with skillful and accurate graphics, illustrations, and engaging typography. Visits to doctors would be brief, targeted, interactive, and designed to achieve specific changes in prescribing practice—exactly like a sales rep's presentation. Because those reps are known as detailers, I named this new approach "academic detailing," reflecting its hybrid origins as a user-friendly educational outreach program sponsored from a medical school base.

If the pharmaceutical industry could change doctors' prescribing patterns this way to increase sales, why couldn't the same method be used to improve the *appropriateness* of drug use? If successful, such a program

could be economically self-sufficient; the drug industry had long ago concluded that although it was costly to deploy a fleet of sales reps, the effort
more than paid for itself in terms of greater revenues. In view of the large
sums being paid for drugs that were more expensive than necessary, a program to reduce silly prescribing should be able to more than pay for itself
through what it saved on prescription costs.

It was less clear who would be willing to underwrite such a program.
Unlike many countries, the United States didn't have a universal publicly
funded drug benefit system that would have the motivation and financial
wherewithal to establish this kind of activity. But the public did pay for the
state Medicaid programs that covered the care of the poor, including their
drug costs. By the early 1980s, several of these programs were starting to
feel the bite of rising pharmaceutical expenditures—a mild foretaste of the
fiscal crisis these programs face today. The abortive attempt to address this
problem in New Hampshire had been one response to those pressures. I
called several state Medicaid programs to see if any were interested in my
idea. But much as they were hurting from rising pharmacy expenses, their
managers weren't comfortable stepping out of the role of bill payer and
into the more complicated role of medical educator. If I could just jump-
start a prototype program and show that it improved prescribing as well as
covered its own costs, it might come to be widely adopted. But I still needed
funding to build the prototype.

A SPARK FROM WASHINGTON

In 1978, I was a year out of my residency when a small pamphlet crossed
my desk from the federal agency then known as the National Center for
Health Services Research. It announced a new initiative to fund innovative
research on improving medication use. I had never written a grant proposal
before, and had no one at Harvard to turn to for advice on how to begin. So
I set forth the argument as clearly as I could and proposed the "academic
detailing" idea in as much depth as I could make up.

The study would be built on three conceptual pillars. The first was
evidence-based medicine, though that term wasn't much in use then. That
is, all clinical content would be driven by findings from well-performed clinical trials or other peer-reviewed data sources. The second was the academic detailing idea itself, which would draw on the disciplines of
behavioral science and educational theory to develop its methods, with generous borrowing from the real-world practices of the drug companies
themselves.

The third main element of that initial study was a commitment to evaluate the new approach in a randomized controlled trial of its own—testing

not the drugs but the intervention. We've seen that clinical pharmacology began to make progress only when it adopted the randomized trial as its indispensable tool for distinguishing drugs that worked from those that didn't. This made it possible to discard thousands of treatments that turned out to be useless when subjected to scientific scrutiny. It was time for health services research and health policy to make a similar methodological leap, to drag these fields out of their own dark ages. The study would use hundreds of doctors, not patients, as the experimental subjects.

The treatments advocated by Galen, Paracelsus, and their followers fit neatly into their ornate logical structures, but usually didn't work and often harmed the patient. Yet for many hundreds of years no one knew it, because those outcomes were never evaluated. The same problem exists in our day for health care delivery. Based on received wisdom and their own intuition, policy makers come up with ideas for restructuring some aspect of the system, such as the way drugs are to be prescribed or paid for, and then implement them without ever studying their effects. Many of the resulting programs are the policy equivalents of the purging, bleeding, and cathartics that were the staples and the shame of prescientific medicine.

A good randomized trial must have its outcome measures specified in advance, and here it would be the prescriptions our doctor subjects wrote before, during, and after the experimental program. The Medicaid programs might not have been willing to subsidize my idea, but their paid-claims files could be a good source of such data. Taken together, all these filled-prescription claims forms could provide rich and accurate documentation of the prescribing patterns of thousands of doctors—if I could just get access to them. At that time, in the late 1970s and early 1980s, some state programs were just beginning to use computer records instead of little slips of paper to process their voluminous pharmacy bills. I had to find out which states had converted to this new technology, and of these, which were willing to copy all their paid-claims tapes and ship them to Boston for analysis.

Not many states met both criteria. One that did was Arkansas, which had just elected a charismatic young governor who was encouraging his state agencies to adopt innovative programs that could lead to creative policy reforms. Three other Medicaid programs also had their pharmacy charges on computer tapes and were willing to share them: Vermont, the District of Columbia, and the eventually notorious New Hampshire.

The grant application required a budget, so I guessed what it might cost to set up the demonstration program: how much the new breed of educators would be paid by the hour, the travel time they'd need, the number of physicians they might see in a day, what a graphic artist might charge to help develop the print materials, how much programmer and computer resources it would take to evaluate the outcomes. I would also need to account for a portion of my own salary, as Harvard and the Beth Israel Hospital, where I did my clinical work, were willing to pay me only for the time I spent teaching medical students or seeing patients, respectively—not for doing idealistic research projects. The total budget for establishing and running the whole program and then evaluating it came to just $80,000 a year over two years, to which Harvard added its standard overhead charge of 71.5 percent. I mailed the grant request in to the National Institutes of Health, which handled the peer-review evaluation process, and forgot about it.

Unrelated to any of this, a few months later the Pan American Health Organization (PAHO) mailed a form letter to several U.S. medical schools announcing the First Inter-American Conference on the Social and Clinical Aspects of Coca and Cocaine, to be held in Peru. PAHO wanted to bring together policy makers, clinicians, and researchers from all over the Americas to discuss topics ranging from the anthropology of coca leaf use in the Andean highlands to the problems caused in U.S. cities by its evil crystallized twin. Abstracts on any topic were invited; the authors of those that were accepted would be flown to the meeting at PAHO's expense. The invitation filtered down to my desk because, as I was later told, "it was about drugs, and we knew you were into drugs." As an intern and resident, going on an overnight excursion to the nearby Berkshire Hills had been a major journey, so a free junket to the Andes seemed pretty appealing. I put together an abstract on the history of the therapeutic use of cocaine in analgesic compounds; to my astonishment, it was accepted for presentation. So it came to be that my wife and I were sipping pisco sours and chewing coca leaves with Dr. Andy Weil at the Hotel Bolívar in Lima when word arrived that the academic detailing grant had been approved for funding.

On returning from Peru I began setting up the study, and as the project grew I needed to bring on additional help. One talented applicant was Steve Soumerai, then a master's degree student at the Harvard School of Public Health. Originally signing on as a research assistant, he went on to make very important contributions to the development and evaluation of the project. Soumerai became a coauthor with me of our eventual publications, and later a prolific researcher in his own right in the area of drug policy.

In the initial grant submission I had proposed three drug groups as targets for the new de-marketing program. Two were categories we have met before: the Darvon-type analgesics that worked no better than aspirin or Tylenol; and the useless cerebral and peripheral vasodilators. The third target was somewhat different, in that it worked quite well. It was Keflex, the brand name for an antibiotic (cephalexin) that was a cousin of penicillin. The problem with Keflex was not that it was ineffective, but that it was often prescribed wantonly to many people who didn't need it, or any antibiotic at all.

LEARNING FROM THE PROS

The project began by studying the promotional approaches taken by the drugs' manufacturers, who had faced formidable marketing challenges. After all, the peripheral vasodilators didn't work, Darvon had bad side effects and was no better than inexpensive over-the-counter products, and if Keflex had been used only by those patients who really needed it, its copious sales would have plunged. If we could understand how use of these drugs had become inflated far beyond their usefulness, perhaps we could counter that trend. What we learned could then be applied to reduce use of other products that were ineffective, dangerous, or unnecessarily costly—as well as to encourage the prescribing of drugs that were effective but underutilized.

It became clear that the vasodilators were doing so well because they filled an unpleasant crater in the therapeutic landscape: there simply were no satisfactory drugs to treat either senility or peripheral vascular disease. (Sadly, that statement is nearly as true today as it was in the early 1980s.) As a result, a slightly reasonable physiological story and a strong marketing program were enough to get a product to be widely prescribed, whether or not it worked. Anguished demand by patients and their families, coupled with the frustration that physicians felt at having nothing to offer, provided considerable pressure to use any product that seemed remotely plausible.

Where's the harm in that? All over the place. First is our version of Gresham's law: bad clinical decisions could drive out good clinical decisions. Some older patients with confusion or forgetfulness might have a reversible medical cause for the problem. The list of possible suspects is long, and includes thyroid disease, vitamin B_{12} deficiency, depression, and the side effects of many medications. Giving a patient an ineffective "anti-senility" drug could preempt a more thoughtful search for underlying causes, some of which might be treatable. In addition, these drugs weren't cheap; the dollars spent on them by patients, government programs, or private insurance policies became unavailable for other medications or services that really worked. A similar argument applied to Darvon. Was it ethical to offer a patient a prescription medication that was far more expensive but no more effective than aspirin or Tylenol? The problem was compounded further if the drug in question was also one of the most common causes of intentional and inadvertent overdose death.

A different set of problems surrounded Keflex. Although it was an effective antibiotic, a large proportion of Keflex prescriptions were being written for patients who probably had a viral infection and needed symptomatic relief but no antibiotic. Besides the costs involved—it was an expensive product for those days—the drug also subjected patients to the risk of side effects ranging from rash, diarrhea, and fungal vaginitis to an allergic reaction that could sometimes be fatal. These are risks we are willing to take in fighting a real bacterial infection, but no risk is worth it if there's no benefit. Keflex also posed a problem unique to this category of drug: its misuse affected not just the person being treated but the larger population as well, since haphazard deployment of antibiotics encourages the emergence of resistant bacteria, both in a particular patient and in the community as a whole.

The clinical and pharmacological evidence in place, the next step was to flesh out the details of the intervention itself. Whenever a question came up in creating the academic detailing program I would ask myself, "What would a drug company do?" We had no interest in emulating the more unseemly strategies of some manufacturers, like Wyeth's frequent prescriber bonus miles program, in which each prescription written for one of its drugs generated points a doctor could trade in for trips to vacation destinations. (When this scam came to light, Wyeth was forced to pay large settlements to Medicaid programs around the country for bribing physicians.) But there was still much to learn about the less slimy aspects of the marketing and behavior-change acumen the industry had sharpened so impressively over its many years of investment, practice, and internal evaluation.

In crafting the educational content, I had to get over the academic's assumption that we knew all the answers and it was the responsibility of the learner (even if he was a seasoned practitioner) to figure out what we were trying to communicate and how to apply it. The drug makers knew better: it was the educator who had to do the homework and figure out where the learner was coming from—his baseline knowledge, attitudes, and behavior—and meet him there. The very geography of the two teaching methods mirrored our different perspectives: we professors remained inside or close to our academic medical centers and expected the practitioner to come around to us, both spatially and cognitively. By contrast, the companies went out to meet doctors where they were, both in place and in thought. Interactivity was key: a good sales rep asked the doctor for his or her opinions about a given problem. Once a physician's baseline knowledge and attitudes were known, it was easier to reshape them to conform to the desired mind-set. It was solid adult learning theory—nothing revolutionary, just a topic that most medical school faculty never paid attention to in those days. Many still don't.

UNDERSTANDING THE PRESCRIBER

Throughout the evolution of the project, we studied the techniques the companies used to persuade doctors to use their products. We read their training manuals, analyzed their compelling ads, and convinced a few former sales reps to reveal some tricks of the trade. The physician focus group became our dissecting microscope in formulating the educational-outreach messages. Doctors are often invited to participate in such company-sponsored sessions, and as our own program developed I started to accept as many such invitations as I could. In exchange for a fee ranging from $50 to $250, groups of five to ten physicians meet with a facilitator to chat about a given clinical problem: urinary tract infections, the management of hypertension, treating depression. Drug manufacturers often farm out the conduct and interpretation of these sessions to specialized consumer research companies that do similar work for purveyors of cars, soft drinks, and tampons. Lacking the substantial resources necessary to pay a real market research company to do the work, we turned instead to Roberta Clark, a Harvard Business School researcher with an interest in nonprofit organizations. Her work provided an essential window on how primary-care physicians made their decisions about the drugs we were targeting.

One typical lesson concerned apparently irrational antibiotic use. We asked our focus group doctors whether they thought antibiotics were useful in treating upper respiratory infections caused by viruses rather than bacteria. The participants divided themselves into two camps. Some voiced positions that bore little resemblance to modern science. Even if a patient has a viral infection, they said, "covering" them with antibiotics would prevent complications later on. Others declared that a sore throat with all the hallmarks of a virus (runny nose, muscle aches, exhaustion, low-grade fever, absence of swollen glands) would still get better quicker with an antibiotic. These were the kinds of practitioners who would need some basic lessons in differential diagnosis and microbiology.

On the other hand, other focus group doctors voiced a very different perspective that went like this:

> *Look, just because I don't teach at Harvard doesn't mean that I don't know the difference between a bacterium and a virus. But I have a big practice to run, and a very busy waiting room. Patients come in demanding antibiotics. If somebody has an obvious viral infection, I can give them a long lecture on Microbiology 101, haggle with them, refuse to write a prescription for an antibiotic, and then find that they went down*

the street to another doc who is trying to build up his practice, and got the prescription from him. Or I can just give them an antibiotic then and there, and have them on their way in four or five minutes as satisfied patients. You give me a way I can get them out of my office quickly and happily without an antibiotic, and maybe I'll try it. Otherwise, forget it.

We heard about this "termination strategy" often, and it was valuable advice as we shaped the Keflex de-marketing campaign. The insight led us to develop one of the first direct-to-consumer un-advertisements. It was a leaflet called *Common Sense About the Common Cold* that a doctor could hand to the patient at the end of a visit instead of a prescription. In layman's language, it explained why someone with a viral infection was better off leaving the doctor's office without an antibiotic: the prescription wouldn't have helped anyway, and there would be no risk of developing an unpleasant side effect or growing drug-resistant bugs inside your own body.

Discussions with physicians about their use of the vasodilators also yielded insights into what I came to think of as "sociopharmacology." Faced with a patient whose memory is deteriorating, or who develops leg cramps after walking a block, it's hard for a doctor to say, "I'm sorry, I don't know of any treatment that will help you." After all, most of us went into medicine because of our desire to help people who are suffering, and our eagerness to use science to do so. Admitting that we aren't aware of anything useful for a given problem means we fail on both counts. During my training in primary care a wise clinician once said, "One of the best and hardest things to put into practice in caring for a difficult patient is the precept, *'Don't just do something—sit there!'*"

By contrast, saying "Here's a medication that is designed to open up your arteries and could help relieve those symptoms" enables the doctor to feel he is offering the patient the hope of improvement through a modern, science-based intervention. So our message about avoiding vasodilators for patients with memory problems suggested this tactic: instead of writing a prescription for an ineffective drug, you can be more scientific *and* more helpful by doing a simple workup to look for reversible causes of mental impairment. We'd then teach them exactly which laboratory tests to order to diagnose these treatable problems.

THE POWER OF ADVERTISING

If we were going to train a staff of de-marketers to go out to doctors' offices on un-sales calls, they'd need some un-advertisements to back them up. They would hand them to the doctors directly, both because we wanted to make sure only the experimental-group doctors saw them, and because we couldn't afford to run them in medical journals anyway. The un-ad we created for the vasodilators showed a pensive-looking physician reading a medical journal. At the top of the page was the headline "SKEPTICAL ABOUT 'VASODILATORS' FOR THE TREATMENT OF SENILITY?" And at the bottom, "YOU HAVE EVERY REASON TO BE." Its flip side presented clinical trial data showing the drugs' ineffectiveness, and a summary of how to identify a potentially treatable cause of the problem by checking for some simple clues in the history and physical exam and obtaining some common lab tests. This became the basis for our de-marketing of the cerebral vasodilators. (This and other un-advertisements can be seen on the book's website, www.powerfulmedicines.org.)

It was less clear at first what to recommend when those same drugs were being used (with equal ineffectiveness) to treat the painful cramping symptoms of constricted arteries in the legs. I went back to the medical literature and found studies in which such patients were put on gently graded exercise programs. That enabled their muscles to gradually increase the efficiency with which they used whatever limited oxygen their clogged arteries provided. Studies had shown that this improved the distance patients could walk and reduced their pain. We doctors are notoriously bad at suggesting behavioral solutions to clinical problems, and we give short shrift to teaching patients about topics like exercise, nutrition, and smoking cessation. Because we aren't taught much about this in medical school, we don't do it very effectively and therefore it often doesn't work; we're much more comfortable resorting first to pharmacological solutions like diet pills, nicotine patches, lipid-lowering drugs, or vasodilators.

It struck me that our outreach program could give the doctor some belated help here. One real ad for a vasodilator had featured a photo of a smiling elderly woman labeled "ACTUAL PATIENT" with the headline "AMY IS DOING WELL ON CYCLOSPASMOL." I was happy for Amy, but all the evidence indicated that if she was doing well, it wasn't because of her Cyclospasmol. I wanted to run a similar photo of an old woman under the headline "AMY IS DOING WELL WITHOUT CYCLOSPASMOL." But my geriatrician friends pointed out that you shouldn't call an older patient by the first name unless invited to, and my lawyer friends worried about using a trade name to make fun of a product. We also had trouble locating a photographer who would work for the paltry sum we had available to pay for illustrations. So we found a local graphic artist who drew us a picture of a healthy-looking older woman hoeing in her garden; we ran it under the headline "MRS. R. IS DOING WELL WITHOUT VASODILATORS." The flip side of the un-ad reviewed the clinical literature about how useless these drugs were and provided some basic suggestions for alternative nondrug approaches, including mild exercise. We also put together a leaflet for patients recommending a short walk each day, increasing the distance as tolerated. A doctor could customize the leaflet by writing the patient's name on it, indicating how far to walk each day, and signing it. The urge for a tangible product of the medical encounter, deeply felt by doctor and patient alike, could be satisfied by giving the patient her own "exercise prescription" at the end of the visit.

Another real advertisement I had seen inspired one of the antibiotic un-ads. The ad was for Keflex and showed photos of active-looking people under the headline "CERTAIN PATIENTS CAN'T AFFORD TO BE SICK." Now, I had never had a patient who *could* afford to be sick, but the idea led to our own version, based on the idea that certain patients couldn't afford Keflex. We depicted a wan-looking woman, a skinny toddler slung over her shoulder, handing a wad of cash to a pharmacist. This drug's high cost, we pointed out, was "a troublesome side effect for many patients." On the reverse side, we explained to doctors what it cost each time they wrote a prescription for Keflex, and compared it with the prices of more appropriate antibiotics if any were needed to treat a bacterial infection. (Our de-marketers would later report that physicians were fascinated by these numbers—no one had ever told them the prices of any of the drugs they prescribed.)

Some of our un-ads were a little more fanciful. To persuade doctors to recommend old reliable aspirin over the less effective, less safe, but newer Darvon (this was in the time before nonsteroidals like Motrin were on the market), we had our artist divide the page diagonally in two. On one side was a drawing of wholesome-looking cows, grazing bucolically in a bright green pasture; on the other, a plastic container of nondairy creamer drawn in the pink-and-gray colors of a Darvon capsule. "WE'VE COME A LONG WAY," the headline read, "BUT IS IT PROGRESS?" The flip side of the page updated the clinical trial literature I had first discovered in my earlier survey on prescribing, and reminded physicians about the risks and costs of the newer, fancier product.

When it came time to hire the academic detailers who would deliver the program to the front lines of physicians, we found several bright young pharmacists from each of the study regions who were eager to test-pilot this new kind of work. We brought them to Boston for an orientation program modeled on the training sessions drug manufacturers provide for their sales reps. The first topic was how to get in the door to talk to doctors. (In rural Arkansas, a great icebreaker was "Hello, I've been sent here by the Harvard Medical School Drug Information Program.") Like good regional sales managers, Soumerai and I developed tools for our reps to track their waiting time, contact time, and travel time—data that would be invaluable in a formal benefit-cost analysis later on. We checked in with our de-marketers regularly for troubleshooting, encouragement, and debriefing.

TESTING THE ANTIDOTE FOR EFFICACY

Just as drug companies use reports purchased from local pharmacies to help their sales reps target the doctors they see, we used the records of Medicaid pharmacy claims to find all the moderate-to-high prescribers of the three drug groups we were de-marketing. We identified 435 physicians in the four study states, and randomly assigned each to get the experimental intervention or to be in a control group. A pleasant early surprise was the enthusiasm with which the new program was accepted. Fully 92 percent of the doctors randomly assigned to the academic detailing group agreed to meet with our pharmacists. Frequently, doctors would have their receptionists usher in "the people from that Harvard program" between patients, letting the big-company reps linger in the waiting room until our educators finished their presentations. My original hunch was right: primary-care doctors genuinely welcomed neutral, evidence-based, noncommercial information about the prescriptions they were writing every day. Some asked our pharmacists for advice about other drugs beyond the ones we targeted, and we were happy to have them comply.

But we still didn't know whether the program was having any effect on prescribing. As in a clinical trial of a drug, anecdotal observations of apparent success are no substitute for real data. Until we had processed the final batch of tapes from each of the four Medicaid programs we wouldn't know whether the program was actually influencing how these physicians were prescribing drugs.

Along the way came that glitch in the New Hampshire data, recounted in Part Three. Once that was figured out and Soumerai and I had analyzed the last set of tapes, the final numbers proved my initial hypothesis. To be conservative, we used a classic "intention to treat" analysis. That meant that the few physicians in the experimental group who refused our educational outreach visits were still analyzed with that group even though they hadn't gotten the intervention. We found that after only two visits, the doctors randomly (and unwittingly) assigned to the academic detailing program had significantly reduced their excessive use of the targeted drugs compared to the control-group doctors. The program was a success, and we had proven its effectiveness with a methodology as rigorous as the kind used to test a new drug. Our findings met the ultimate test of respectability when they were published in the *New England Journal of Medicine*.

THE SKEPTICS were on our case almost immediately. Even if such a program could be piloted with a federal research grant, how could it have any relevance to the real world? How could it be run without constant and costly infusion of government money to keep it going? The answer had seemed clear from the beginning: the drug companies knew that dollars spent to keep their sales reps in the field were repaid many times over by the resulting changes in prescribing practices; why should our experience be any different? We knew we had substantially reduced use of a number of overprescribed drugs; these savings should have covered the relatively modest sums needed to run the program. But more formal proof would help, and Soumerai used our field data in a formal benefit-cost analysis that turned into his doctoral dissertation at the Harvard School of Public Health.

We had tracked every dollar spent on our academic detailing staff, as well as all the travel costs, graphic artist fees, and printing expenditures the program required. The Medicaid tapes provided accurate measures of the amounts each state program was spending on the targeted drugs in both the experimental and control groups. His analysis found that even if the economics were restricted to the perspective of the Medicaid payers alone (which accounted for only a portion of each physician's prescribing), the states' expenditures on target drugs prescribed by doctors in the experimental group went down by an amount that was twice what it cost to run the program. And this was based on only two visits over a six-month time span, conducted by people who had never done this kind of work before and targeting only three drug groups. If we had had the resources to continue the program beyond its demonstration phase, the savings would have continued to increase further.

Several months after our 1983 paper came out, a research group at Vanderbilt University, funded by the same federal grant initiative, reported a similar intervention in the *Journal of the American Medical Association,* also with positive results. In the years that followed, other programs patterned on this approach were developed and put into place throughout the United States and the world, with similar outcomes. Hard evidence was accumulating that it was indeed possible to provide evidence-based, pro bono educational outreach to physicians that improved their use of drugs and paid for itself.

EXPANDING THE APPROACH

Energized by the outcome of that first project, I wondered whether the academic detailing idea could also work in a part of the health care system where some of the most egregious use of medications was occurring— nursing homes. Years of caring for older patients had taught me that sedating drugs of all kinds were commonly overprescribed in this setting.

The problem would hit the public consciousness about once a decade; each time, a shocking report would be followed by outrage, government hearings, a few reforms, and then societal amnesia until the next such discovery. Nursing homes would be a tough neighborhood to work in, full of layers of clinical and organizational complexity more daunting than office-based prescribing.

These institutions are our highly medicalized solutions to the often non-medical problems of old people too frail to live alone. More than any other industrialized nation, the United States addresses frailty in old age as a problem that requires a clinical solution, one that is often provided by large facilities based on a hospital-like model of care. (Other countries are more in tune with the sociological aspects of geriatrics; they place proportionately fewer of their parents and grandparents in such quasi-medical institutions, preferring community-based solutions that have lower costs and considerably greater warmth.) As part of the American vision of "the public use of private interests," most U.S. nursing homes are owned and operated as profit-making businesses. Like their nonprofit counterparts struggling to make ends meet, most of them rely heavily on limited payments from state Medicaid programs. As a result all nursing homes, whether set up for profit or run by charitable institutions, are forced to watch every penny.

These economic forces create powerful incentives to manage large numbers of impaired elderly people with a bare minimum of staff. Geriatricians and public health authorities frown upon tying down confused, agitated, or wandering patients, and the practice makes a bad impression on visitors. Less visible means of crowd control are preferable—particularly if they can be thought of as medicines. In the trade, such sedatives are referred to as "chemical restraints." The problem is compounded by the fact that most of the nation's medical students finish their training without ever having set foot in a nursing home. Add the dearth of training in practical pharmacology, and for most graduates the proper use of medications in frail elderly patients becomes the overlapping of two voids, creating a particularly dense black hole in their clinical knowledge.

With these organizational constraints and the knowledge vacuum in place, ready solutions are offered by the makers of sedating drugs, eager to point out how their tranquilizer or sleeping pill can transform a pesky oldster into a docile institutional denizen. One of my favorites was an ad for Haldol (haloperidol), the effective but overused antipsychotic drug widely employed to sedate agitated geriatric patients. (For a time it was so popular in teaching hospitals that interns called it "Vitamin H.") One Haldol ad showed a demure, smiling, white-haired elderly lady holding a daisy made of cloth and pipe cleaners. It carried the caption "I MADE A FLOWER TODAY."

As I thought about designing possible un-advertisements for the nursing home project, I considered trying to find that same model (she wasn't a real patient, of course) and using the same photo and caption on the cover, but on the other side showing her dressed in a white lab coat, saying, "BUT YESTERDAY I WAS A NEUROSCIENTIST!"

Prescribed carefully, sedatives and tranquilizers in the elderly can be helpful drugs. A confused, agitated patient with Alzheimer's disease can be a risk to himself or to other patients or staff, and wise use of these medicines can provide effective, humane treatment in the right situations. But when we began our work in this area in the mid-1980s, the sheer volume in which these drugs were being dispensed in nursing homes suggested that only a portion of that use was thoughtful and sparing. Defining the scope and nature of the existing problem was our first job; to do this I called on Dr. Mark Beers, then a research fellow working with me, who later went on to become director of geriatric medicine for Merck and editor of its *Merck Manual*. I asked him to review the existing clinical literature to define the nature of psychoactive drug use in nursing homes: the products most commonly prescribed, their doses and clinical outcomes. After several tries, he kept coming back from the library empty-handed. (These were the days when we still went to the library to look up stuff.) There was nothing current in the medical literature.

A TOUGH NEIGHBORHOOD TO WORK IN

Nursing homes represent the largest collection of complex patients in the country, with more people in long-term care beds on any given day than in acute-care hospitals. These patients are gathered together and marinated in some of the most highly concentrated drug regimens used in medicine, often with minimal physician involvement. But hardly anything systematic was known then about the quantities and doses of the drugs being used, no less what effects they were having. It was nobody's job to know. All those medical students who finished their training without ever seeing the inside of a nursing home weren't likely to spend much time later as researchers trying to understand what was going on there. The baseline data we collected for our study became a paper in its own right, which Beers published in *JAMA*.

To test the intervention I planned, we enlisted a dozen typical nursing homes in Massachusetts. We equipped a research assistant with a newfangled oddity called a portable computer and sent her into each facility to record all the drugs taken by every resident—about 850 people across the twelve homes. We measured how many were using sleeping pills, antipsychotics, tranquilizers, and mood-altering drugs. It turned out that fully half of all residents were on some kind of psychoactive drug to quiet them down, get them to sleep, relax them, make them happier, or otherwise render them more manageable. The majority of those on sleeping pills or tranquilizers took them every day, often in high doses, despite what was known at the time about the need for less intense use in frail elderly patients. Doctors' choices of drugs revealed a slender grasp of the principles of geriatric pharmacology, such as the problems caused by long-half-life drugs that older patients have trouble clearing from their bodies. These initial findings, and others that followed from other researchers, helped lead to federal regulations that tightened suveillance over some of these drugs in such settings.

The doctors who made those prescribing decisions were rarely on-site, and the nurses and aides who were there felt overworked and underrespected. Could the gentle approach of academic detailing be effective in such a tough environment? And if it were, would lifting this chemical miasma cause all hell to break loose when the patients were no longer so heavily sedated? I didn't think so, but there was hardly any data to back up that hunch and it went against the grain of many institutional care traditions. Some of the concerns we heard sounded like dim echoes of the objections made to Dr. Philippe Pinel, the nineteenth-century French physician who removed the chains from the lunatics in the insane asylums of Paris. His colleagues were convinced that doing so would put both the inmates and staff at mortal risk.

My research unit was somewhat larger by then, and we had the benefit of our earlier experience to guide the new work. As before, the "market research" phase of the study was both crucial and fascinating. We started out trying to understand why so many nursing home residents were being given sleeping pills every night. There was good evidence that after months of daily use such drugs didn't really improve sleep, but they did cause an ongoing risk of falls and hip fractures. Our new perspective of sociopharmacology proved helpful in tackling this problem. We learned that in many homes the night shift was staffed so thinly that the day workers had to get the residents ready for sleep before leaving. As a consequence the residents were put to bed early, in some cases before 9 p.m. Many of them weren't ready to doze off at that hour, so they needed a little pharmacologic nudge. Worried staff told us that failing to administer such chemical assistance could mean that when the lone night nurse came on duty, she might be confronted with wards full of wandering demented old people making more demands than one person could possibly meet. (Scenes from the cult film classic *Night of the Living Dead* flashed through my mind when I heard about these fears.)

Chronobiology haunted the night staff in other ways as well. Residents who regularly awakened at 3 a.m. could earn themselves a diagnosis of chronic insomnia and the virtual guarantee of a prescription for a "sleeper"—or an increase in dose if they already had one. But do the math: if someone is used to six hours of sleep and is put to bed at 9 p.m., she'll be awake, fresh as a daisy and raring to go, at 3 a.m. A slide I show medical students in discussing this problem reads simply, "9 + 6 = 3." Does this problem require more sleeping pills, or a rethinking of nursing home schedules and staffing patterns? What would be the benefit-risk relationship of writing a prescription to watch *The Late Show* instead?

To understand the tranquilizer-use problem from the patients' perspective, we went to talk to some of them. I remember one pleasant lady who admitted that she requested a sleeping pill every single night. We asked if she really thought she needed it that often.

"Of course I do, dear," she responded. And how did she know? "Around here, if they have a pill for you around bedtime, the nurse comes in and gives it to you along with some juice or milk to help it go down. Then she tucks you in and says, 'Good night, sleep well.' If you don't have a pill, nobody comes around to tuck you in or say good night."

That woman taught us a vital lesson on the nonpharmacologic role of medications, and inspired one of the project's un-advertisements. The grant supporting this project, from the John A. Hartford Foundation, was bigger than my first one. As a result, we could afford to commission a photographer to shoot a soft-focus portrait of a nurse tucking in an elderly model we hired. To this we added a headline: "YOUR GENTLE TOUCH MAY BE ALL SHE NEEDS AT BEDTIME." The text pointed out that a few kind words and a fluffed-up pillow were a risk-free way to help an elderly nursing home patient fall asleep. It went on to present data on the hazards of prescribing sleeping pills for every-night use, and the side effects that could result.

ENFORCED TRANQUILLITY

Another goal of the project was to reduce overuse of antipsychotic drugs, motivated by our previous research on their Parkinson's-like side effects. In a separate project done in rest homes with the Massachusetts Department of Public Health, I had found that many staff in those settings didn't know that the medications they were administering could mimic parkinsonian symptoms. We had presented rest home staff throughout the state with a clinical vignette depicting a patient with this very problem; fully half the staff members missed the connection altogether and said that the abnormal movements were probably signs that the patient was having a stroke, was mentally ill, or just wanted more attention. So for the current study, we created an un-ad illustrating the movement disorders such drugs could cause so that staff could recognize them more easily. We then pointed out how little these drugs had been studied in the elderly and proposed safer alternatives, including nondrug person-to-person interventions.

My favorite un-ad for this study was one I had doodled on a napkin while listening to a boring lecture. It depicted a road forking off in multiple directions into a psychedelic-colored landscape; each fork led to a dead end. One was labeled CONFUSION, another FALLS, others DISORIENTATION and FORGETFULNESS. The headline read, "IN THE ELDERLY, THE SIDE EFFECTS OF SEDATIVES ARE ALL OVER THE MAP." The accompanying text reminded doctors and nurses that although the benefits of sedating an elderly patient may often be small, the risks were not.

As before, we implemented and evaluated the program as a randomized controlled trial. We grouped the twelve nursing homes into six matched pairs. A random-number generator assigned one home in each pair to get the experimental program, and the other to serve as a comparison home. This time I hoped to do more than just change prescribing; I also wanted to see whether we could improve patients' clinical condition. That would help address the fears of some in the nursing home industry that their residents "would start bouncing off the walls" if their sedation were reduced, as one skeptic put it. To the contrary, I felt that lifting the chemical burden might improve the patients' level of function. But we couldn't know which would occur, because no one had ever tried to reduce drug use in this setting on such a large scale. To find out, we sent another research assistant into each home to measure the level of function of every patient getting a psychoactive drug. Neither of the two assistants knew what the other had recorded, or which home was in which group, or even what the study hypothesis was.

Next we trained our academic detailer, a talented pharmacist with years of nursing home experience, and launched him into the six homes that were assigned to get the experimental program. All prescribing decisions remained in the hands of the doctors who normally cared for each patient. Our man was sent to visit each of the prescribing physicians in their off-site offices, using the un-ads as a mini-curriculum on the proper use of psychoactive drugs in the elderly. More important, he ran training sessions for the nurses in the target homes as well. In the face of the near-total absence of doctors, it was the nurses or sometimes even the aides who often initiated the chain of decision making that led to sedative overuse. ("Dr. Jones, it's Nurse Smith. The aides tell me that Mr. Jackson's been getting a little randy on the late shift, so I started him on some Haldol rather than call you in the middle of the night. Make sure you sign the order when you're here next week.")

I worried that because these women's jobs were so grueling they might not want to stay after work to sit through extra training sessions put together by some university doctors. Quite the opposite; they were delighted that someone from a medical school was willing to come into their forsaken workplaces to talk to them about the tough problems they faced every day. ("No one *ever* comes out here to teach us about anything!" said one delighted nursing supervisor.) Building on what we had learned about the sociology of medical decision making in these facilities, we also set up separate training sessions for the aides, and special sessions after midnight for the late shift. Six months later, once all the educational outreach sessions were completed and all the un-ads distributed, our research assistants went back into each experimental and control home. One captured information on all the medications now being used by every resident; the other reassessed their functional status.

Even in this difficult setting, the academic detailing approach worked as we had hoped. The homes randomized to get the program saw a significant drop in the overuse of sedating medications in each of the drug groups we targeted; our measure of staff stress did not deteriorate at all. As for clinical outcomes, there was no evidence that the residents had become more agitated or disruptive once their sedative medications were reduced or eliminated.

A particularly encouraging clinical outcome turned up in the before-and-after test of memory function in patients who had been taking antipsychotic drugs prior to the intervention. In the control homes, memory function deteriorated in about half the patients during the course of the project, and remained stable or improved slightly in the other half—about what one would expect in such an elderly group. But in the homes that had the educational outreach program, memory test performance remained stable or improved in about 70 percent of these patients, and deteriorated in only about 30 percent, a significant difference. That result was at least as good as what's seen with the current crop of drugs for Alzheimer's disease in most patients. If the intervention that wrought this change had been a new biotech product someone would have quickly patented it, spun off a public stock offering, and made a fortune. But it wasn't a new drug; this powerful medicine was just a new way of thinking about how to use the drugs we already had. All we did was lift the burden of oversedation that had been making some of these patients appear more senile than they actually were.

One of the clinical outcomes we measured did give me pause. When we administered a standard test of depression, some residents in the experimental homes scored slightly worse after the program ended. The withdrawn drugs didn't have any important antidepressant properties; why would reducing their use make patients more likely to report sad feelings? I have my own guess: as the doses of sedatives were lowered, more patients became alert and said, in effect, "Hey, I hate living here!" Was this awakening a bad result? Or were these patients better off in an existential sense, being more fully aware of their predicament? Fortunately, when the *New England Journal of Medicine* published our paper, the editors did not require us to venture into these Sartrean waters.

BRINGING IT ALL BACK HOME

A thirty-five-year-old kindergarten teacher is brought to the emergency room of a major academic medical center at 2:30 a.m. with a temperature of 104, rapidly dropping blood pressure, acute kidney failure, and an extremely elevated white blood count. Her medical history is notable for a bleeding ulcer five years earlier. The intern diagnoses septic shock. He considers using a newly introduced drug that can improve the chances of survival in this situation; but it can also cause severe hemorrhage, particularly in patients with her history. Timing is critical, as her condition is deteriorating quickly. Because the drug has been on the market for only a few months, the two senior physicians he consults have not had much experience with it and disagree about what to do.

The intern logs on to the hospital's computer system. It guides him through a decision tree that prompts him to enter specific data on the patient's history and details of her clinical status. At its end, the program indicates that based on the patient's situation and the latest available evidence, her chances of survival will increase if she is given the new drug. It recommends the optimal dose.

Two weeks later the patient is discharged to her home in excellent condition.

The benefits, risks, and costs of drugs loom particularly large in academic medical centers, home to teaching hospitals, medical schools, and the intense complex of research, training, and state-of-the-art practice that constitutes their intertwined missions. In tertiary-care medical centers like the one at which I work, our patients are often much sicker and more complicated, and the care we provide is more intense and costly. Each year brings with it exciting and expensive new drugs, and teaching hospital faculty and trainees cherish their prerogative to try the latest cutting-edge products. Because our research physicians often participate in the pivotal clinical trials for these discoveries, in doing so they frequently become internal advocates for their use. Yet payers are intent on aggressively constraining what hospitals are reimbursed to provide that care.

In 1998, the Brigham and Women's Hospital gave me the opportunity to create a new Division of Pharmacoepidemiology and Pharmacoeconomics, which would grapple with these problems using all the analytic and educational tools described above. Dr. Victor Dzau, chairman of Harvard's Department of Medicine at the Brigham, was enthusiastic about establishing a program in his department to explore these areas rigorously. The new division would pursue research on the benefits, risks, and costs of medications while developing a curriculum on these topics for medical students and other trainees. We would also provide in-house expertise about appropriate medication use to help the hospital remain on the forefront of research and practice while containing our billowing drug budget within reasonable bounds. Dr. Dzau acted as a strong advocate for this vision, as did Dr. Gary Gottlieb, the hospital's CEO.

Early on, we began to refer to our Division of Pharmacoepidemiology simply as DOPE. The teaching materials we produced, "Data on Prescribing Effectively," were designed to give our colleagues "the straight DOPE on drugs." To match the disciplined academic tone of a Harvard teaching hospital, they weren't as glossy or profusely illustrated as our earlier unadvertisements, but like their predecessors each provided a neutral, evidence-based assessment of drug choices in a given area, delivered in a concise user-friendly format. We wanted to be seen as a disinterested resource for this kind of information, representing neither the commercial interests of the pharmaceutical manufacturers nor the narrow cost containment motivations of insurance companies, HMOs, or other payers. At the division's inception, to guard against even the appearance of conflicts of interest, I instituted a policy that is uncommon in academic medical centers: neither I nor my faculty would accept honoraria, consultancies, or other personal remuneration from any pharmaceutical company.

In the most research-intensive medical community on the planet, fulfilling this honest-broker role would not be easy. The Brigham's medical internship is among the most selective in the country; a number of our trainees have already earned Ph.D. degrees along with their M.D. before entering the program. Many of these young doctors have gotten an A or A+ in every course they have taken since childhood; giving them pointers on prescribing can be a challenging task. One tool we use is an online computer-based order-entry system through which all drugs in the hospital are prescribed. As in the vignette above, this makes it possible for us to provide instantaneous guidance, warnings, and reminders that pop up when a doctor enters an order for a particular drug.

Besides consigning the illegible scrawl to the dustbin of history, the order-entry system enables us to provide data-driven teaching to the physician writing a prescription at the moment the decision is being made. We can program the computer to ask the prescriber for more information on why a drug is needed, or propose a more appropriate alternative, or send an alert about a potential problem before the order is completed. This makes it possible to give interns and residents real-time expert guidance about their actions as they occur; I think of it as "just-in-time education."

In the end the ordering physician retains the prerogative of making the final decision in most cases. This is based on our belief that as clever as any computer may be, it is ultimately the responsibility of the doctor at the patient's bedside to make the final choice of a drug. When the system allows the doctor to override a recommendation, it asks the prescriber to explain why in a free-text entry. We occasionally download these to get some feedback on how our messages are being received. One of my favorite typed-in reasons for ignoring the system's advice: "Because I'm the doctor, and you're the computer."

Like many medical centers, we also employ other strategies to ensure that our drug use remains evidence-based and not wasteful. In considering a new drug for our formulary, or list of approved medications, we try to include a cost-effectiveness assessment, to hold the line on agents that are costly clones of existing products but have no advantage over those alternatives. Equally important, this can also pave the way for adopting an expensive new product with a huge sticker price, as long as we can demonstrate that its cost is likely to result in better efficacy, greater patient comfort, shorter length of stay, or a reduction in adverse events.

My division's broad mandate forces us to grapple daily with ground-level application of the benefit-risk-cost trade-offs explored in earlier chapters. For example, the anticoagulant heparin has been a mainstay for hospitalized patients for decades. Its use in humans dates back to the 1930s, when it was extracted from the liver, lungs, and intestines of cows. Given intravenously, it immediately puts the body's clotting mechanism in check, a vital step in caring for patients in whom abnormal coagulation poses a risk: those who might develop blood clots in the veins of the legs or in the lung, or those with atrial fibrillation or coronary artery disease.

Manufacturers have now synthesized several new molecules in attempts to build a better anticoagulant. Some of the new products cost tens or even hundreds of times the price of the old standby. Clinical trials indicate that some of them may slightly reduce the risk of bleeding that comes with any anticoagulant, or may keep arteries open just a little bit better if given to patients with severe angina. How much of an increase in safety or efficacy should warrant what multiple of cost? The question is far from academic when our Pharmacy and Therapeutics Committee tries to make these decisions for the hospital for specific new drugs.

In earlier years, before budgets were so tight, it was easy to yield to the opinion of a clinician-advocate that "we really should have a new product like that available in a cutting-edge place like this." But we can't any longer afford to take that easy way out for every new medication that comes along, especially those that are many times more expensive than currently used drugs but offer only a questionable or theoretical clinical advantage. With growing economic pressures, we would inevitably need to decide what other products we would have to forgo or what services we'd curtail in order to afford the costly new addition to our drug list. A logical source of advice for such questions is the local clinical expert in a given field, even though in many teaching hospitals the best experts are also likely to have their research funded by the manufacturer of one of the competing drugs. Our division's goal is to review critically all the data we can find about a drug's performance, try to factor in the economics, and present the findings and trade-offs to the hospital's Pharmacy and Therapeutics Committee to inform its final decision.

We also take on another function that often goes unperformed in many hospitals: ongoing surveillance of how well we're using existing drugs. Doctors in one department may be prescribing more of a given medication than seems necessary. Others may be underutilizing another therapeutic category, suggesting a quality-of-care problem. Here, too, the hospital's computer system can help us identify which departments and which physicians might need some educational feedback about the uses of a given product, or about the way they are managing a particular diagnosis.

We physicians hear from all sides that we must "practice cost-effectively," but most of us have never been given the tools and feedback we need to follow this dictum. So we established a curriculum on benefit-risk-cost analysis for the medical residents and students who pass through the Brigham's training programs. I realized that we had gained some measure of credibility when the residents asked the hospital to stop allowing drug company sales reps to host the traditional Friday afternoon "pizza rounds," and have our division buy the pizzas instead. Winning the pizza wars meant winning the hearts and minds of young doctors.

In rolling out our division's multipronged approach to improving drug use, I was unsure how well the academic detailing model would work in the critical environment of one of Harvard's most elite teaching hospitals: Brigham interns and residents may be brilliant, but they're not known for their humility. But the idea seemed worth a try. An area of special concern was the overuse of broad-spectrum antibiotics, drugs that kill a wide variety of bacteria; the interns sometimes refer to them as "gorillacillins." They can be lifesaving for a sick patient who has an infection of unknown cause, but using them too often, especially when more narrowly targeted antibiotics would work as well, can breed bacterial resistance in the patient and in the hospital as a whole. We had audited our utilization patterns and found that some of the more heavily promoted broad-spectrum drugs were probably being used too liberally. This was not a cost issue; the more precise narrow-spectrum drugs were sometimes more expensive. The larger problem was that in our hospital, as in most others around the country, the proportion of bacteria resistant to specific antibiotics was increasing each year.

A computerized order-entry fix didn't seem like the best solution, because choosing an antibiotic is often more complex than the kind of algorithm that could be fit onto a computer screen. Academic detailing seemed like a promising way to go if we could tailor it to specific patient-related decisions. I had never used the approach in this way, or in a teaching hospital setting. So before implementing a full-scale program, Dr. Dan Solomon and I tested it out—in a controlled trial, of course. We randomly assigned existing teams of interns and residents either to be "detailed" by specially trained Brigham clinicians or to serve as controls. A research assistant in our division came in early each morning to scan the hospital computer system and find all the previous day's orders for the targeted antibiotics. She then ran the patients' clinical information (also drawn from the computer) through a simple decision tree to see if there was an obvious reason to justify use of these drugs. If none was found, she'd send the patient's name and data to one of our three staff detailers, who reviewed the medical record. If there was still no apparent reason to explain use of the drugs, one of them would page the intern and provide an educational intervention on the spot.

Solomon's study found that the teams we randomized to the detailing intervention substantially reduced their overuse of these drugs, with no evidence of any adverse clinical outcomes. We also noted that as the year went on and interns rotated off the experimental teams and onto the control teams, use of the targeted antibiotics came down there as well. The education they had received had become contagious as they spread the word to their colleagues. Perfect. Microbiologists had shown years earlier that bacterial resistance to antibiotics spreads so quickly because fragments of the DNA of resistant bacteria can jump from bug to bug, carrying with them vital information on how to overcome the effects of a given drug. Now we had shown that information on how best to overcome bacteria could jump from doctor to doctor, increasing the interns' resistance to the problematic antibiotics. We implemented the program on an operational basis.

THE BEST TEST of an idea, like a gene, is whether it proliferates when given the chance. Academic detailing has done well by this standard. As with any new idea that "takes," the concept had probably become inevitable by the early 1980s. Even if our studies had never been done, others would likely have gone down the same road, as many now have; the conceptual vacuum of the drug information marketplace was just begging to be filled. Since those early stirrings, such programs have proliferated, providing physicians with evidence-based alternatives to mere sales promotion. I had the chance to help a Dutch team apply the approach to groups of physicians who met on a regular basis with pharmacist-educators. The British National Health Service now hires squads of pharmacists to visit general practitioners and offer guidance on how to improve their prescribing. Prescription benefit managers and HMOs throughout the United States have set up physician education programs based on our initial work. Canadian provinces from coast to coast set up their own academic detailing programs to enable their governments to continue to offer broad-based drug entitlement programs without going broke. To assess the growing worldwide literature describing such activities, the Cochrane Collaboration, an international consortium that reviews evidence on the effectiveness of clinical interventions, made "educational outreach visits" a review topic in its own right. And by the century's close, I had the privilege of helping develop the groundwork for a program in Australia in which academic detailing was established throughout the continent. That effort is described in a later chapter.

The scientific grounding on which all these activities are based is an insistence upon distinguishing science from promotion. Each academic detailing program around the world assesses the evidence about a drug's effectiveness with a perspective of open-minded skepticism, taking the perspective of the controlled trial to the next logical level. Collectively, we are asking much tougher questions than "Is this new drug better than placebo in achieving a surrogate outcome in a modest number of people over a few months?" We are instead demanding to know whether a treatment is more effective *and* safer *and* more cost-effective than alternative choices when used in typical patients over a period of years.

These are tough questions, but they are precisely the ones that doctors and patients and those who pay the bills need to have answered. Asking them takes Popper's falsificationism to its next logical stage. The new "null hypothesis" to evaluate isn't "Drug X is no better than placebo." Instead, it's "Drug X is no better than what we're currently using." As if this were not threatening enough, many of us who are asking this new generation of questions go on to actively disseminate our conclusions to all who will listen. This movement, if we dare call it that, is the latest incarnation of a noble tradition in medicine that stretches back over a century. It makes for bracing science and improved medical care. But it doesn't necessarily make for popularity.

19: THE EMPEROR'S
FASHION CRITICS

Men become civilized, not in proportion to their willingness to believe, but in proportion to their readiness
to doubt.

—H. L. MENCKEN

Every schoolchild has heard of the heroes who invented wonderful new treatments: Louis Pasteur, Alexander Fleming, Jonas Salk. Literature offers similar examples, from Shaw's *Doctor's Dilemma* to Sinclair Lewis' *Arrowsmith*. There is an equally fascinating dark side to this history: the people who discovered not the benefits of therapies but their downsides. They are the clinical equivalents of the little boy who pointed out that the Emperor's gorgeous new clothes weren't real. In life and in literature, the fates of these people have been less happy. Yet we also need these medical whistle-blowers to hold up an unflattering mirror to the healing enterprise when needed, revealing its excesses and its hazards. That process, too, is powerful medicine.

Scientific progress isn't just about splendid breakthroughs; insight also comes from the systematic demolition of attractive ideas that happen to be wrong. This is how bones grow. Cells called osteoblasts make new bone tissue, but their output would be useless were it not for their sister cells, the osteoclasts, which break down old bone no longer needed in that precise location. (The word shares a root with "iconoclast," "one who destroys religious images or opposes their veneration.") The coordinated action of both kinds of cell is necessary for normal bone growth. The osteoclasts' "creative destruction" turns out to be crucial for maintaining strong bones during adulthood as well. Vital as their role is, if osteoclasts were on the faculties of most medical schools, few of them would ever get promoted.

THE TOXIC SPA

Just as some surgeons delight in collecting ancient scalpels and retractors, my work has drawn me to collect stories of Popperian heroes, human osteoclasts—people who made major contributions to health by discovering treatment-induced illness. One of my favorites is the fictional Dr. Thomas Stockmann, a small-town Norwegian physician in Henrik Ibsen's 1882 play, *An Enemy of the People.*

The plot will appeal to anyone prone to both idealism and paranoia, and illustrates several of the themes we've been considering. As a young man, Stockmann comes to believe that the waters of his town's natural baths might have healing properties. The concept leads his brother the Mayor to set up a lucrative private consortium to commercialize the baths. The town's waters become renowned for their power to combat disease and restore vitality, and everyone prospers. But Dr. Stockmann, hired as the new spa's physician, soon notices that some visitors are coming down with typhoid fever and gastrointestinal infections. Analysis of a water sample reveals that the baths are contaminated by industrial pollution near their source; the spa's treatments turn out to be spreading rather than alleviating disease.

Using language that could have come from a modern-day class-action lawsuit, Stockmann declares that the water "is poison for internal or external use! And it's foisted on poor, suffering creatures who turn to us in good faith and pay us exorbitant fees to gain their health back again!" After his initial shock, the doctor feels privileged to have discovered the source of so much preventable disease. We learn that Stockmann had tried to warn the authorities at the start of the project that putting the baths' intake pipes too close to the source of pollution was a bad idea. But economic considerations took precedence, and shorter pipes were used to minimize cost and maximize profit.

Like any dedicated epidemiologist, Stockmann expects that his discovery will be welcomed by all, including the Mayor: "Undoubtedly he has to be glad that a fact of such importance is brought to light." A local journalist declares that the discovery makes the doctor the town's leading citizen, and proposes a parade in his honor.

Act Two: The Mayor points out that if word of the pollution gets out it could spell economic ruin for the town, since so much of its commerce is based on tourism centering on the spa. Revenues would shrivel, jobs would be lost, and the townspeople would have to bear a large tax increase to reroute the water supply. If everything were just kept quiet, the Mayor suggests, his brother could use his medical knowledge to control the problem more inexpensively (an early risk-management approach). No way, the doctor responds; facts are facts, and as a man of science he must make them public. In one of the first recorded examples of a fiscally driven hazard assessment, the Mayor retorts, "What's involved here isn't a purely scientific problem. It's a mixture of both technical and economic considerations."

The business argument carries the day, and the local paper refuses to publish the doctor's discovery. Instead, it runs a brief press release from the Mayor explaining that the supposed risk is minor, and its importance greatly exaggerated. Dr. Stockmann refuses to agree to the deception and is summarily fired. When he persists in warning of the waters' sickening effects, the townsfolk brand him an enemy of the people. His discovery is ridiculed, and the baths stay open; he ends the play a crushed, embittered man. There is no parade.

As someone who spends much of his life studying the potential adverse effects of health-related interventions, I feel a warm glow inside each time I reread this play. It's not pride—it's acid reflux.

DEADLY DELIVERIES

Ibsen's plot bears a striking resemblance to the biography of a real-world doctor of the same era. Dr. Ignaz Semmelweis (1818–1865), a Hungarian physician, also discovered that an intervention meant to be therapeutic can be lethal. In the mid-nineteenth century, it was not unusual for a pregnant woman to have a normal delivery, give birth to a healthy child, and then develop a horrendous illness in the first postpartum days. In this condition, known as childbed or puerperal fever, the temperature rose uncontrollably as the patient alternated between chills, drenching sweats, and delirium. She might go on to bleed uncontrollably from multiple sites as her blood pressure plummeted. Vital organs shut down one by one. The condition, whose cause was unknown, was usually fatal.

Authorities of the day attributed childbed fever to miasma, that same vague toxic presence in the atmosphere that John Snow's colleagues during that period thought was the cause of cholera. Few doctors then believed that either condition was infectious in origin; wide acceptance of the germ theory of disease was still decades in the future. But just as Snow was able to discern a pattern that connected a home's drinking water with the occurrence of cholera, Semmelweis made a similar key observation. He noted that women whose babies were delivered by physicians came down with puerperal fever far more often than those attended by midwives.

Semmelweis worked in a teaching facility, the charity obstetric hospital of Vienna. It admitted indigent women and unwed mothers free of charge as long as they made themselves available for educational purposes and agreed to serve as wet nurses after delivery. The death rate from childbed fever there was appallingly high, over 12 percent of all deliveries. By contrast, Semmelweis found that the comparable figure was only 2 percent at the adjacent maternity hospital, where nearly all deliveries were handled by midwives-in-training. Today, we might worry about "case-mix differences"—the possibility that the women at one hospital may have been sicker or weaker to begin with. But he made another key observation: the death rate at his hospital was lower for women who arrived after giving birth at home or even on the street, compared to those who made it to the hospital in time and delivered there. Something was being done to these patients at the hospital that was killing them.

Looking into the problem further, he found that medical students and physicians often examined patients or performed deliveries right after they finished dissecting cadavers in the autopsy room; the midwifery students didn't have such an advanced component in their curriculum. Maintaining sterility or even cleanliness was still not a value in medicine; the basic discoveries in this field would not be made until more than a decade later. Semmelweis doubted that the cause of childbed fever was a miasma, or constipation, or becoming chilled, or the position in which the woman lay while delivering—all explanations current at the time. What if the physicians themselves were bringing the disease from the corpses to the women they were caring for? Germs were still unknown, so Semmelweis called his hypothesized substance "cadaveric particles." Whatever it was, he reasoned that doctors and medical students could rid themselves of it by washing their hands in a chlorinated water solution. As chief of service, Semmelweis had the power to require that the students and physicians in his hospital engage in this odd ritual before delivering or even examining a pregnant woman—particularly if they had just been slicing into cadavers. He issued this edict in 1847. Some senior physicians objected, saying that the procedure was undignified, but most complied. Within a year, the death rate from childbed fever at his institution was reduced from 12 percent to under 1 percent of cases.

Like Ibsen's character, Semmelweis was delighted that he had found the cause of a terrible and now preventable disease, even if that cause was the health care system itself. He became a missionary for his theory, presenting it to audiences of physicians whenever he could. But as Dr. Stockmann found, those who deliver treatments to improve health don't like to hear that they can occasionally cause disease. The academic authorities of the day decreed that Semmelweis' science was not very good, and that he was a troublemaker. Senior professors at his institution blocked his promotion. His citizenship did not help; in Vienna, a Hungarian who declared that the city's medical establishment was killing its patients was vulnerable to xenophobia as well. Eventually, he was dismissed from his post and forced to return to Hungary. His successor at the university proclaimed that the radical new theory about the cause and preventability of childbed fever had been "discredited and universally rejected."

Semmelweis' next position was at the University of Pest (today part of Budapest). When he introduced his chlorine hand-washing procedure there, he reported that the hospital's high postpartum death rate also dropped to under 1 percent. In 1861 he assembled his findings into a book, *The Cause, Concept, and Prophylaxis of Childbed Fever*. It received terrible reviews from the medical establishment and from his fellow faculty members, most of whom dismissed it as unsound science. Enraged that the medical authorities refused to pay attention to information that could prevent so many deaths, Semmelweis wrote a furious open letter to the professors of obstetrics: "Your teaching . . . is based on the dead bodies of . . . women slaughtered through ignorance. . . . [If] you continue to teach your students and midwives that [childbed] fever is an ordinary epidemic disease, I proclaim you before God and the world to be assassins." Tact was not his major strength.

Increasingly marginalized, Semmelweis by the summer of 1865 had taken to walking the streets of the city handing out leaflets, particularly to those who appeared to be pregnant: "Beware of doctors, for they will kill you. . . . Unless everything that touches you is washed with soap and water and then chlorine solution, you will die and your child with you!" His upsetting predictions and innovative educational outreach were seen as the work of a madman, which perhaps Semmelweis had become. In August 1865, his colleagues had him confined to a mental hospital. The admission was disastrous. He tried to escape, was restrained in a straitjacket, isolated in a darkened cell, and beaten by the guards. Within thirteen days he was dead, probably of the same kind of invasive bacterial infection we now know to be the cause of childbed fever and septic shock, which he contracted following his beatings. The autopsy report concluded, "It is obvious that these horrible injuries were . . . the consequences of brutal beating, tying down, trampling underfoot." Grotesquely, he died a victim of the medical care system that he had tried to reform.

Decades before the discovery of the bacterium that causes childbed fever, and well before the acceptance of the germ theory, the straightforward observational studies of Semmelweis yielded insights into the cause of a dread disease and offered an effective means of preventing it. Medical authorities eventually came to accept the idea that the clinical enterprise itself could harm patients, and that such harm could be reduced to nearly zero by a simple, low-tech intervention—however demeaning it might seem to some doctors. Wherever his insights were implemented, they saved the lives of hundreds of thousands of pregnant women, long after he was written off as a madman and a threat to the medical establishment. At the time of his death, Ignaz Semmelweis, the father of three small children, was forty-seven years old.

A LOCAL HERO

To counterbalance these stories of whistle-blower physicians trampled underfoot both figuratively and literally, I set out to find a less depressing role model and discovered one right in my own backyard. The man had died seventy-five years before I got there, but in my line of work you embrace any mentors you can find, dead or alive. He was Dr. Oliver Wendell Holmes, Sr. (1809–1894), the physician cited in Chapter 1 for his comment about throwing all available medicines into the sea. Dr. Holmes' therapeutic skepticism was not limited to pharmaceuticals. Like Semmelweis, who was just nine years younger, he suspected that doctors were a key risk factor for childbed fever. Fortunately, Holmes' work in this area led to a happier outcome. In an 1843 treatise, *The Contagiousness of Puerperal Fever,* he carefully collected patient histories and made deductions about the role of doctors in transmitting the disease. After analyzing thirty "strings of cases" comprising 250 episodes of illness and 130 deaths, he concluded that the attending physician was often the likeliest cause of the condition.

Holmes was less astute than Semmelweis as to the mode of transmission; he knew it was a contagion of some kind, but wasn't sure "whether it be by the atmosphere the physician carries about him into the sick-chamber, or by the direct application of the virus to the absorbing surfaces with which his hand comes in contact." It was, of course, the latter, though we would now use the term "bacterium" instead of "virus." The clinical vignettes he collected included stories of doctors who used the same gloves to care for women with the dreaded fever and then to deliver the babies of healthy women; and the reuse of the same enema instruments (totally unnecessary in any case) for the deliveries of both sick and healthy women.

The histories Holmes presented made it clear that the answer had been there all along for all to see, if only the adverse-event data had been evaluated with an open mind. Consider this episode reported by Holmes that had occurred over twenty years earlier:

> Dr. Campbell of Edinburgh states that in October 1821 he assisted at the post-mortem examination of a patient who died with puerperal fever. He carried the pelvic viscera in his pocket to the class-room. The same evening he attended a woman in labor without previously changing his clothes; this patient died. The next morning he delivered a woman with the forceps; she died also, and of many who were seized with the disease within a few weeks, three showed the same fate in succession.

Not all cases of childbed fever developed after a doctor had performed an autopsy; caring for living patients with bacterial infections would work as well. Holmes' reports provide a humbling window on the prevailing standards of care among highly respected practitioners in Boston, even then a medically sophisticated part of the country. One doctor recalled that just before the first case in a puerperal fever outbreak, he "was attending and dressing a limb extensively mortified from erysipelas [a streptococcal skin infection often accompanied by copious pus] and went immediately to the *accouchement* [delivery room] with his clothes and gloves most thoroughly imbued with its effluvia." Reading these accounts makes me wonder what practices of twenty-first-century medicine will appall our own descendants. I envision twenty-second-century authors writing with similar revulsion about our nearly random use of antibiotics to treat viral infections ("This was, of course, just before the devastating epidemics of resistant bacteria that killed so many during the 2020s . . .") or our failure to implement the lessons of our own clinical trial data ("As late as 2015, thousands of Americans died each year of preventable strokes and heart attacks because they were never provided with the medications that had been shown to prevent these needless events . . .").

The gift of good writing is not common among physicians, but Holmes had it. He had composed the poem "Old Ironsides" in 1830 when he was twenty-one, and now used his skills to exhort his fellow physicians to see how their own therapeutic habits were transmitting the very illnesses they sought to treat. The evidence from both America and Europe, he argued, must lead clinicians "to accept the solemn truth knelled into their ears by the funeral bells from both sides of the ocean—the plain conclusion that the physician and the disease entered, hand in hand, into the chamber of the unsuspecting patient." His papers convey a keen understanding of the problem of adverse-event underreporting that we considered in Part Two: "Behind the fearful array of published facts there lies a dark list of similar events, unwritten in the records of science, but long remembered by many a desolated fireside."

The study of medically induced illness seems to bring out rage in those who study it. Elegant as he was, Holmes could also be ferocious, although not as combative as poor Dr. Semmelweis. "Whatever indulgence may be granted to those who have heretofore been the ignorant causes of so much misery," he wrote, "the time has come when the existence of a private pestilence in the sphere of a single physician should be looked upon, not as a misfortune, but a crime." He saw how reluctant the medical profession was to admit its role in causing such misery, but had an optimistic New World view of how that would be handled: "Whenever and wherever [physicians] can be shown to carry disease and death instead of health and safety, the common instincts of humanity will silence every attempt to explain away their responsibility."

Perhaps because of his foggier grasp of the means of infection, Holmes' clinical advice was less to the point than his European counterpart's: he recommended hand-washing but did not mention an antiseptic solution, a key precaution. He suggested instead that a physician with one or more cases of puerperal fever should cease practice for a month or so to ensure that he did not spread the disease. That may have worked, but no better than a quick change of clothes and a chlorinated scrub, after which the doctor could have gone on immediately to care for his next patient.

Perhaps it was the greater openness on this side of the ocean to antiauthoritarian insights in medicine, or the fact that the Bostonian was more diplomatic than the Hungarian. In any case, Holmes was not driven from his post, and did not end his career or his life disgracefully in an insane asylum. Quite the opposite: he was made the dean of Harvard Medical School. American physicians were not universally hostile to the new ideas, but they also did not rush to embrace the implications of Holmes' discovery. The idea that medical care itself could spread illness continued to meet with resistance; for years to come, paintings of great professors performing surgery under the respectful gaze of students and colleagues still often depicted them in street clothes, with no evidence of modern antiseptic hygiene apparent.

THE BOSTON LYING-IN HOSPITAL, named with the now-archaic term for childbirth, was one of the nation's first obstetrics hospitals and one of the first to translate Holmes' research into practice on a large scale. By the end of the nineteenth century, it required doctors and medical students to wash their hands and use antiseptic technique when examining pregnant women and performing deliveries. Long affiliated with Harvard Medical School, it was eventually merged into the Brigham and Women's Hospital complex. One hundred and fifty years after Holmes published his seminal work, our research unit moved into renovated space in "the Old Lying-In" that had long since been converted to offices and labs. The building's exterior is still adorned with stone medallions of babies and storks (yes, storks). They remind me that each day I come to work is another day to try to end up more like Holmes than Semmelweis.

THE ABILITY TO DETECT and reduce clinically induced illness is a vital tool for alleviating human misery, both in daily clinical practice and in public health. It keeps the medical care system on track by enabling us to contain one important cause of human disease; it also ensures that our profession's humility does not fall to dangerously low levels. As nature perfected the structure and function of bones, it must have taken millions of years of evolution to get the right balance between osteoblasts and osteoclasts. In the case of drugs, we're still working on that balance. Popper's sour-tasting falsificationism is the powerful medicine twenty-first-century health care will need if it is to nurture a vibrant, effective, and affordable approach to therapeutics—indeed to all of medical care. Whenever the Emperor is sold a bill of goods by an overly entrepreneurial merchant, we need that little boy to speak out as loudly as he can. This insight is alive and well at the edges of our medical research community, although not always at its center. As we will see in the next chapter, it is a bit closer to the medical mainstream beyond our borders.

20: SAME LANGUAGE, DIFFERENT ACCENTS

Much is excellent and even wonderful about medicine in the United States. But we are a bit too quick in leaping to the conclusion that Americans get By Far the Best Health Care on Earth. For those who can afford to pay top dollar, U.S. medicine is as good as can be found anywhere. But for the population as a whole, the quality of our care is not substantially better than that in most advanced nations, even if we pay about 50 percent per capita more for it. And of course for those without adequate insurance, things are much worse. If we are to grapple successfully with the problems besetting our system, we'll have to consider the possibility that some aspects of health care are just handled better elsewhere.

Most industrialized nations face the same medical challenges we do. Even in systems that pay less per capita for pharmaceuticals (i.e., virtually all of them), rising drug costs pose a major problem. Price controls aside, many of those countries have been creative in developing programs to gather and disseminate information to doctors and patients to improve their drug choices. Before considering specific policy options for our own system, we can learn a great deal by looking at how other nations are grappling with the same issues. For a quick overview, we'll restrict ourselves to innovative programs in Australia, Britain, and Canada.

ADAPTIVE MUTATIONS

I've become most personally involved in the program that is farthest away, in Australia. Like the continent itself, some aspects of Australian medicine long ago drifted away from the conceptual landmasses of older health care systems, even though the profession maintained its roots in the British scientific tradition. Starting from conventional origins, Australian medical culture has traveled down its own quirky evolutionary path. The absence of a predatory indigenous pharmaceutical industry spared it from the selection pressures that helped shape the drug policies of other advanced nations. As a result, the country was able to establish some unusual medication programs that are both odd and endearing—health policy equivalents of the platypus and koala.

The country was a pioneer in the critical assessment of drugs, introducing a controversial requirement in 1993 that before a company could market a new medication there it had to provide evidence about its cost-effectiveness, along with the usual data on efficacy and safety. Policy in this area took another innovative leap in the late 1990s with the creation of the National Prescribing Service, a consortium of over thirty organizations representing clinicians, consumer groups, researchers, the health care and pharmaceutical industries, and the government. Together, these groups identified the need for "an organization that could coordinate and provide independent information on new and existing drugs, and comparative information on drugs within a class." The NPS was established "to make sure practitioners have access to the information and support they need to make good prescribing decisions, ensuring the best and most cost-effective treatment for patients." Its mission requires that the focus be "on quality rather than cost containment. . . . We do not presume that quality prescribing always means less prescribing, and expect that some programs will lead to increased prescription of medications."

The service is controlled by an independent group representing all of these stakeholders and not by the government, whose role is confined to paying the bill for its educational activities. This costs only about 11 million Australian dollars per year, about one quarter of 1 percent of the $4–$5 billion the government spends each year on its universal drug entitlement. The program commissions evidence-based reviews of competing drugs within a class, performed by experts external to both the government and the drug industry. In its first years of operation, NPS more than paid for itself in reduced unnecessary drug expenditures, not counting the benefits of improved quality of prescribing.

The Australians have long been interested in how best to teach doctors about drugs, and were among the first to pick up on our initial work on academic detailing. One early adopter was Dr. Ken Harvey, a spunky and intense microbiologist from Victoria who took on the problem of antibiotic misuse as a personal crusade in the 1980s. He traveled about his region making one-on-one visits to local general practitioners, trying to persuade them to reduce their excessive use of antibiotics. Initially he met with considerable resistance; on a visit to America, he came by to discuss his project. I asked him how he presented the information to the doctors he visited.

"Well, I drive 'round to their practice; we discuss their heavy antibiotic use. I talk a bit about the problem of bacterial resistance, and after that I tell them to stop prescribing like a fuckwit."

I had never heard the term "fuckwit" before, but was able to guess at its meaning. I complimented Dr. Harvey on his interactive approach and we discussed his program in detail, covering both its microbiological and interpersonal aspects. I suggested he might want to rethink the confrontational style. In any case, I urged him to take pains to avoid using the term "fuckwit" at all costs. He went back home, continued his work in a mellower manner, and his project became a model for several similar start-up programs in Australia over the coming years.

One project that became particularly influential was initiated by Frank May, a burly, genial man who had planned a career as a concert organist before becoming a pharmacist. Working in the state of New South Wales, May, too, had read our papers on improving medication use as well as those from the group at Vanderbilt, and used them to establish his own program. He persuaded the government to provide some seed money to enable him to visit general practitioners in his area and present them with evidence-based, noncommercial information about medications. To document the effect of what he was doing, he identified an adjacent part of the country with comparable patterns of drug use to serve as a control group. Although prescribing had been similar in both regions before his program began, he found that doctors in the test area substantially improved their prescribing after his educational visits, compared to doctors in the neighboring territory. More government support followed, and over the years May succeeded in building up a model program that gained national attention.

As Australia struggled in the mid-1990s with an increasingly costly national drug benefit program, word of these innovative local activities percolated up to the federal government. One day I got a call from May. "Good news, mate!" he bellowed. "They may want to expand this work to the whole country." He asked me to help review the worldwide evidence (by then substantial) that operational-size academic detailing programs could improve prescribing, and then to help think about how the idea could be implemented throughout that continent. Working with Professor Chris Silagy, we reviewed everything we could find about how such programs had fared since publication of those early papers.

May and Silagy summarized programs in Europe and Australasia; I was assigned the Western Hemisphere. We knew that much valuable experience was accumulating in small, isolated programs all over the world, even if the people who ran them never submitted descriptions of their work to medical journals for publication. Working with colleagues in my division, we supplemented a formal literature review with phone calls to the growing but diffuse collection of academic detailing programs throughout North America. Our work was combined with that of our Australian colleagues and submitted to the federal authorities in Canberra. It helped provide the rationale for the first continentwide program of educational outreach to improve the use of medications. This was a dream come true for any academic—to see the concepts set forth in my original grant proposal of 1979 put into practice on such a large scale.

Much additional work by Australian physicians, pharmacists, and policy makers led to the creation of an "action arm" of the National Prescribing Service. In 1998, NPS established an ambitious and creative program that used academic detailing to bring the results of its drug assessments right to practitioners in their offices. Most of the general-practice regions in that huge country came to be covered by academic detailers, known as "facilitators"—pharmacists and other health professionals trained in educational outreach using an approach similar to the one we developed in Boston. The NPS provides each facilitator with advanced training on the pharmacology to be covered, and equips them with engaging print materials to convey the key messages. The content of all NPS materials, courses, and academic detailing visits is developed by a staff of physicians and pharmacists independent of the government.

NPS also publishes concise reviews of common medication-related problems; these are delivered to practitioners in person and used as teaching tools by the facilitators. Between visits, physicians can phone in for advice on new prescribing issues that arise; NPS staffs a hotline to respond to these queries. Patients have their own call-in service that provides answers in lay language to questions about their medicines. Because doctors are used to learning by the case study method, most NPS reviews also contain vignettes describing patients who presented a prescribing dilemma, followed by five or six key questions. Physicians review these with the facilitator during the visit, or can fill in the sheets themselves and send them into NPS offices. A few weeks later, responses of practitioners from all over the country are summarized on the NPS website along with commentaries by experts.

If they choose to, practitioners can participate in a self-study program known as a clinical audit. Doctors review the drugs they've prescribed for a group of patients with a given medical problem; an NPS facilitator then evaluates their prescribing in light of evidence-based standards, and suggests areas for potential improvement. Involvement in any of these programs is completely voluntary. There is no charge, and physicians can even be paid for participating. A doctor who takes part in a modest number of group or individual academic detailing visits, a clinical audit, and other educational activities can earn a salary bonus that averages about $1,000 per year. The rationale is that if a bonus is to be given to physicians based on how they prescribe, it should be for learning how to take better care of their patients, not for avoiding expensive drugs.

A NICE IDEA

On the other side of the globe, the British National Health Service has long both fascinated and appalled foreign observers. Founded in the pain-ridden years after World War II, it was rooted in the premise that the nation had a social responsibility to provide decent medical care to every citizen regardless of the ability to pay. In the decades since, the NHS has served as a model that has inspired many other countries, although few have chosen to replicate its socialized structure and financing. It remains severely underfunded, with Britain spending less of its gross domestic product on medical care (only about 6 percent) than nearly any other advanced nation. This has put added pressure on the NHS' growing medication expenditures, and has resulted in some interesting attempts to fix the British drug problem.

The rationing that this degree of underfunding has required could only work in a nation that formed orderly queues to file into air-raid shelters during the blitz, and where *The Highway Code,* a national compendium of traffic regulations, is a perennial best-seller. Delay or outright denial of medicines or of services like dialysis or hip replacement might be more tolerable if all royal subjects faced the same fate; in a nation that helped invent class differences, NHS defenders like to point out that their single system provides the same care for princes as for paupers. (Only about 4 percent of total British health expenditures are paid for through private insurance.)

But in the 1990s, the use of medications became an embarrassingly visible scar on this image of equality. Uneven distribution of NHS funds across the country meant that local health authorities in some parts of Britain could afford certain costly drugs while other areas could not. Newspapers carried stories of doctors in poorer areas who didn't even write prescriptions for some expensive drugs because they knew the local budget couldn't provide them. Patients' addresses rather than their clinical needs seemed to determine the medicines they got; this geographic variation in care came to be known as "post-code prescribing." General underfunding of the NHS might be something the British could grudgingly accept, as they had for decades, but blatant evidence of variations in care based on one's hometown (i.e., wealth) was unacceptable.

Consensus emerged that if the NHS was going to cover a medicine, everyone should have access to it. If a drug was too expensive to provide, then everyone should face that burden equally (except, of course, for the well-off citizens who could always pay for it privately). But how to decide which drugs should be made available to all, and which were too costly for any? The question came to the public's attention at the same time that the system's overall drug budget was rising inexorably. Some proposed that equity and cost containment could both be served if the nation developed a uniform way to measure the clinical and economic value of all medical interventions.

To accomplish this, in 1999 Britain established the National Institute for Clinical Excellence, known as NICE. It was set up as an independent organization within the NHS that would make judgments about what the health service would cover; it would also provide guidance for physicians, patients, and caregivers about which drugs and other medical interventions are worth using. NICE is a lean organization: with only about thirty-five core staff, it works closely with existing reservoirs of expertise throughout the country in medical schools and professional groups like the Royal Colleges of Physicians, of Surgeons, of General Practitioners, of Psychiatrists, and so on. The program draws on these experts to form "appraisal committees" that assess controversial treatments. In sharp contrast to FDA policy, no one with any conflict of interest may participate in this process.

The committees review every available bit of published or unpublished information concerning a treatment's efficacy, safety, and cost-effectiveness, with minutes of all discussions publicly posted on the NICE website. After several iterations for comment and feedback, the panel assigns the product to one of four categories: (1) approved for unrestricted use; (2) restricted to defined patients; (3) for use in clinical trials only; and (4) not to be used. If the final NICE recommendation is to fund a given treatment, the NHS must cover its cost for all patients in the system. Copies of each NICE report are sent to every primary-care physician and relevant specialist in the country, and posted on the net.

Interestingly, some of the first NICE assessments called for *greater* use of several costly medicines, adding millions of pounds to the NHS budget. Other assessments found particular treatments to be grossly overused, or to represent very poor value in relation to their cost. A good illustration of the process is the NICE treatment given to proton pump inhibitors, or PPIs, the heartburn drugs that alleviate that condition in patients and tended to cause it in anyone paying for them. The category includes the costly "purple pills" Prilosec and Nexium, which at the time of the British assessment were being extravagantly advertised and used in the United States at $4 to

$6 per dose, even though much less expensive alternatives would work as well for many patients. The NICE assessment concluded:

> The majority of patients should not be prescribed PPIs on a long-term basis, the dose should be reduced where appropriate, and the least expensive PPI that is most appropriate for the patient should be used. This advice will have real benefits for patients because there is no advantage in having more of a drug than is needed.

Implementing this one policy throughout the NHS resulted in savings of £40–£50 million (around U.S. $75 million) per year.

Another interesting component of the NHS/NICE effort is a suite of decision-support software developed for primary-care physicians. If we expect doctors to practice high-quality medicine cost-effectively, the reasoning went, we need to make sure that they have the tools to do so. So the NHS and NICE created a user-friendly interactive computer-consultant called Prodigy and put it into the public domain on a website accessible by anyone at no charge. It presents the best current information on optimal management of over 130 conditions, from Adverse Drug Reactions to Wound Care. It also provides information on the reasoning behind the recommendations, what tests to order, and when to call in a specialist. Click on a drug and you are linked to an electronic version of the British National Formulary, a publicly available listing of all the nation's medications that displays their uses, proper dosing, side effects, and interactions. Click on another part of the site and you can print out a patient-education leaflet explaining the condition and the treatment chosen, in English or Welsh.

In the year following publication of the first NIH hormone replacement trial, troubled by my surf through commonly used American sites, I logged on to the NHS site to see what a perplexed doctor or patient might find there to guide decision making. I was directed to its Menopause section (a good thing, since the British persistently spell "oestrogen" with that superfluous *o* in front). For patients, it offered an accurate and detailed laylanguage summary of the risks and benefits of estrogen replacement; for physicians, it provided a good summary of data about the strength and implications of the evidence, drugs currently in use, and clinical alternatives—quite different from the informational debris my chaotic Google and WebMD searches produced on the same topic.

A FEW MILES TO THE NORTH

When it comes to human services, Canada looks more like Britain than like the United States. Most of its provinces provide drug benefit programs that help cover the cost of prescriptions—some for all their citizens, others just for the elderly and poor. With government paying such a large share of pharmaceutical bills, Canada has also embraced the idea of comparing the effectiveness, safety, and value of competing products. Ironically, it was the nation's socialized approach to drug coverage that prompted it to encourage the careful product comparisons that are (or should be) the lifeblood of free enterprise systems. Many of these assessments are done in universities or other nongovernmental settings; the efforts are united under a loose umbrella by the federal government's Canadian Coordinating Office for Health Technology Assessment, or CCOHTA. That agency collects, synthesizes, and critically evaluates studies of drugs and other technologies. For each product it seeks to measure its "safety, efficacy, effectiveness, cost-effectiveness, quality of life and/or patient use, and ethical and social implications." This mission is similar to that of the U.S. FDA, except that the FDA eschews the last six of these eight topics, limiting its purview to just the first two—safety and efficacy. Like Britain's NICE, the Canadian analyses obsessively evaluate all available data according to the ground rules of evidence-based medicine, prohibit any potential conflicts of interest by evaluators, and solicit exhaustive review by outside experts before the assessment is finalized.

CCOHTA's early years were traumatic. One American pharmaceutical manufacturer didn't like the way its drug fared in the review of cholesterol-lowering products, and tried to take the government to court to block it from issuing its report. (The attempt eventually failed.) Like NICE, the effort slowly earned itself a place in the health care system. It recently established a program to get a jump on new product developments that won't hit the clinical front lines for years to come, "a national horizon-scanning program developed to alert health care planners and practitioners" about the technology assessment issues of tomorrow. Staff scour the internet and medical journals to uncover reports of new drugs and other interventions that are still far from regulatory approval or clinical acceptance, but will likely raise important questions in the future. Canadian physicians and regulators can then begin to develop the expertise needed to put the new drug into perspective, assemble the necessary evidence, and figure out how the treatment should be used and further evaluated when it is ready for prime time.

With a system like that in place, the first notice a doctor or patient gets of a new drug need not be through promotional channels. Instead, it can be an evenhanded appraisal by experts unrelated to the company selling the product. This would be a marked departure from the way most doctors and patients usually learn about a new medication—through a marketing blitz from the manufacturer. That can leave evaluators, payers, and practitioners scurrying to try to assess the product once the horse is out of the barn. The Canadian system capitalizes on the edge that those of us in academia or government ought to have over our colleagues in industry. In most countries, including the United States, the law forbids companies to communicate with practitioners about a new medication until it has won regulatory approval. But the rest of us could begin the discussion as soon as we have enough information to perform an evaluation—often months before a drug is released for use. All too often we don't take advantage of this prerogative, instead leaping into reactive mode only after the ads are in the journals, the reps are in the offices, and the commercials are on TV.

The coordinating function of CCOHTA is being broadened so that it can also serve as a central resource for Canada's evolving locally based academic detailing programs. Provinces that had been developing their own reviews of the literature, educational materials, and outreach interventions for physicians will soon be able to exchange their information and experiences with one another through a clearinghouse in Ottawa. This should make it possible for all the programs to benefit from what the others have done, while enabling each province to maintain local control of its own policies and initiatives.

THE UNITED STATES, Britain, Canada, and Australia—four great nations, as the saying goes, divided by a common language. As with health care delivery, each country has developed a different way of assessing medications and disseminating that knowledge to clinicians and patients. America has the most extensively developed pharmaceutical industry and research infrastructure, but the Commonwealth nations seem to do a better job of evenhanded, evidence-based drug assessment and information transfer, perhaps for that very reason. As the power, risks, and prices of drugs rise, all participants in the health care enterprise will need ready access to drug information shaped solely by the best available evidence; this is one of the most powerful medicines we have for improving the quality of drug use and keeping it affordable. Informed by our brief world tour and all that came before, we are now ready to propose some practical ways to get to this goal here at home.

PART FIVE: POLICY

21: PULLING THE FACTS TOGETHER

In grappling with all the challenges that face us in relation to prescription drugs, it seems we're making more progress on the hard problems than on the easier ones. Here are some of the hard problems: blocking the tiny transformations that make normal cells become malignant; repairing the deranged neurochemistry of schizophrenics' brains; and calming the hyperactive immune responses that produce debilitating conditions from rheumatoid arthritis to inflammatory bowel disease. Exciting work is also going forward on developing new ways to treat AIDS and even prevent Alzheimer's disease. But we aren't doing as well with the easier problems: learning about a drug's side effects before it comes into widespread use; knowing which treatments work better than others for the same condition; getting that information to doctors and patients; ensuring that people actually take the drugs they require; and figuring out how to pay for it all, so the cost of medications doesn't become an economic iceberg threatening the rest of our titanic health care enterprise.

If I had a chance to drive my own Faustian bargain, I'd want to be the doctor who solves one of the hard problems. But no devils have come along to make me a proposition like that, and there are plenty of talented scientists around the world who would be far more able to make good on (and off) such a deal if it were offered to them. Failing that, we can try to build on all the earlier chapters and propose solutions to the easier problems, the ones I understand better. Implementing some of these ideas will require us to reclaim the scientific and humanitarian goals that have traditionally guided medicine. If we could accomplish that, it would be a deal even better than Faust's: gaining awesome new powers and winning back our souls at the same time.

. . . .

WE CAN BEGIN by asking why there is such a contrast between the robust success of biomedical science and the lame disarray with which we sometimes deploy that science. Part of the problem can be explained by an odd little word that E. O. Wilson chose for the title of one of his books: "consilience." It refers to the coming together of different disciplines and different modes of inquiry to create gorgeous and powerful synergies. Scientists working on the hard problems in biomedicine long ago grasped the power of consilience, though they don't call it that. Physiology and molecular genetics came together to yield insights that would be impossible if each field plowed ahead in blind isolation; a biophysicist studying membranes collaborates with a pharmacologist who is trying to learn how drugs get into cells; a protein chemist exploring what a particular gene does finds a statistician to calculate which traits sit near each other on a particular chromosome. These basic scientists have even been seen consorting openly with epidemiologists, to learn how molecular differences manifest themselves in large populations of people with and without a certain disease.

But once a new drug is discovered and let loose into the health care system, its use is less likely to be subjected to such boundary-crossing approaches to solving problems. If consilience is the intellectual skill of "working and playing well with others," our health care system would get a C– when it comes to the way we use drugs. Ideas, like genes, flourish through cross-pollination; hybrid vigor results when plants, animals, or fields intermix. By contrast, we all know what too much inbreeding can do. At its best, the process may yield thoroughbreds with impeccable pedigrees. But overbreeding in any single discipline can also create genetic or conceptual progeny that are lovely to behold but frail and even neurotic. At worst, debilitating recessive traits can manifest themselves, producing grotesque offspring with limited functional potential.

Inbreeding in medical care delivery has produced both kinds of offspring. Excessive "keeping to your own kind" deprives us of badly needed hybrid vigor. Clinicians don't talk to pharmacologists much; economists and epidemiologists seem to live on their own separate planets; policy analysts, behavioral scientists, and anthropologists each study the way people use medicines but usually don't have much to say to one another about it. Intercourse between any of these people and those who actually run the health care system sometimes occurs, but only rarely. At many universities the social scientists and economists work on one side of the campus and the doctors on another, and they have all too little to say to one another.

Because of these schisms, a doctor's decision to use a given drug can become totally uncoupled from a grasp of its underlying physiology; economic prescribing incentives are put in place that would make Adam Smith blush and Albert Schweitzer weep; systems in which doctor and patient interact are designed without the most basic insights into behavioral science; population-oriented researchers who measure numerators and denominators rarely connect with the doctors and hospitals that take care of patients one at a time; and sophisticated information technology is used more to schedule appointments and send out bills than to guide complex clinical strategies.

There is good news too. Consilience could yield the same synergies for drug use as it has for drug discovery and development. As with the laboratory sciences, this will require people from different fields to learn from one another, across disciplines.

On a modest scale, I have seen in my own division what can result from bringing together smart, committed people with expertise in epidemiology, pharmacology, biostatistics, management, informatics, health policy and economics, psychiatry, decision science, and internal medicine with its various specialties. As a group, we can consider research problems and practical issues that would stymie any one of us working from a single professional perspective. It's demanding and sometimes humbling work, far harder than spending every day with people who have the same training and perspective as you do. But the stimulation and synergy are worth it. The following thoughts on the practical options before us are guided by this interdisciplinary vision.

WHAT WE CAN DO NOW

Prospects may be dim for sweeping, definitive action in health policy at the federal or state level, but we could still make progress on several fronts by facilitating the emergence of the "swarm intelligence" that already exists in abundance among practitioners at ground level inside the health care system. Many of the options below are presented as potential stand-alone components that could be put in place in modular fashion right now. Several of these ideas are already in use in other industrialized countries, or exist on a small scale in innovative programs here at home. Many of the interventions proposed will not require large doses of altruism, insight, or funding from lawmakers, because these may continue to be in short supply for the foreseeable future. In fact, much of what follows could be implemented even in the face of continuing gridlock in both houses of Congress and the entire executive branch; we will have to work toward some constructive solutions even if the limiting political conditions of recent years persist indefinitely.

Most medical students have heard the classic spoof of career choices that goes like this: If you become a surgeon, you won't understand much about your patients' diseases, but you'll do a lot to help them. If you become an internist, you'll understand a great deal about their diseases, but you'll only be able to help a little. Or you can become a pathologist; once you've completed the autopsy you'll know absolutely everything about what's wrong with the patient, but it will be too late to do anything about it.

When it comes to fixing the health care system, many of my physician-activist friends adopt the surgical perspective parodied above ("A chance to cut is a chance to cure"), even though few of them are surgeons. By contrast, my academic colleagues who study the health care system fit more into the pathologist's role, forced to trade off policy influence for scholarly precision. For me, the internist's worldview seems right for dealing with our health care system. Internists who have worked as primary-care doctors are used to managing multiple interacting chronic problems, to losing as many battles as we win, to gleaning satisfaction from partial victories that would drive others mad with frustration. (Being a Red Sox fan helps here as well.) Sure, I've had my flirtations with more invasive approaches. The most engaging one involved getting a binding referendum for universal health care put on the Massachusetts ballot in 2000, which led to an electoral battle that we almost won. But the rest of the time I'm temperamentally a policy internist, looking for conceptually elegant and nonlethal ways to get the body to heal itself over time, or at least to stop destroying itself. Don't mistake this for wimpiness; at both the policy and patient levels this measured approach can be its own very powerful medicine, and dangerous if handled poorly.

Granted, some aspects of the U.S. health care system do need major surgery: the absurd way we pay for medical care on a piecework basis, the shame of over 40 million citizens lacking health insurance, the bleeding off of such a large proportion of scarce resources by managers, bureaucrats, and profiteers who do nothing for patients. These are all areas in which policy change could use some cold hard steel rather than the internist's measured touch. A few well-placed scalpel strokes will also be necessary as we address medication use policy as well, but nothing that will require general anesthesia. This isn't because the problem is benign or well contained—quite the opposite. It isn't pushing the metaphor too far to consider a lesson from oncology: once a disease has spread throughout the body, it's often best to prescribe a treatment that tries to make use of the patient's own mechanisms for healing, instead of performing a potentially mutilative operation to try to "cut it all out." In widely metastatic disease, it's often impossible to use a knife to differentiate the diseased "it" from the patient. This is the problem that faces us in many areas of medication policy.

What follows mirrors the kind of approach I've often taken in caring for patients with slow worsening of a long-standing illness. First, identify some immediate steps to stop the deterioration and avert a crisis. Then, devise a sustainable regimen to correct the underlying derangements and restore some normal function. In the case of drug policy, this will not require any amputations, organ transplants, or eviscerating surgery. Instead, we need the most radical kind of change there is: an alteration in the way we think about things.

The agenda can be divided into five components: (1) pulling together existing drug information; (2) generating the missing data we need to use drugs more effectively, safely, and affordably; (3) getting that information to prescribers and patients through an innovative knowledge delivery system; (4) realigning incentives so that only quality and value drive prescribing practices; and (5) tackling the cost problem that makes medicines unaffordable for many.

Some of the developments described here have already begun. There is a growing understanding that the best way to improve the use of prescription drugs—or any other components of the health care system—is not to treat them atomistically like isolated widgets in a marketplace free-for-all. A sea change has started to occur on several fronts, and we can't yet know where it will lead us. But that also means there's still time to influence the direction and impact of these changes.

PULLING TOGETHER EXISTING DRUG INFORMATION

Studying drugs is what I do for a living, and I still have trouble finding a reliable way to compare a given medicine with its alternatives in terms of effectiveness, safety, and price. I can ask a junior faculty or research assistant in my division to do a literature search and try to summarize its results, but that's not an option for the busy practitioner. The most damning evidence of this problem is the fact that the most commonly used source of prescription drug information in the country is still the *Physicians' Desk Reference,* the dense, 3,500-page tome that's simply a compilation of indigestible industry-produced package inserts. Technophilic doctors refer to electronic databases that can be stored on their palm-top computers; these are useful listings of a drug's doses, indications, and side effects, but they are not as helpful in providing the higher-level information needed to choose *which* drug to prescribe.

We've seen that in the United States it is presently no one's responsibility to pull together and synthesize that kind of comparative information on an ongoing basis. Most physicians in independent practice are left to try to piece together the enormous patchwork of disparate findings for ourselves as best we can. The task of doing this more systematically and proactively has been taken up in small islands of effort throughout the nation, and more broadly in other countries. Many of the modules to help do this are already in place. The problem is that they operate in splendid isolation from one another, or cover just a small piece of clinical or geographic territory, or do great work that is virtually unknown outside their own programs.

It is ironic that marketplace advocates in medicine have not been leading the charge in calling for and performing such comparative work, since this is precisely the information that would be needed to turn their implausible visions into reality. To the contrary, most of the output of conservative think tanks has instead focused on defending the prerogatives of the pharmaceutical industry, which itself has been a major opponent of requiring comparative data about effectiveness and pricing.

Malcolm Maclure is a virtual member of our division's "extended family" of researchers. A Canadian epidemiologist who has taught at Harvard and worked for the Ministry of Health of British Columbia, he now runs a program on drug policy at the University of Victoria. Maclure has argued compellingly for using epidemiology and health services research to inform and evaluate policy decisions. In one of our e-mail exchanges, he likened the current situation to the gradual arrival of dawn:

> Until recently, providing drug coverage was like watering your garden in the dark. You knew that some plants needed less water and some more, but weren't sure where to point your hose, so you directed your "flow of liquidity" indiscriminately. But with morning's light, we can now see what we're doing and witness the consequences. It's quite messy: we've been overwatering here and underwatering there. Now we can be more efficient and get better results with the water we have. But change is slow. Policymakers are so used to the dark that they're just beginning to open their eyes and make use of the evidence they need for their decisions.

Let's return one last time to our comparison of medications and information technology. The pills and IV solutions are the hardware, analogous to computers; the information needed to use them optimally is the clinical version of software. The relationship is deeper than metaphor; analyzed a bit more, it can illuminate our search for answers to some vexing drug problems. In several important ways, the techies have already been down this road, and their experience can help show us the way.

In the very early days of computers, the programming needed to run them came free with the hardware, akin to a fancy user's manual. It took years for software to be seen as a product in its own right, something that could be developed by companies other than computer makers and sold separately at a profit. Similarly, medication's software, the information needed to guide the use of drugs, can have an importance comparable to that of the drugs themselves.

The world of prescription drugs today is like the world of computers before Microsoft. Nearly all the focus is on the tangible goods, with much less attention paid to the value of the knowledge needed to use those goods optimally. In the gargantuan scale of health care expenditures, the cost of synthesizing and managing that information would be relatively small. In other nations, governments provide public funding to perform this information management function. Should the United States do the same?

Probably not; the odds are we wouldn't get it right.

There are several worries about having the government try to do this work itself. The FDA struggles mightily just to answer the much easier question of whether a drug is probably better than nothing, ignoring all considerations of comparison and cost in doing so. For subtler questions of *comparative* risk-benefit ratio, and even more so of relative cost-effectiveness, the rules of evidence are much less well worked out. In the present climate, a federal program whose judgments on such matters offended a powerful lobbying group could well be paralyzed—and that's if it got off easy. If it were very effective, the agency would more likely be done in altogether, as occurred to several of the now-defunct entities we considered earlier. Apart from NIH and the National Science Foundation we don't have a reassuring track record of support for innovative federal programs that do not involve weaponry.

Appropriate judgments about any technology will require periodic proclamations of the Emperor's nakedness. Billions of dollars in sales may ride on whether a drug truly brings a new clinical advantage, and whether that advantage is worth its price. Imagine the reaction of a manufacturer that invested hundreds of millions of dollars to bring a product to market, only to have it doomed by the following revenue-crippling government evaluation:

> This new medication has not been shown to be any better than currently available products, and has a much more limited safety record. There is no evidence that its higher price is accompanied by any demonstrated therapeutic advantage.

That may be the most appropriate assessment for many new drugs, but a federal agency making such pronouncements might not last long. To survive, its evaluations would have to become so cautious and innocuous as to make antacid seem like Tabasco sauce. Yet the capacity to make that kind of statement is just what we need.

One circumscribed aspect of the problem will require a role for government. The FDA should be given a mandate to prosecute any manufacturer of a pill, liquid, or powder that makes unfounded claims about its product's medicinal properties, even if it's labeled a supplement or an herbal remedy. The nutraceutical lobby has blocked such legislation for a decade.

FINDING A HOME FOR THIS WORK

While we wait for the day that common sense and the needs of the citizenry influence public policy more than lobbying dollars and campaign contributions, we can move on to consider practical solutions that could be put into place without waiting for action from Washington. Happily, a number of solutions are possible even in the face of Capitol gridlock.

We can start by putting some existing pieces together. One instructive example is the Cochrane Collaborative, a decentralized international consortium of researchers who regularly assess all the evidence in a given area of medical practice to evaluate what works and what doesn't. Similarly, the *British Medical Journal* publishes and frequently updates a publication-cum-website called *Clinical Evidence,* an evidence-based summary describing which treatments have been shown to work and which have not; the National Health Service there provides it at no cost to all its physicians. On this side of the Atlantic, the United Health Group, the vast American HMO network, sends subscriptions to *Clinical Evidence* free to tens of thousands of American physicians. There are also the country-specific drug assessment activities based in the three nations we visited in Part Four. Fortunately for us, their work is posted on the web, and is in English.

Experience has started to accumulate with other technology assessment services; several such programs are listed in the Notes. The best of them apply a rigorous evidence-based approach to assessing a given intervention. But pharmaceutical products are not covered thoroughly by many, and cost-effectiveness may be ignored. Some reports are available freely to anyone; other services are by subscription only, and primarily serve large institutions. A few update their results on an ongoing basis as new data emerge; others continue to publish assessments that are years old and no longer relevant. Even when they are current and accurate, many of these reports would be numbingly boring for a practitioner or patient to read. A promising recent entrant in this field is a program of drug assessment that the state of Oregon has mounted. Reasoning that it could spend its scarce drug dollars more effectively if it had a guide to which drugs in a category offered the best value for its money, the state has begun its own drug assessment program and plans to post its results on the internet for public scrutiny. Consumers Union has recently joined forces with the Oregon effort and now provides summaries of their findings for patients.

The nation could benefit greatly from a structure to apply all these disparate approaches systematically to commonly used drugs, fill in the missing components as needed, pull the pieces together into a coherent whole, and then disseminate the package effectively. In a country that collectively spends $200 billion a year on drugs and nearly two trillion dollars on health care overall, it shouldn't be hard to come up with the modest sums needed to support a solid drug evaluation process from nonfederal sources. Core support from one or two foundations could be supplemented if necessary with minuscule fractions of the health care budgets of a few employers, insurance companies, or HMOs. Less than one-quarter of a percent would be plenty, the size of rounding error on most of their annual budgets. The minute annual costs of the programs in Britain, Canada, and Australia prove that this work can be done with modest funding.

Support from these health care payers would be based on the understanding that a small annual amount of cash is an investment necessary to generate the information-rich environment on which their continued viability depends. The new information organizations created in this way would be analogous to the programs we've seen in other nations, and could collaborate with them to reduce duplication of effort. They would employ small staffs of experts from a range of fields, including medicine, pharmacology, economics, epidemiology, and statistics. Also needed would be medical writers with the skill to take arcane issues and make them intelligible to clinical audiences (and to lay audiences—more on that later). Our own experience and that of these other programs make it clear that talented staff would flock to join such a project, so the needed expertise would not be hard to assemble.

The new programs could accept some grant support from government as long as they didn't become dependent upon it as a main revenue source, because of its unique susceptibility to pressure from special interests. Even limited federal dollars would have to be received with suspicion in light of the embarrassing lessons taught by the National Endowment for the Arts and the Corporation for Public Broadcasting—that governmental largesse can be threatened unexpectedly if a few irate congressmen become upset about a controversial program. Similarly, the fledgling organizations would have to avoid accepting any funding from the pharmaceutical industry because of the obvious conflicts of interest, or even the appearance thereof.

These new organizations would issue initial assessments of new drugs before they went on the market. Before a drug reaches the pharmacies, they will have gone over all available data on its efficacy and safety, compared it to the evidence on comparable drugs, considered whether it was worth its projected cost, and put its initial assessment up on the internet for all to see—much as our hospital was able to do with the new drug for septic shock. The main conclusions would be summarized on a single screen or two for busy practitioners; the equivalent of a "translate this page" link would put the content into lay language for patients. A more nuanced evaluation would follow, with hypertext links to detailed analyses and the underlying data, down as many levels as the attentive browser could possibly want. Once a drug is on the market, these services would slog through reams of often-obscure data, staying alert to new information that can turn up at any moment and reveal new advantages about an existing product or turn a high-flying prospect into a dead duck.

If we're looking for a typically American solution to this problem, we probably would not want to stop with only one national drug evaluation program. After all, we don't have one national newspaper, or television network, or religion. If our nation's strength has been in its pluralism, perhaps we'd do better with several such not-for-profit information services, each competing for credibility in the knowledge marketplace. This would introduce more noise, as pluralism always does, but it would also protect the public from having any single organization fall under the sway of either end of the pharmaceutical continuum: manufacturers who tend to see any new patented product as God's gift to medicine whatever its price, as well as insurance industry cost containers, who could have an opposite bias against costly new advances.

LEARNING FROM WALL STREET?

Some might argue that the most truly American approach would be to do what the nation does best: turn the whole thing into a business. What would be wrong with competing for-profit drug assessment services? If the corporate sector is part of the problem, couldn't it also be part of the solution? At first glance, the argument appears to make some sense if we consider a precedent in the world of finance. When a corporation or government agency wants to borrow money, it must persuade lenders that it is creditworthy. But it's not possible for every potential lender to come in and audit the books of XYZ Inc. or the Placid County Turnpike Authority before investing in a bond issue. That would be duplicative and wasteful, even if each lender (including individual investors) had the expertise to dig deep into the details of a balance sheet, and many don't. So bond rating services developed to perform this function; Standard & Poor's and Moody's are the two best-known examples. A worker contemplating the investment of part of her 401(k) plan or a bank seeking to place several million dollars of cash can look up the credit rating of the company or governmental entity issuing the bonds. If Moody's or S&P rates the issuer AAA, then the investment is very safe; a much lower rating would mean that the bond is not investment grade, and your principal could disappear like an investment in Enron. Neither Standard & Poor's nor Moody's was created as a government watchdog agency, and neither is supported by grants from Washington or any foundation. Both are private corporations that came into being to provide an information service for which they could charge handsomely.

This solution to our drug assessment deficit could emerge by default if no foundations or enlightened health care payers come forward to support noncommercial evaluation organizations, and if the federal government remains in its continuing spasm. According to this vision, those drug evaluation services that perform their function well would prosper, as they would provide a valuable information product; those that do their work poorly would in theory lose their client base and wither away—the Arthur Andersens of pharmacology.

But the mention of Enron and Andersen reveals the most serious objection to this plan. We must have learned something from the collapse of the technology bubble, the accounting fiascoes and stock analyst travesties that were revealed in its wake, and the deregulated energy market ripoffs of the same period. By now, it should sound unbearably glib to suggest that the marketplace is all that's needed to provide critical evaluation of complex issues when billions of dollars are at stake. Medicines are not balance sheets, and sick people are not megawatts on the spot market. For one thing, there is a rather important ethical difference. If energy companies miscalculate or lie about the supply of power for California, the price of electricity goes through the roof in Los Angeles. If an accounting company fudges the books for a large corporation, its stock price tanks when the deception is uncovered. But these lapses don't directly cause anyone to get sick or die. Because of that vital difference, matters related to health ought to be treated in a way that can protect them from the inevitable excesses of corporate miscalculation and worse.

Medicine is also orders of magnitude more complex than energy, autos, or even the most exotic financial instruments and as we have seen, our tools for assessing drugs are still in their adolescence. Even the simpler analyses of the financial world can be skewed or falsified and escape detection for a long time, as these corporate crises made clear. The problem is far greater for the more difficult calculations and interpretations needed to define medication benefits, risks, and value. An analyst with an attitude or an ax to grind can put considerable spin onto pronouncements about particular medicines, and the bias will barely be noticed by most audiences.

If we opt then for noncommercial drug evaluation organizations, should they be established in medical schools and their academic medical centers? Not necessarily. The reason relates to another lesson learned from Wall Street. It's now well understood how some brokerage firms used their analysts' rosy company evaluations to attract or reward lucrative investment

banking business from those firms. In medicine we have our own version of
the stock analyst whose optimistic view of a company is colored by the
"externalities" that can be bestowed by that firm. For us, it's the researcher
whose lab prospers by virtue of large research grants from a drug maker, or
who is a highly paid consultant to a particular manufacturer. Just as a technology company's future earnings stream may exist only in the eye of the
beholder, so the view of a new drug's presumed advantages can be colored
by corporate allegiances—sometimes even unconsciously. Trivial differences can be perceived and then hyped as major advances. The bias could
operate in the opposite direction as well: a commercial evaluation organization dominated by a payer (perhaps a large health insurance company trying to contain its drug spending) could tend toward excessive skepticism,
downplaying the important advantages of a costly new drug.

We live at a time when marketplace solutions are put forward as the
answer to nearly every problem. The main policy agenda for the coming
decades will be to rediscover which human affairs are too fragile or precious to leave exclusively in commercial hands. Robert Kuttner described
these issues cogently in his book *Everything for Sale,* whose title conveys
both the cynicism of the marketplace worldview and the desperation of a
going-out-of-business closeout. To be believable, the work of an analyst—
of stocks or of drugs—must be uncoupled from any lucrative links that he
or his employer may have with the company whose product is being evaluated, or those who pay for it. If drug evaluations were put into the wrong
setting, it would be almost impossible to protect them from influence by the
billions of dollars at stake on all sides. There may well be a role for free-
market competition further along in the information transfer process—but
not at its origin, where a NICEr solution will be needed.

In the end, there is one final reason for these new drug assessment organizations to be nonprofit: their work would inevitably enter the public
domain as soon as it was disseminated. If a report found, for example, that
all available drugs of a given category were therapeutically equivalent,
though some were much cheaper and therefore more cost-effective than
others, that insight could become available across the country the day it was
generated. "Information wants to be free," the saying goes. This property
may render it less appealing as a product to be owned and sold, but makes it
quite wonderful in other, more important ways.

DIGGING OUT THE DATA ON RISK

It makes little sense to assess a drug's comparative effectiveness without
also considering its comparative safety. Here, too, our present system needs

an upgrade. Some pharmaceutical companies run conscientious, effective, proactive surveillance programs to monitor the adverse events their products cause. But we've seen that others do the minimum that is legally required: they passively await the receipt of spontaneous reports that doctors or patients may or may not send in, and then pass the raw reports along to the FDA to the minimum extent required by law. A very few others handle data about potentially lethal side effects even more shabbily, resisting attempts to warn patients and practitioners about known dangers. Like financial wrongdoing, epidemiological misbehavior can stretch all the way from sluggish compliance to outright fraud.

Epidemiologists who work within pharmaceutical companies can play a pivotal role in ensuring the safety of the nation's drugs, and many do this well. For the occasional bad actors, intentional malfeasance or reckless negligence in suppressing evidence about important drug hazards should lead to the prospect of substantial civil or even criminal penalties. After all, there aren't many kinds of white-collar crime in which a person can sit behind a desk, manipulate some numbers on a spreadsheet, and in doing so increase the risk of severe illness or death for substantial numbers of people. The response to another kind of corporate scandal might provide a lesson here as well. Just as CEOs are now required to vouch personally for the accuracy of their firms' accounting data, perhaps we should also expect the CEOs of pharmaceutical manufacturers to certify the accuracy of the safety data their staff submit in the company's name.

THINGS MUST BE PRETTY BAD IF WE NEED TORT LAWYERS TO SAVE THE DAY

Another part of the legal profession has brought an unconventional kind of quality control policy to many companies. For all their excesses, tort lawyers have had effectiveness comparable to that of government, academics, and corporate ethics officers in motivating the creation of active postmarketing surveillance efforts. Facing a cluster of worrisome adverse events, responsible company officers ideally will ask themselves, "How can we learn more about this potentially important problem?" Unfortunately, this is not the universal response. In its absence, the pursuit of knowledge is also served by a less lofty reaction: "Could we get sued if we don't look into this?" Sadly, one of the nation's best strategies for ensuring careful postmarketing safety surveillance is the prospect of a deposition in which the medical director of a large firm is asked by a plaintiff's lawyer, "Doctor, do you mean to tell the jury that even though your company kept receiving reports of this serious side effect in patients taking your drug, you never initiated a comprehensive study to determine how widespread the problem was?"

Like most people, I shudder at the more bizarre extremes of the tort law industry. But if the governmental drug regulatory apparatus has undergone administrative orchiectomy, the fear of huge liability settlements may be the only compelling reason left at some companies for doing the right thing. The financial consequences of doing otherwise make rigorous pharmacoepidemiology look much more attractive in comparison.

A similar extreme quality control function is served by Ralph Nader's Health Research Group, headed by Dr. Sidney Wolfe, a dedicated and merciless industry critic. Wolfe and colleagues were the first to sound the alarm on many excesses of the pharmaceutical industry in both the clinical and commercial domains. The focus on hazards in his best-selling book *Worst Pills, Best Pills* occasionally terrifies its readers. But many of Dr. Wolfe's critiques have been on the mark and have had a bracing effect in shaping the expectations of both the FDA and industry. I've attended a number of closed-door meetings in which drug company officials made statements like "I'd rather not pursue that problem, but if things turn sour, imagine what Sid Wolfe would do with it . . . so we'd better look at this more closely." It's the same as with the lawyers: the more one worries that regulatory capture can turn federal watchdogs into lap pets, the more one is willing to keep a pit bull around.

LINING UP THE THREE Ms

The Vioxx–heart disease debacle awakened the public to the need to deal with three key deficiencies in the present system: mandate, money, and methodology. Some of these tasks may prove to be beyond the scope or the will of the FDA, but they'll still need to be done.

MANDATE

The string of unanticipated drug withdrawals in recent years led some to suggest that tracking medication risks is too important to be left in the hands of the manufacturers and a single federal agency. When the industry put pressure on the FDA throughout the 1990s to speed the process of drug approval, most of the agency's energy became focused on that goal, and far less on uncovering and addressing the problems drugs could cause once they are in routine use. Revivifying this part of the agency will require ardent rehab work for years to come.

The industry has succeeded in keeping federal requirements for postmarketing surveillance to a minimum. Shortly after a new FDA commissioner was named, a manufacturers' trade group met with him to express their concern that the burden of tracking their products' adverse effects more carefully could have a chilling effect on business and prevent the discovery of new medicines. With the FDA's epidemiology budget chronically inadequate, the industry itself became the main source of financial support for these analyses. Companies commission the studies they want, to focus on selected problems in their own product or occasionally to demonstrate safety problems with a competitor's medication. Sometimes this results in good science; our own research group has accepted such grants, provided that we could study a problem as we saw fit and publish our findings without any restrictions. But not all researchers demand these terms, and there is little public-sector funding for such studies.

What would work better? There are several possible scenarios for risk assessment policy that are not mutually exclusive.

The FDA Gets It Right

The agency could choose to enforce its power to require that companies perform thorough postmarketing safety surveillance of the drugs they sell. Its pharmacoepidemiology branch would be resuscitated, and receive enough funding to commission numerous outside studies of pressing risk questions. If the FDA's new orientation toward risk management succeeds, it could lead to a vigorous agenda that helps define and reduce the inevitable downsides of good products.

Other Governmental Agencies Get Involved

If that doesn't work (and it hasn't for years), some suggest that the nation could embrace the same model used in another industry that produces important benefits and occasional hazards: air travel. There, the organization that investigates lapses in safety (the National Transportation Safety Board) is separate from the body that regulates the industry (the Federal Aviation Agency). This could also help address a problem in organizational politics and psychology, since the entity that decides a drug is safe enough for widespread use would not be the one to determine whether that decision was wrong. The safety surveillance function could be taken on by the Centers for Disease Control and Prevention, a separate part of government that already functions as a public health–oriented agency rather than a regulatory one; its mission is the reduction of preventable disease. The Agency for Health Care Research and Quality is another logical possibility, but its tiny size and annual near-death experience during the budget process would have to be addressed so it could provide stable support for this key function. Other options include the creation of a new institute within NIH, or a totally new unit in the Department of Health and Human Services.

Nonprofit Groups Outside Government Fill the Gap

Given the pervasive concerns about the influence of industry over government, drug safety assessment might flourish better in a freestanding nongovernmental organization. A new foundation created for this purpose could remain aloof from the two sectors with the most deeply vested interests, the FDA and the industry. In this vision, studies of adverse drug events would be sponsored by a non-governmental program specially created for this purpose or by one that already exists, such as the Institute of Medicine of the National Academy of Sciences. Exclusive reliance on this approach would be an acknowledgment that the government was unable to perform a vital public health function adequately on its own.

The Marketplace Alone Makes Everything Work

This Tooth Fairy scenario would be a poor substitute for effective public policy in this area, but for completeness, here's how it goes: Drug purchasers in the private and public sectors demand better safety information to inform their decisions about which drugs to use, and require companies to develop better evidence on adverse effects in order to win market share. Alternatively, these large payers might directly commission the studies themselves to get the information they need to guide their billion-dollar purchases. At the same time the drug companies, reeling from enormous settlements of cases in which they failed to address a safety problem promptly, expand the size and effectiveness of their own internal and extramural surveillance studies to protect their own bottom lines. Those that do this well prosper and expand; those that don't go out of business.

The abject failure of such misguided industrial Darwinism at the start of the last century created the obscene excesses and tragic lapses that made the Progressive movement inevitable, and led to creation of the FDA in the first place. The fact that this naive vision has never been adequate by itself to ensure drug safety should dismiss it from any further consideration.

MONEY

Discover a new drug and you can profit from doing so; the same is not true for the discovery of a new drug side effect, and this creates a chronic problem for the funding of such work. While the latest renewal of the federal Prescription Drug User Fee Act did allow for some of its dollars to support the FDA's surveillance of adverse effects, some worry that if industry helps to pay those evaluators it will also call their tune, as it has increasingly done in the drug approval process since PDUFA began. Requiring industry to underwrite the FDA's drug safety work may save the government a little money, just as letting the industry pay for all those lunchtime lectures helps a teaching hospital save on its meal expenses—but at what price?

An alternative view would consider medical research on adverse side effects a public good that merits public funding, just like any other preventable cause of disease and death. Drug safety studies are far cheaper to perform than clinical trials or molecular biology laboratory work. Much important information can be collected through computer-assisted analysis of large-scale automated databases like those we use in our work, supplemented as needed by review of primary medical records or targeted patient interviews. Dozens of health care organizations routinely collect this information: HMOs, the Veterans Administration, state Medicaid programs and other drugs-for-the-aged plans, whole Canadian provinces. Research groups skilled in this kind of work can assess drug exposures and clinical outcomes with great efficiency in large populations of patients, with only modest financial investment.

METHODOLOGY

Study design issues are far more problematic in assessing adverse drug effects than they are in determining efficacy in randomized clinical trials. For the latter, the rules of the road are older and more established; in the younger discipline of pharmacoepidemiology, the way you ask the question can have a great deal to do with the answer you get. Such methodological fragility makes this a poor arena to leave primarily in the hands of the organizations that have the most to lose from unwanted findings. Much more work is needed in refining the ground rules of observational studies, just as the methods of clinical trials required years of refinement in mid-century before they became the durable and powerful tools they now are. The problem with estrogen's "heart-protective effect" made it clear how wrong we can be if such observational studies are not performed impeccably. This refinement is possible; cutting-edge work is moving forward on a variety of arcane epidemiological and statistical methods to get us there. Some of these studies are even being supported by NIH, which correctly sees this as the basic-science work of our field.

Since World War II, NIH has helped build the nation's awesome biomedical science infrastructure by committing funds to training programs. That piece is still missing in the evolution of the fields of pharmacoepidemiology and its cousin, pharmacoeconomics. The FDA, academic programs, health care systems, and the drug industry are all starved for well-trained scientists in these disciplines, yet the university programs that turn out such professionals are tiny and often poorly supported. A modest number of training grants from the public and private sectors could generate the personpower needed to populate the field with the talented people who are in such short supply. This would make a big difference in enhancing how well drug risks can be measured in both the private and public sectors.

GENERATING THE NEW KNOWLEDGE WE NEED

So far, we've considered ways to assemble and analyze drug information that presently exists, because we could be doing much more with data that are already out there. But some of the most pressing questions—such as those that compare one treatment against another—can best be answered only through new clinical trials. This will require us to get beyond the false economy that assumes pharmaceutical companies will perform all the drug evaluations the nation requires.

It would be ideal if all new drugs were routinely compared in randomized studies to the existing treatments with which they'll compete. But these are often the very projects a wise manufacturer will try to avoid undertaking. Such comparative trials would address the questions we most need answered, but they are appallingly rare; there is simply too little budget and no mandate to do them. The policy question is not "How expensive would it be to pay for such head-to-head studies?" It is, rather, "How expensive is it for us to lack the information these studies would provide?" Medicaid, health maintenance organizations, the Veterans Administration, insurance companies, and soon Medicare all face unnecessarily high drug bills because we don't have this information. Fixing this problem will require addressing the same three issues we confronted in defining drug risks: methodology, mandate, and money.

METHODOLOGY

This research is not brain surgery, and the necessary participants are all around us. Head-to-head drug trials require large numbers of subjects, and sick people who need drugs are in ample supply. The administrators who run large health care systems usually don't have much patience for research, but they have plenty of patients for research—as well as the doctors who prescribe their drugs and evaluate their outcomes every day. Whether it's raising a barn or generating clinical data, many hands (or hearts, or kidneys, or colons) can make light work. Randomized trials don't have to cost thousands of dollars per patient enrolled, as they do in many conventional studies. That may be what contract research companies charge drug makers for the modest-sized pivotal trials necessary to win FDA approval of a new product, in which an obsessive level of detail must be collected. But a simpler alternative is increasingly considered by drug researchers; it's known as the pragmatic clinical trial. The method was designed to generate key information about treatments quickly and cheaply, by stripping down the question to its bare essentials—sort of a Volkswagen randomized study.

First, an ethics review committee would determine that equipoise is present—that each of the two or three medications to be tested would be an acceptable clinical choice, given the state of current knowledge. The criteria for including and excluding subjects are kept straightforward, minimal, and easy to administer; this also has the advantage of ensuring that the results will be relevant to typical practice. If screening indicates that a patient qualifies, he or she is invited to join the study, usually in the context of routine care. For each consenting subject the participating doctor (often the patient's regular physician) opens a sealed envelope or logs on to a website to learn which treatment the next study participant has been randomly assigned to receive. These are usually coded, to make sure neither physician nor subject knows who is getting what. Criteria for study outcomes are likewise simple and clearly specified (stroke, hip fracture, heart attack, death). As patients are cared for over time, when outcomes occur the data are sent to a central coordinating center, a process made even more practical through the internet. Or they may be recorded automatically as a routine part of the health system's normal record-keeping activities.

Expanding the capacity to conduct such pragmatic clinical trials could be an affordable way to get the answers we need to many unresolved questions about how particular drugs stack up against each other.

MANDATE

You'd expect that any entity paying big drug bills would have a natural interest in mounting these trials: large health maintenance organizations, employers, insurance companies, governmental drug benefit programs— the usual list of suspects. Despite some interesting exceptions, that promise is far from being realized. Many private-sector organizations remain stymied by their own self-image. They usually started out as insurance companies rather than in the clinical world; as a result, their leaders often see health care primarily as a task of calculating premiums and avoiding payouts. Facilitating medical research just doesn't feel right to many of these executives, even if it could save them huge sums of money. In both government and the private sector most still define their role as bill payers and rule makers, not as people who help generate new knowledge. (There are some notable exceptions here, such as the large clinical trial activities of the Department of Veterans Affairs, or the research arms of some HMOs like United Healthcare and California's Kaiser and Seattle's Group Health Cooperative, or the collaborations our group has begun with Pennsylvania's PACE program and the Canadian province of British Columbia.) For their part, beleaguered physicians see their job as taking care of patients, not conducting studies. And patients want to get medical care more than they want to push back the frontiers of knowledge.

Those who pay for health care in both the public and private sectors will have to get over this limited vision of their role, as well as the fiscal myopia that defines long-range planning as thinking about the quarter after next. Ironically, the stress of out-of-control drug expenditures has made it even harder for them to take the long view, worsening their vision problem instead of correcting it. (Stress releases adrenaline into the circulation and dilates the pupils; as in a camera, the widened aperture limits the range in which objects remain in focus.)

Allowing for the inviolable right of any patient to opt out of any study, we can think of the health care system as one enormous learning machine in applied pharmacology (and many other clinical disciplines as well): every practitioner a part-time researcher, every delivery system a laboratory, every consenting patient a participant in one or more important trials. Of course we will have to protect the privacy of patients' information, as well as their safety and autonomy. There will have to be adequate compensation for the extra time spent by doctors and other clinicians in doing this work. We might even have to pay patients for their participation. If these requirements can be met, the vital frontline research we need so desperately could be performed with considerable efficiency and power, in the very settings where typical doctors deliver care to regular patients. The resulting findings about which drugs work best (and most cost-effectively) could be immediately fed back into those same practices, improving the quality and efficiency of patient care, and more than covering the cost of the studies.

MONEY

Who would underwrite such research in an increasingly market-driven health care system? One problem here is the issue of competitive advantage. Years before the ALLHAT study was completed, I asked a senior executive of a large HMO why his organization didn't run its own trial of the costly calcium-channel blockers versus the cheaper thiazides for managing high blood pressure. Such a study could be readily conducted in the hundreds of practices it controlled. After all, the HMO was paying for the more expensive drugs for hundreds of thousands of its patients, employed all the doctors who prescribed the drugs, and had access to all the medical records.

"But where's the competitive advantage for us?" the executive asked. I didn't understand. "Let's say we spend all that money to do the study, and we prove that the less expensive drug works just as well, at a fraction of the cost. Would we publish that information in a medical journal?"

"Of course," I said. "It would be a great study. Its results would have huge implications for care."

"But then *everyone* would have that information," he replied. "It wouldn't give us any competitive advantage over the other HMOs. What good would that do for us? The other managed care companies could just take those findings and use them for their own benefit. In business we call that 'the free rider problem.'"

Funny, I thought. In universities we call that "discovering something important."

In a way, he was perfectly right. The knowledge gained through such a large trial could not be patented or copyrighted or trademarked. It would immediately become the common property of humankind, and anyone could use it. Why would a large company want to spend money to generate knowledge that it couldn't own? In the old days we used to think of such knowledge as a public good. It would be natural for the public sector to support such research, just as it supports the basic science that underlies so many drug discoveries.

In fits and starts the public sector does on occasion commission such trials, but not systematically. We've seen some examples of isolated, heroic studies initiated by the National Institutes of Health or another governmental body to evaluate commonly used drugs. These trials often yielded important findings that had major implications for medical practice and costs. It's remarkable how few of them there have been. NIH and those who shape its policy perceive that this would drain scarce dollars away from their core mission of supporting more basic research; they'd prefer to leave such applied studies to be paid for from the deeper pockets of the pharmaceutical industry. And we know where that leads.

To move this idea forward, a practical next step would be to create an agenda-setting catalyst, perhaps a blue-ribbon panel supported by some very modest core funding from one or more foundations. The group would represent clinical experts, health care payers, and consumer groups. It would identify the top ten unresolved frontline medication choice questions. Picking them would generate some hearty debate, but a few topics would probably bubble to the top of most people's lists: congestive heart failure, cholesterol, insomnia, depression, adult-onset diabetes, blood pressure (again), Parkinson's disease, Alzheimer's disease. Conducting the relevant head-to-head drug studies as pragmatic clinical trials would require considerable work, but wouldn't have to break new methodological ground. The research could be funded by modest contributions from a broad group of participating HMOs, other insurers, employers, and governmental sources. Within a few years, the savings resulting from more appropriate drug expenditures by each funder would almost certainly exceed their contribution to the cost of the research. A portion of such savings would be recirculated into the funding pool for subsequent studies. The fact that modest proposals on this topic have begun to appear in Congress suggests that this is an idea whose time has come, even if those initial proposals can't yet take the nation as far as it needs to go. Senator Hillary Clinton included funds for the comparative study of drugs in the late-2003 Medicare prescription benefit legislation, but President Bush deleted them when he sent his budget to Congress.

A MORE SUBTLE APPROACH TO DRUG APPROVAL

Spurred by the antidepressant and analgesic crises, the FDA has started to take some tentative steps beyond the YES/NO binary thinking that traditionally guided all its decisions; it needs help in moving much farther in that direction. The agency has to reassess its singleminded reliance on the lowest possible standard: that a new drug must merely be slightly better than placebo in achieving a surrogate outcome over a few months, in modest numbers of highly selected patients. This just doesn't provide the information that doctors, patients, and payers require to make the best possible decisions about the drugs we use. It's sobering to recall the well-documented beneficial effect that estrogen replacement has on a patient's blood cholesterol levels. Achieving that surrogate outcome is all that is presently required by the FDA to approve drugs in the lipid-lowering category. If estrogens were judged by those criteria, they could be approved tomorrow for that indication and promoted widely to prevent cardiac disease, even though they have the opposite effect.

There are some important countervailing arguments here. The first can be called the brute force argument: the FDA's enabling legislation states that a drug shall be approved for sale if the agency determines that it is safe and effective. The law makes no mention of "more effective than . . ." or "safer than . . ." And it certainly says nothing about cost-effectiveness, a topic that the FDA studiously avoids. The pharmaceutical industry argues that holding the FDA (and therefore them) to a higher standard would quite literally take an Act of Congress. Whether or not this is true, Congress does occasionally Act. Should it create new legislation requiring the FDA to make judgments about *relative* efficacy and safety? Or require it to approve only products that work better or are safer than existing products? Or insist that all clinical trials must last long enough to show an impact on real clinical events, like heart attacks in a study of a new cholesterol-lowering drug? Should all these trials also be required to include enough people to detect a side effect that occurs in one in ten thousand patients? And should the FDA be responsible for assessing a new drug's cost-effectiveness as well? If one could wave a magic wand even more powerful than the industry's inside-the-Beltway influence, would we *want* Congress to make all these changes in the way the FDA approves new drugs? Probably not.

TIERS OF ACCEPTANCE

Competing social goods are in play here; the desire to know nearly everything about a drug before it is launched could have important public health downsides, as well as economic ones. Clinical trials would have to enroll implausibly large numbers of people to detect all rare adverse events before marketing, and include enough randomized groups to permit comparisons with standard therapies. Studies of preventive medications would have to last years longer in order to show a reduction in the rate of real clinical events rather than surrogate measures. All this could double or triple the time before a new drug becomes available for general use; that would create a new problem if the drug truly provides an important advantage for patients. It would also add substantially to the price of such trials, and to the opportunity cost of tied-up research capital; that in turn could raise high drug prices even further. At first glance, this looks like a zero-sum problem, a kind of pharmacologic Heisenberg uncertainty principle in which the more we know in one domain, the more we have to give up in another. But that needn't be the case.

The Gordian knot can be cut if we move beyond binary thinking. A decade ago I coauthored an essay in the *New England Journal of Medicine* with Drs. Wayne Ray and Marie Griffin of Vanderbilt University in which we proposed a two-step approach to evaluating new drugs. A related proposal was presented five years later in the same journal by Alistair Wood, a respected clinical pharmacologist also based at Vanderbilt, and two colleagues. Like ours, their piece pointed out how such a system could be a boon to the detection and prevention of unanticipated adverse drug effects. (Wood was close to being nominated in 2002 by President Bush for the long-vacant job of FDA commissioner. But some in the drug industry found this essay objectionable enough that it helped end his candidacy. Senator Bill Frist, also a physician, was asked why Wood was dropped from consideration for the top FDA job. He explained that "there was a great deal of concern that he put too much emphasis on safety.") Since several years have passed since the last publication, and I never expect to be nominated for an FDA job, it may be time to bring back some of these ideas again.

Just as no coins in the ancient world were stamped "100 B.C.," some key facts can be known only in retrospect. We often cannot determine that a drug will turn out to be more effective or safe than its alternatives until it's been used for some time by large numbers of typical patients. Colleagues in the industry often tell me that no company ever sets out with the primary goal of developing just a "me too" drug. While that's not true, it is correct that many of our current therapeutic mainstays were the second or third similar product to enter the market, with advantages that became clear only after a few years of widespread use.

A start to reconciling these competing social goals would be a two-tier system of initial drug approval, an extension of the same classification the FDA currently employs in its review process. At present, the agency puts the most promising new drug applications on a fast track for evaluation, while the numerous more-of-the-same drugs are reviewed at the regular pace. This distinction could well be applied to the final approval itself. As at present, existing advisory committees of outside experts would review the results of the premarketing clinical trials submitted to win approval. For approved drugs, the final designation could then be put in one of two categories. For now, we can think of these categories as Meaningful or Exceptional Advance in Therapy *(MEAT)* versus Fundamentally Average Treatment *(FAT)*. The *MEAT* approval label could be conferred on products like a novel treatment for AIDS or cancer; the *FAT* designation would go to a drug that looks like just another entrant into an already populated class, such as yet another statin to lower cholesterol or another calcium-channel blocker to lower blood pressure.

It's true that even within the nonbreakthrough category, a new drug could still have a small edge over available products, such as marginally better efficacy, or once-a-day dosing. To recognize this, the *FAT* designation could be divided into two subcategories. A promising drug that appears to have a small increment in benefit could be provisionally put into a subcategory that reflected its modest advantage: Treatment Optimization Foreseeable with Use, or *TOFU*. Drugs that show no evidence of any superiority at all would be relegated to a lower *FAT* category, which we can for now call Likely Advantage Really Doubtful, or *LARD*. A drug's designation could change over time as more experience with it yields additional data. Of course, more appropriately official-sounding terms would have to replace these examples, preferably without food pyramid overtones. An appealing aspect of this idea is that it wouldn't require any new legislation. The *MEAT/FAT* designation could be assigned by the FDA commissioner on advice from the existing advisory committees that already evaluate drugs for approval. The new designations would be required to appear on all promotional materials.

It also ought to be within the FDA's current mandate to hold manufacturers to a higher standard of inclusiveness in the trials they submit for initial approval. This would mean requiring adequate numbers of truly elderly subjects in all premarketing studies of drugs likely to be used by older people. The "over sixty-five" category must not be populated primarily with sixty-six-year-old golfers, as it sometimes is now; it must extend deep into the age range of patients who will actually use the drug, and include frail older subjects as well. This will introduce some statistical noise, and cost a bit more. But those are not reasons to avoid doing so; it would be far better than learning things the hard way, when bad things happen to sick elderly patients in the course of routine medical care.

A SECOND LOOK

The initial FDA approval of a drug should be seen as the beginning of an intensive period of assessment, not the end. Those competing social goals could be reconciled if we adopted a plan of two-phase evaluation. The idea is rooted in a simple understanding of how clinical decision making works. In medical practice as in life, few decisions can be made optimally at a single point in time. In prescribing a new drug for a patient, I would always schedule a follow-up visit to find out how well it was working and whether any problems had developed; all good doctors do. No physician would ever say, "Mrs. Smith, giving you this medication seemed like a fine idea when I first wrote the prescription eight months ago, based on the information we had then. So even if it's not working, or is making you sick, let's just stick with that plan."

We need to be able to meld such real-world clinical thinking about drugs into the regulatory decision process. New information emerges constantly about the performance of a recently marketed drug, as well as about alternatives to it. From both a clinical and a policy perspective, good decision making requires flexibility about new evidence. This could be accomplished if the approval process moved beyond a single YES/NO decision made at one point in time, and added in a mandatory reevaluation step.

Such a change would have to be implemented in a way that did not wreak havoc on manufacturers' expectations. The year the international pharmacoepidemiology conference was held in Edinburgh, my family and I took some time before the meeting to visit some old castles in the north of Scotland. Climbing a number of helical tower staircases, I learned the hard way about "trip steps"—randomly placed treads purposely made much deeper or shorter than all the others. The idea was that marauding invaders (or visiting tourists) running up the stairs would be thrown off their stride by the occasional unpredictable step, knocking them off balance. The drug approval process shouldn't contain any trip steps; the FDA should not resemble a castle booby-trapped against invaders. These new rules will have to be concrete and predictable.

The first day a new drug is on the market should mark the start of a systematic ongoing evaluation of how wisely doctors are prescribing it, how thoroughly patients are taking it, what adverse events it causes in routine care, and (eventually) whether its promised benefits are actually being realized with routine use. To accomplish this, these new questions would be specified in advance and their answers required by a certain date three or so years after a new drug is launched, when a mandatory reassessment would be done. That reassessment would bring together rigorous studies of the drug's utilization and outcomes in a variety of settings; its goal would be to reveal how well the product actually performs in the health care system.

If a new statin drug was approved solely on the basis that it could lower cholesterol, has it achieved this goal in routine use? Did any unexpected safety problems arise? Has its use been associated with the hoped-for reduction in cardiac events? (The methodological aspects of this last determination are daunting, but by no means impossible.) If a company's drug was initially labeled as *FAT/LARD* by the FDA advisory committee that first reviewed it, postmarketing data could be assembled to justify its elevation to the better *FAT/TOFU* ranking; that could be useful in gaining market share among savvy large purchasers. A manufacturer could also have its product graduate at this stage from a *FAT* categorization to *MEAT* if it presented convincing new information on effectiveness or a major unexpected safety advantage.

Such postmarketing studies could be conducted in HMOs, academic medical centers, governmental programs, and practices covered by large employers or private insurers. Why would these institutions do all that work? The simple, but wrong, answer would be that they need such information to understand what they're getting for their billions of dollars of annual drug expenditure. No, they would do this under contract, with funds provided either by a federal agency such as the FDA, CDC, or NIH, or by the drug's manufacturer, who would have to assemble such a dossier for the drug to remain on the market. Universities don't have the financial wherewithal to initiate the studies on their own, and as we've seen most HMOs may not choose to spend their money in this way, but both would be quite willing to perform the work if paid to do so. In addition, a large network of contract research organizations (CROs) currently perform drug evaluation studies routinely. At present most of their business comes from pharmaceutical companies required to perform premarketing trials to win regulatory approval. But the CROs are entrepreneurial organizations that would no doubt be pleased to bid on such reassessment studies as well, whoever is paying for them.

Any new information-gathering activity in health care has to justify its cost, even if we don't require the same standard for new medications. This wouldn't be hard to do; the economics are compelling. The nation is spending enormous sums to pay for our lavish use of drugs; a small fraction of that expenditure would cover the cost of a very ambitious real-world comparative evaluation program. Just a half-percent of the $200 billion we annually spend on drugs could help us find out what that expenditure is buying and how those dollars could be deployed more effectively. The resulting $1 billion a year would support a substantial amount of evaluative research.

A stable line item in the federal budget would spread out responsibility for such funding. But support from general revenues is always at the pleasure of Congress and the executive branch, a fact that has so far worked to the great disadvantage of this kind of research. Some have instead suggested a dime-per-prescription fee to cover these costs. Americans fill about three billion prescriptions a year; that would yield a respectable $300 million annually to support this work. This would put the funding burden disproportionately on the shoulders of patients, but it would be a light one compared to most current tax-the-sick methods of paying for health care. A per-prescription system of support would make it easier to require that all funds collected could be earmarked solely for public-sector research on the effectiveness, use, and safety of medications.

An alternative strategy would have the studies funded federally with resources extracted from the private sector, including insurers and HMOs. It may seem odd to expect private entities to help fund the work of a federal agency, but this is precisely what happens now at the FDA through its user fees. These payers, along with the employers and governmental programs that provide drugs to patients, could be required—in their own self-interest, we must note—to pay a "user's user fee" to support such evaluations; the fee could be charged on a per-person-covered basis. Or we might extend the existing FDA user fee by requiring pharmaceutical companies to pay for the reassessment of the drugs they produce, just as they do for their initial assessment—as long as the conduct of such studies was managed independently.

One important bottleneck relates to the privacy of all that rich existing data about drug taking and clinical events in millions of typical patients. Protection of patient confidentiality is supremely important, but need not be an insurmountable barrier to getting this work done. Well-developed methods exist for converting personal identifiers into untraceable code numbers that enable researchers to track the medication use and subsequent outcomes in millions of patients individually, without ever knowing who any of them are. The HMOs have learned that this information is a valuable commodity, and have become adept at selling it to the highest bidder—usually drug companies rather than university-based researchers. The public sector—Medicaid, Medicare, the VA—already has this data in electronic form and could serve as a unique national resource for information on millions more people, particularly the elderly and the poor, vulnerable populations often underrepresented in drug trials. We have for years worked with Medicare and Medicaid data in performing this work, despite daunting and often painful bureaucratic hurdles.

Unfortunately, access by researchers to this valuable information has recently been made far more difficult. Growing paranoia warns that any access to data beyond the medical team caring for a patient constitutes an invasion of privacy, and new legislation that took effect in 2003 made it much harder for researchers to get access to the data needed for these studies. Ironically, this restriction of access was not prompted by its misuse at the hands of evil epidemiologists or rogue medical researchers. It was in part a response to some very real abuses by insurers who denied health care coverage on the basis of information about a person's medical history. That continues apace.

As long as proper safeguards are in place to protect confidentiality, the government's restriction of access to these vital data for approved studies makes as much sense as putting the human genome project under the control of the CIA. Yet each year researchers find the legal sphincter around this priceless resource tightening further. A less paranoid policy could still protect patients' privacy while permitting university groups throughout the country to tackle vital questions about how well the health care system is using its drugs, how patients are or aren't taking them, the side effects they cause, and the illnesses they are helping to prevent.

Assuming we can find a way beyond the current privacy hysteria, we will still need to identify a safe organizational home for such work. The issues here are identical to those we considered earlier, and so are all the same potential organizational solutions. As long as the drug reassessment process is conducted rigorously, the FDA would be expected to accept the recommendations it generates, just as it nearly always accepted the conclusions of the National Academy of Sciences during the DESI process in the 1960s and 1970s. If a drug successfully passes its three-year reassessment, the FDA would require the manufacturer to summarize these results prominently in all official statements about the product, including all promotion. This could be a boon as well as a curse for a drug's sales—that's the point. An ad for a cholesterol-lowering drug could boast: "Postmarketing reassessment of this drug has been based on studies of its use in over 600,000 patients in numerous health care settings. The evidence demonstrates that this product is effective in preventing heart attack and stroke, and has a rate of adverse effects lower than that of other comparable drugs in this category." By contrast, another cholesterol-lowering medication that had won approval based only on its ability to improve numbers on patients' lab tests might be given three years to demonstrate an association between its use and reduced rates of the outcomes just listed. If it failed to do so, it could be taken off the market.

A devotee of the free market might object that all that's really needed would be to inform doctors and patients that a drug in use for years had been shown only to improve surrogate markers, but had never demonstrated any beneficial effect on actual clinical events. In the competitive pharmaceutical environment, they might argue, a product obliged to confess this fact in every advertisement would eventually lose out to medications that produced improvement in real clinical outcomes in large controlled trials. Tooth Fairy thinking strikes again. Pfizer's Lipitor (atorvastatin) was a late entrant into the cholesterol-lowering market, and for years no major trial was published demonstrating that it reduced cardiac events rather than just improving the outcomes of lab tests. Throughout this period, the FDA required that every Lipitor ad and television commercial report that fact prominently. During this time, Lipitor became the best-selling cholesterol-lowering drug, as well as one of the most widely prescribed products in America, far outselling older, similar medications whose manufacturers had invested millions of dollars in large randomized trials that proved their clinical effectiveness. Lipitor isn't the only sobering example. Pfizer's Norvasc became the best-selling drug to treat high blood pressure in the United States despite the very thin clinical credentials of the calcium-channel blockers until 2000. And millions of women still take lifelong estrogen replacement despite its occasionally fatal side effects.

(In 2003, after billions of dollars in sales, a study did finally appear in *Lancet* documenting that Lipitor indeed reduces the risk of cardiac disease. The story took an ironic additional turn in early 2004 when another randomized clinical trial showed that Lipitor in high doses was actually much *more* effective at preventing heart attacks than usual doses of another widely used statin. That important difference could represent thousands of preventable hospitalizations each year—but it took nearly a decade for the comparison to be made.)

FOR A PERSON who spends his life trying to generate data about drugs, it smarts to admit that those data are only the start of the road to optimal drug use—necessary, but not sufficient. There is much work to do to assemble the information we need about drugs' effectiveness and risks. But even once that task is complete, we will still have to figure out how to feed all that knowledge back into the health care system and make sure that it is acted upon appropriately. The goal should be nothing less than to ensure that every prescription is based on the very best information available on the day it is written. That job will require us to confront a very different set of challenges.

22: TURNING KNOWLEDGE
INTO ACTION

In practical matters, the end is not mere speculative
knowledge of what is to be done, but rather the doing
of it.

— ARISTOTLE, *Nichomachean Ethics* 6.13.1 (350 B.C.)

What we have here is a failure to communicate.

— *Cool Hand Luke* (1967)

My unruly home office houses a shaggy collection of mass media
articles on the high cost of prescription drugs, clipped over the
years from dozens of magazines and newspapers. Typically, the
stories spotlight patients ground down by unbearable pharmacy bills that
cost them thousands of dollars annually. To pay for their medicines, some
had to take a second job, or lower the thermostat to save on heating bills, or
skimp at the supermarket. The pieces elicit sympathy and frustration, occasionally rage. Once in a while the actual drug bills are enumerated in a side-
bar. When that happens I sometimes find myself reacting instead with
astonishment: *"What were their doctors thinking?"*

The lists often include high-priced brand-name products that have inexpensive generic equivalents, or are in a class containing similar drugs that
would have been much cheaper and work just as well. The significance of
these vital pharmacological details is usually inapparent to nonphysicians,
but for me they mean that one big problem some of these patients had is

thoughtless prescribing. Their predicament is different from that of others whose health really does require multiple high-priced medicines for which no affordable substitutes exist. A key agenda for individual patients and their doctors, as well as for the health care system as a whole, is to understand when each cause is at work, since their solutions are quite different. Yet most public debate fails to take on these fertile questions about doctors' prescribing choices.

Instead, most current policy discussions have dwelled more on green-eyeshade issues like the right levels for deductibles or copayments, or what expenditure should trigger what degree of coverage, or how large the druggist's dispensing fee should be. These are important questions, and make good discussion topics for policy analysts because they require no medical background. But such debates ignore the appealing solution of smarter prescribing. That won't address all our access and affordability problems, but it would take care of many of them.

You could fill rooms with tens of thousands of studies that elegantly define the benefits, risks, and cost-effectiveness of specific drugs but have had only a modest impact on how medicine is practiced. I know this because I have been in such rooms; they are called medical libraries. The situation is a little like that of AIDS in the developing world. For an African with that disease, it's not enough that drugs have been discovered that could treat it, if those medicines are never delivered to the people who need them. If the companies that produce the drugs insist on excessively high prices, or if the infrastructure is too fragmented to get the pills distributed, or if patients don't believe that taking them will make any difference, then it is as if those important breakthroughs had never been made.

In the United States, we have our own infrastructure problems. We can't deliver enough of the powerful medicine of information to doctors or to patients. Even if our patients could afford all the drugs in the world (a topic we'll take up in the next and final chapter), we doctors would still need more help in knowing which ones to prescribe. Implementing the proposals of the last chapter would mean that even more trials would be conducted to answer our numerous head-to-head comparison questions, yielding even more complex facts to communicate to us and to our patients accurately, comprehensively, and efficiently. If that knowledge doesn't influence how drugs are used, it will do us little good.

Our information transfer solutions will have to begin at the beginning, in medical school. This is where we doctors lay the foundation for all our future learning and where we absorb our sense of what matters, what kinds of ideas are important, what approaches make a difference. The soil prepared or soiled in those years will determine which ideas will grow in it for the rest of a doctor's life. Yet most students hear precious little about the measuring and balancing of benefits, risks, and costs. When I give talks on these topics, many superbly trained doctors are surprised to learn about the prevailing "probably better than nothing" standard for drug approval, or the level of unmeasured risk associated with many new products, or the utter lack of cost-effectiveness of many of the medications they prescribe every day. That scantiness of exposure explains how readily some of my colleagues fall prey to the data-thin claims pitched to us by sales reps, persuasive ads, and insistent patients.

They are equally astonished about the epidemic of drug underuse in our health care system because patients cannot afford their medicines, or comply poorly with them, or never receive the prescriptions they need because their illnesses are undertreated or never even diagnosed. Just one or two dozen hours devoted to these topics in the medical school and residency years could confer lifelong immunity to some of the worst of these misperceptions, and make us more intelligent consumers of the endless education we will all need.

RECLAIMING THE POSTGRADUATE YEARS

Those of us who have finished our formal training (no one should ever really "finish" training in this line of work) desperately need more noncommercial sources of information to enrich the informational space in which we practice. When I first started thinking about academic detailing in the late 1970s, I naively assumed that if we could show that it worked and was at least cost-neutral, similar programs would be set up by universities all over the country. Medical schools seemed then to be the most logical sponsors of such activities. After all, they had reservoirs of expertise in all areas of clinical medicine, pharmacology, and epidemiology, and ties to the communities of practicing physicians around them. Many had links to other university divisions with know-how in economics and management as well. And their mission was, at least in part, medical education. We had even shown that such programs could easily be economically self-sustaining or even revenue-generating. When I wrote that initial grant there weren't many HMOs around, but I expected that even if future sponsorship came only from state Medicaid programs and the Veterans Administration health care system, that could provide enough funding to set up educational outreach programs in hundreds of communities across the country.

Granted, it would have taken some out-of-the-box thinking for medical schools to take on this mission. But the same deans who brought their institutions into the large-scale health care delivery business in the 1990s, often with disastrous results, had much less interest in becoming large-scale pur-veyors of medical knowledge. Medical schools continued to offer post-graduate education in the traditional mold of one- to three-day didactic courses, usually requiring practitioners to travel to their respective Meccas. This established a small presence in the community and a modest revenue stream, and most schools felt that was enough to satisfy their mission. It didn't come close to meeting the need for ongoing education about medica-tion use, but it was no one's job to meet that need systematically.

Similarly, throughout the 1980s and 1990s most state Medicaid pro-grams and private-sector insurers remained stuck in the mind-set of bill payers rather than care improvers—an orientation that persisted even when they could no longer afford to pay those bills. At that point they assumed the role of bill deniers or obstacle creators, with the hope that doctors would be intimidated by all the hassles and therefore prescribe fewer expen-sive drugs. This didn't provide much of a fiscal or intellectual demand for unbiased education about drugs, and the pharmaceutical companies con-tinued to fill the educational vacuum themselves. As a result, nearly two thirds of all continuing medical education for physicians is funded by the pharmaceutical industry—with predictable results. Some HMOs and pre-scription benefit management companies did establish their own academic detailing programs, and as we've seen, other countries began to implement the approach on a much larger scale. But there was much less innovation here at home in the predominant fee-for-service piecework medical market-place. With the sharp rise in medication expenditures of the last few years, interest in providing non-product-driven drug information to these doctors has now started to increase.

I no longer reflexively assume that medical schools would be the best organizations to host such knowledge transfer systems. In some institu-tions, the growing reliance on industry funding doesn't lend itself well to the skeptical arm's-length posture required to evaluate any therapy effec-tively. Many individual faculty still execute this role admirably, but they often find themselves swimming upstream. The mixed allegiances of others will require looking for other homes for this process, at least in the current climate.

Might government be a likely sponsor of such large-scale educational outreach activities, as it was for the agricultural extension service that helped inspire my first project? If the availability of accurate, timely, evidence-based drug information is a public good like clean air, mass tran-sit, and homeland security, shouldn't the public sector help provide it? We've seen that some national governments have taken on the role of underwriting these activities boldly and effectively. But the United States has a more checkered record in government-sponsored technology assessment, particularly in health care. As with some medical schools, some governmental entities could rise to the occasion and perform this function quite well within their respective domains: a given state drug benefit program here, a particular Veterans Affairs region there. But if we need to supply a wide constituency of physicians and patients with the vigorous programs that are needed all over the country, we'd be unwise to rely solely on government.

The good news follows, even if its verb tense for now is somewhere between subjunctive and future perfect. In the preceding chapter, I argued that the easily biased process of comparative drug assessment needed to be protected by a noncommercial context. The costs of doing that evaluative work would be relatively modest and not hard to come by—a small price to pay for insulation from the powerful pressures of insurers, manufacturers, and politicians. But the larger industrial-strength programs that will be needed to reach every practitioner in the country are unlikely to be supported by either foundations or government, nor need they be. Getting this work done on the scale required may well call for old-fashioned American entrepreneurialism. Indeed, those billions of dollars coursing around in the pharmaceutical marketplace could help pay for the creation of a new drug information service industry.

Public health aside (another typically American approach), it would be worth a lot of money to insurers, employers, state and federal governments, HMOs, doctors, and patients to have access to a reliable and independent medication information delivery service. This in turn will require that indispensable American ingredient, the business plan. (Note to my friends from the 1960s: "It would be a neat idea and help a lot of people" is *not* a business plan.) If government and academia are unable or unwilling to do this work on a national scale, we need to explain how such organizations would survive. The answer: they will be paid for their services.

This isn't the first time such an idea has been put forward, and its last incarnation was not comforting. In the 1980s and 1990s, a new industry arose that promised to improve the use and contain the escalating costs of medications: prescription benefit management companies, or PBMs. Employers, HMOs, and other large insurers contracted with these companies with the expectation that they would control rising drug expenses by getting better prices from manufacturers and moving utilization to the most cost-effective products. A few PBMs set up physician education divisions that emphasized appropriate clinical decision making, and several of those interventions provided a useful service. But subsequent litigation has revealed that the profits of some PBMs also came from kickbacks paid by the manufacturers whose drugs they favored; it appears that sometimes they passed along only a portion of those rebates to the insurers or employers for whom they were ostensibly working, and kept the rest. Some PBMs secretly contracted with drug companies to protect their products' market share in return for lucrative payments—a kind of pharmaceutical protection racket. The fact that several of the largest PBMs were for a time owned by drug companies made these relationships even more complicated. Given this recent history, it ought not to seem paranoid to propose that the new information transfer businesses would have to be prohibited from having any financial relationships with pharmaceutical manufacturers. They will have credibility only if they are free of influence from those whose products they are advising about.

The economic opportunities are impressive. Dr. Michael Fischer and I undertook an analysis of what the nation would be paying to treat high blood pressure if physicians' prescribing were influenced solely by clinical trial evidence and not by marketing pressures. Fischer went into our anonymized database of pharmacy claims and diagnoses, identified over 130,000 such patients over the age of sixty-five, and ran a simulation. Person by person, he had the computer theoretically "replace" their actual medication use with the prescriptions they would have been given if their doctors had been prescribing according to evidence-based guidelines. In this virtual world of ideal decision making, we found that the high use of calcium-channel blockers declined sharply, and that of thiazides rose. When he calculated the resulting costs, we found that the drug bill for those patients would have been tens of millions of dollars lower. Projected to the United States as a whole, such evidence-based prescribing would have lowered the nation's costs for treating hypertension by about $1.2 billion a year, just for patients over sixty-five. And according to the clinical trial evidence, their health would have been better as well.

So it seems that on both economic and medical grounds, implementing such information transfer services could do a great deal of good. Some of the parts are already in place as freestanding components—isolated outreach programs, newsletters, occasional literature reviews, sporadic cost-effectiveness analyses. In the United States, a few managed care organizations and other health systems have established programs that subsume several of these functions, and we've seen that the entire package is deployed impressively in a number of other countries. It's interesting to speculate about what could be done on a larger scale in the United States if we could just pull all the pieces together in one convenient tamper-proof package.

A NEW KIND OF INFORMATION TRANSFER ORGANIZATION

WHAT WOULD THESE GROUPS DO? They would contract to provide evidence-based drug information services to physicians or groups of them, such as doctors working in a given health care delivery system or in a particular geographic area. Their mandate would be to give physicians the data they need to help them prescribe according to the best current information, and cost-effectively.

WHERE WOULD SUCH CRITERIA COME FROM? Literally dozens of criteria for optimal medication use already exist, developed after extensive review of the literature by panels of experts. Most of them are quite good. The problem isn't developing the criteria, it's getting them into the hands of doctors and persuading them to follow them.

HOW WOULD THEY ACCOMPLISH THIS? Tools would include computer software, educational outreach (academic detailing) visits, critical overviews of major drug-use topics, and 24/7 phone and e-mail consultation services staffed by drug information experts. These organizations would also perform surveillance of patterns of drug use for quality assurance, feedback, and program targeting.

HOW WOULD THEIR SUCCESS BE MEASURED? The outcome of these activities would be evaluated and compensated based on the clinical quality of the doctors' prescribing—not simply its cheapness.

HOW WOULD THE EVALUATION WORK? With the increasing automation of clinical data, it's possible to perform an electronic "biopsy" of all prescribing by a given physician or group. This can be done today in most programs that pay for medications. More sophisticated assessment would also consider the mix of patient demographics and diagnoses in a given doctor's practice. This is possible now in systems with advanced informatics capacity; it will be nearly universal in the coming years.

WHO WOULD ESTABLISH AND RUN THESE ORGANIZATIONS? The safest path initially would be the approach of "Let a hundred flowers bloom." (Despite Chairman Mao's affection for the slogan, it is after all the founding concept of both capitalism and evolution.) Several start-up companies may be created de novo to fill this niche; others may be offshoots of existing groups such as professional societies or universities. Still others might be subsidiaries of health care delivery organizations, such as health maintenance organizations that have already created their own in-house staffs to perform these functions.

WHERE WOULD THE MONEY COME FROM TO PAY FOR THESE SERVICES? The information delivery services would be paid by those who incur drug costs: employers, insurers, governmental programs, managed care organizations. Tax credits and direct government subsidies for companies that purchase such services could help lighten their economic impact. Our earlier research and much evidence on the economics of drug use make it clear that the cost of better information transfer would be more than offset by the resulting savings in drug expenditures, not even counting the improvements in quality of care.

WOULD THESE NEW ORGANIZATIONS BE NONPROFIT OR FOR-PROFIT? Either, as long as the former are motivated enough to satisfy their clients' needs, and the latter are prohibited from yielding to the easy-money temptations that distort the mission of some "medical education" and PBM companies.

WILL AUDITING BE NECESSARY? Yes. Each organization would be reviewed annually by an outside group to assess the quality and integrity of its work. There are several precedents in health care for such professionally driven certification: the Joint Commission on Accreditation of Healthcare Organizations, the National Committee on Quality Assessment, and all the professional societies that provide voluntary physician certification in medical specialties. Such outside observers would also audit an organization's books to ensure that it receives support only from the clients for whom it works, and not from product manufacturers or drug industry–dominated intermediaries. A clinical dimension of the audit would ensure that the educational content focuses primarily on optimal medication use and not just on reducing drug costs. As with other kinds of certification in the health care system, such a seal of approval would be required to receive government subsidies for these services, and its absence would be a sign of potential quality problems.

DOCTORS ARE UNBEARABLY BUSY; WHY WOULD THEY GO ALONG WITH THIS? Most doctors want to learn how to take better care of our patients, as long as the information is made convenient, accessible, engaging, and relevant; many now set aside a given portion of each week to meet with sales reps. This would work even better if such programs help physicians meet prescribing quality goals or incentives set by their payers or employers, or new competency benchmarks that could be established by accrediting authorities. It would also be smart and cost-effective for payers to reimburse doctors for the modest amounts of time spent on these quality-improvement activities.

COULD THIS EVIDENCE-BASED EDUCATIONAL OUTREACH ALSO BE USED TO IMPROVE OTHER KINDS OF CLINICAL DECISIONS, LIKE USE OF DIAGNOSTIC TESTS OR PROCEDURES OR CONSULTATIONS? Definitely; some academic detailing programs have already expanded in these directions.

GETTING COST INFORMATION WHERE IT'S NEEDED

If prescribers are to think capably about economically rational drug use, we will need better access to price information. Some managed care plans now remind doctors of the relative costs of comparable drugs within a class. But one doctor may see patients covered by dozens of different insurers with different arrangements, and patients with no drug coverage must shoulder the full weight of each prescription we write. Our ability to prescribe cost-effectively for them is severely hampered if we don't have a clue what anything costs. Federal regulations require that the fuel and energy efficiency of cars and appliances be posted prominently on the stickers attached to these products. Why not require that the average cost of a medication be disclosed in every drug advertisement directed at doctors or patients? This would be a common benchmark price, such as the average cost per month for the most commonly prescribed dose of that product. The figure would be data-driven from national prescription information and updated regularly, so it couldn't be fudged the way the often-fictitious "average wholesale price" now is. Of course the price of the same drug will vary widely across payers, but an average U.S. benchmark would still have to be listed in all promotional materials. In principle, one would expect free-market advocates in Congress to get behind this idea as a means of empowering consumers and making pharmaceutical commerce more efficient. Unfortunately, the voting record of most conservative legislators appears to be determined by other inputs instead. Some of them might worry that a requirement that drug ads reveal the purchase price of the medication being promoted could soon be followed by a demand that political ads reveal the purchase price of the candidate being promoted.

WHAT THE PATIENT KNOWS

Medical school commencement speakers like to point out that the root of the word "doctor" is the same as that of the Middle English word for "teacher." As caregivers, one of our most important roles is to educate our patients about their illnesses, and about the medicines needed to treat them. This teaching becomes more important as chronic illnesses and lifelong risk states like high blood pressure or osteoporosis come to define so much of medical care. But shortsighted notions of efficiency are squeezing down the length of each doctor-patient encounter, making it hard to fulfill this role adequately. The abundant evidence that patients frequently don't take the medications they need, even when cost is not a barrier, means that this information transfer function often fails. As a result, millions of prescriptions for useful drugs are never taken. At the same time, patients demand and often get drugs they don't need, such as antibiotics for viral infections—another casualty of the failed doctor-as-teacher mission.

Here, too, we have models for how things could work better, but they have yet to be adopted on a large scale. Ideally, the doctor would have enough time in a clinical encounter to review all medications a patient is taking, explain why each one matters, and answer all of a patient's questions about them. Such "excess" time added to the length of a visit might look like a loss of productivity to the nonclinician managers who increasingly dictate physicians' workloads. But such a change could prevent much of the avoidable illness and hospitalization that result from misuse or nonuse of needed drugs. This function could also be performed well by a nurse or a pharmacist working with the practice. Where this is implemented, the improvements in quality of care can be substantial, and some practices could reap net cost savings as well.

BETTER USE OF INFORMATION TECHNOLOGY

In my last year of medical school in the 1970s, I wrote an article for the *Atlantic Monthly* about information technology and the future of medicine. It seemed then that we were on the brink of a sea change in how computers would help doctors make decisions about a wide range of clinical interventions, particularly drugs. Thirty years later, we still seem to be on that same brink. The evolution has been surprisingly slow, but we're definitely getting there. Computers are now ubiquitous in pharmacies, although their most common use is to verify insurance coverage and enable the store to bill the correct party; some checking for drug interactions is also done. But by the time the patient has brought a paper prescription to the drugstore, the horse is out of the barn. A far more important transition is occurring as more doctors write our prescriptions on a computer. Whether the change is clinically or fiscally driven, it's much better for a patient to get the right prescription the first time rather than to hear at the drugstore that there's a problem and that the doctor has to write a new one. So far, the main driver of this development has been efficiency and legibility, but technology will make its most powerful contribution here in shaping the very content of those decisions. Once a doctor sits at a terminal instead of a pad to write a medication order, the door flings wide open onto a universe of informatics potential.

The transformation began with some simpler applications. The computer can remind a doctor that a given drug isn't covered by a patient's insurer (or would require a much higher copay for the patient) and that a virtually identical product is. Things get more interesting when the computer can also make suggestions to improve clinical decisions. Working with Dr. David Bates and colleagues at the Brigham, we arranged for dosing guidelines appropriate to a given patient's age to appear on the computer screen whenever a prescription is written on the hospital's order-entry system. A doctor prescribing a sleeping pill for an older patient can be reminded that a lower dose is needed for an eighty-year-old, or that a drug with a shorter half-life will be less likely to cause morning-after unsteadiness. Unlike the computer at an outside pharmacy, the doctor's machine could also access information on a patient's diagnoses, so that reminders can pop up if a new prescription is likely to interact with a patient's other medical conditions—such as starting a potassium supplement in a patient who has previously had problems with high potassium levels. As we've learned at the Brigham for several drug categories, more sophisticated messages are also possible.

Today, when a doctor writes a computer-based prescription for a calcium-channel blocker to treat high blood pressure, it's technologically practical for her to receive this response instantaneously before the order is completed:

> A large randomized clinical trial has found that patients using CCBs as initial therapy for hypertension had more strokes and heart failure than patients taking thiazides, and incurred much higher drug costs. Click here —— to receive a download of this paper. Click here —— to change this order to hydrochlorothiazide 12.5 mg daily; this dose is based on the patient's age and weight. Click here —— to continue with your original order.

In a coordinated health care delivery system, the doctor's computer could also be linked to computers servicing other sectors. A link to the clinical laboratory could warn of an early side effect *("This patient's liver enzymes have become elevated; reassess the following prescribed drugs he is taking that can cause this reaction...")*. Feedback from the pharmacy computer system could reveal substance abuse *("This patient is currently getting narcotics prescriptions from three different physicians and filling them at four different pharmacies")* as well as poor compliance *("Thirty-day pre-scriptions for cholesterol-lowering medication are being filled by this patient at an average of 52-day intervals")*. The programming needed is straightfor-ward; in integrated delivery networks like many HMOs and the VA, all that is needed is the commitment to make it happen.

Some systems have made good progress in these directions. For patients and doctors working in the rest of our piecemeal health care enterprise, it will first be necessary to connect the components that currently live in splendid isolation from one another—the doctor's office, the pharmacy, the laboratory, the hospital. Once those linkages are made, software packages will eventually be used routinely to provide immediate feedback to the doctor about how well a given prescription fits with the patient's clinical situation, as well as with the best current knowledge—all at the critical moment a prescribing decision is being made. Installing a computer-based medication-ordering system is still a costly undertaking, but affordable off-the-shelf packages are becoming commonplace.

GETTING STARTED

It's time to think about moving beyond a thousand points of light; after all, that image implies a sea of darkness separating each tiny piece of bright-ness from everything else. Many of these pieces could be pulled together by any organization with the will to move in this direction—group practices, hospitals, insurers, state-run pharmacy benefit programs, employers, even individual practitioners. Sharable evidence-based drug evaluations and educational materials are already out there, developed by innovative pro-grams here and in other English-speaking countries. Although some dig-ging is required, most can be accessed by any individual or organization right now, at the websites listed in the Notes to several chapters.

In earlier, gentler times in medicine, the linkage between knowledge and action came from the concept of professionalism: the sense that as a physi-cian I have a personal responsibility to get and apply the knowledge I need to care for my patients. That's an old-fashioned idea, seen these days as far less efficient than the adrenaline of financial incentives. But in the end, it may be the more powerful medicine. To administer it, we will need to move beyond the Hobbesian all-against-all melee of commercial health care, as we must in so many other aspects of medical policy.

We doctors need to embrace these new tools as a way to reclaim respon-sibility for educating ourselves and each other; after all, our profession has done so for generations. If we do, the organizations in which we increas-ingly find ourselves employed are more likely to respect that professional-ism and nurture it rather than attempt to undercut it with financial bribes, penalties, or demeaning restrictions. Reaffirming our professional identity would require that we not allow salespeople or large health care corporations or any central command-and-control authority to unduly influence the clinical decisions we make. Failing to keep up with the latest evidence from the medical literature, being unaware of the economics of what we prescribe, forgetting that every prescription is inherently an interpersonal transaction—these lapses are undercutting our moral authority as gatekeepers to the sacred world of science-based healing. As we're about to see, if we don't act soon they may prove to be our professional undoing.

23: MARKETS AND MEDICINES

Wh-at can be done when information alone isn't enough to drive change as far as it needs to go? The scent of economic incentive is everywhere in medicine, occasionally rising to the level of stench. In large measure, that's what bound us into the fix we're in. But in small doses, could such incentives also help to fix the bind we're in? Even if the quest for riches has diverted so much of medicine away from its samaritan traditions, can economics also play a role in improving clinical decision making? As our old friend Paracelsus would again remind us, it's all about the dose (and, we might add today, the route of administration).

THE POWERFUL GREEN MEDICINE

My colleagues often complain bitterly that payers are restricting their freedom to prescribe. I remind them that we helped bring this problem on ourselves, through decades of naïveté and indifference about the prices of the drugs we order for our patients. That irresponsibility helped lead HMO managers to the following logic: if doctors neither know nor care what drugs cost, then we'll have to drive their decisions by constraining their choices or manipulating their salaries. I once suggested to a managed care executive that just letting us know what specific drugs cost might help us become more cost-effective prescribers, but he scoffed at the idea. "Doctors will only pay attention to drug costs if they have some skin in the game," he replied.

H. L. Mencken observed that for every complex problem there is one easy solution that is neat, plausible—and wrong. Penalties and bribes can catch a doctor's attention and probably change behavior, but so would electric shocks or corporal punishment. The more a physician's raw "drug

spend" determines his or her salary, the more it will become a personal economic burden to care for patients with complicated or severe illnesses. To
use the business lingo that accompanies this kind of thinking, it could truly
"realign the doctor's incentives" to fit those of the HMO—but not necessarily those of the patient.

There are three kinds of organizational relationship that can shape prescribing. First, the system can employ physicians directly, as occurs in some
health maintenance organizations, the Veterans Affairs medical system,
and Great Britain. The system can influence doctors' actions because it's
their boss.

Second, the doctor may be an independent agent who contracts with the
organizations that pay for health care; this is the arrangement of many
physicians who see patients with managed care insurance. The payer can
promulgate drug-use criteria and incentives through that contractual relationship; this can be done well or poorly.

The third way for clinical decisions to be influenced is for doctor, payer,
and patient to share a common set of values and goals, even though there
may be no concrete mechanism for anyone to control the doctor's decisions
directly. Flaky as it may sound, this is how things work in many non-U.S.
systems, where physicians live with the understanding that all providers and
patients operate within the confines of a single budget, so that excesses in
one area will inevitably cause shortfalls elsewhere.

None of the above arrangements applies to the majority of doctors and
patients in the United States—certainly not to most of those outside
HMOs or the VA system. For nearly all the rest of us, there really is no
"health care system." What we have instead is a collection of lone entrepreneurs, penurious insurers, aggressive multinational companies, beleaguered
government programs, embattled charities, and isolated consumers—all
engaged in hurly-burly piecework transactions. It's hard to monitor and
improve the quality of drug use in this chaotic environment, and even
harder to contain unnecessary expenditures.

For a commodity this complex and with stakes so high, it would help to
find our way back to the old-fashioned notion of informed decision making by an impartial learned intermediary, perhaps leavened with some
gentle incentives to encourage all parties to think about the relation
between cost and value. In systems with the power to impose economic
incentives on physicians, these must relate to the quality and appropriateness of our prescribing, not to its cost. Ordering an unnecessarily expensive
drug to treat depression or high cholesterol before considering an equally
good one that's cheaper could still result in penalties, but so would failing to
prescribe a needed drug, even an expensive one, when the patient's condition requires it.

The clinical benchmarks needed to implement this approach are not ineffable; a great deal of work in recent years has produced some fine standards to define high-quality prescribing. The best of these are based on evidence-driven recommendations crafted by professional organizations, groups of academics, and publicly supported programs. I participated in the development of one set of guidelines for drug use in the elderly, part of an initiative mounted by the RAND Corporation and physicians at UCLA. It was called the ACOVE project: Assessing Care of Vulnerable Elders. With Dr. Eric Knight of my division, we produced one component of a comprehensive, evidence-based "manifesto" that was later published in the *Annals of Internal Medicine*. Built on the best available information in the medical literature, it provides a set of guidelines for the optimal management of particular conditions, as well as criteria for evaluating practices in heath care systems. It is just one example of how the information base of clinical medicine can be turned into an action-oriented tool for informing medication use as well as auditing its quality; many other such road maps exist.

By serving both as benchmarks and as guideposts, such tools can be put to a variety of uses. Medical practices or organizations that perform well can be rewarded with greater esteem, more patients, or higher payment rates. Physicians who perform poorly can be identified for targeted education or for sanctions if they fail to improve. If the criteria are intelligently designed and well implemented, the only way to "game the system" would be to provide better care. Often, simply measuring and displaying the results of these quality audits will be enough to drive behavior all by itself—a fact long known to industrial psychologists.

ECONOMICS AND THE PATIENT

Like doctors, many patients have also moved from economic indifference to rude awakening when it comes to medications. People with comprehensive coverage often developed a blithe insensitivity to drug costs, leading many to demand the expensive drugs they saw in ads even when less costly ones would have worked as well. Insurers worried that too-generous medication insurance coverage was causing patients to lose all touch with their prescription bills. (Of course, many patients bought that insurance primarily because they *wanted* to lose touch with their prescription bills.) In public-sector programs, too, an excessive sense of entitlement threatened to undermine many entitlement programs like Medicaid.

So health system administrators put a different set of economic hurdles in place for patients, often crude ones. The abortive New Hampshire three-drug limit was one attempt. Another strategy was to raise deductibles—the amount patients have to pay on their own each year before their insurance kicks in. Other systems increased participants' copayments—the share paid out-of-pocket for each prescription. The rationale was that obliging people to share in the pain of paying for their drugs could make them better consumers. Even if that didn't work, the policies would at least shift a good part of the drug bill from insurer to patient. Here again, this can be a useful or a terrible idea, depending on how it's implemented.

The goal of cost sharing is analogous to the idea that a higher copay or deductible on your car insurance will make you less likely to bring every little scratch into the body shop for repair. But simpleminded extension of the auto-body model to pharmaceuticals doesn't make much sense. A higher deductible or copayment for fender repairs is a good way to keep auto insurance costs down, but what is the analogue in medicine—having patients think twice before they fill that prescription for a high blood pressure pill or heart medicine? The higher the level of "moral hazard" is set, the less utilization will occur. But do we really want to keep drug expenses down by discouraging people from filling their prescriptions? Such poorly conceived systems of cost sharing also put the heaviest burden on the shoulders of the sickest and poorest: patients who need several costly drugs are hit hardest by one-size-fits-all copay requirements. The poor also suffer disproportionately: a $35 monthly copay for each of six drugs feels very different to a clerk than it does to her CEO.

We need to identify a way of structuring patient copayments that will dampen inappropriate demands for the drugs with the best commercials, while keeping copays low enough so that they don't discourage people from using the medicines they require. We can think of this as the method first proposed by Jagger et al.: "You can't always get what you want / But . . . you get what you need." The best use of copayments is to direct patients away from expensive drugs, as long as similar products exist that are more cost-effective. Several insurers and HMOs have moved sensibly in this direction. They make the copay for a well-priced, cost-effective drug small or zero, while products that are priced higher but are no better require larger copayments. Having to pay a higher bill for a needlessly expensive drug will cause a patient to ask her doctor why she is taking a high-priced blood pressure pill or allergy medicine that requires a stiff copay each month, while her neighbor is taking a similar drug that costs him nothing.

Such gentle economic incentives can bring prescriber and patient into useful discussions about whether a given costly drug is really worth additional hundreds of dollars out-of-pocket per year—a discussion that would be unlikely to occur if all products were covered equally. Ideally, both parties should be aware of these facts *before* the prescribing decision is made. A patient shouldn't have to learn that a costly prescription isn't covered or requires a hefty copayment when he tries to fill it at the drugstore, once it's harder to reverse the economic damage. Ideally, these copays would also be linked to patients' income, and capped at a bearable limit.

Moving in this direction can redirect the attention of both doctor and patient to more cost-effective treatments in a way that is compelling, effective, and safe, to reduce use of those bizarrely overpriced products that now account for such a large fraction of rising drug expenses.

This sensible approach was taken by the Canadian province of British Columbia, which asked Dr. Sebastian Schneeweiss in my division to rigorously evaluate the outcomes of its cost-sharing policies to make sure no patients had been harmed (they weren't). The policy makers took a risk in doing so, but in the end his paper in the *New England Journal of Medicine* vindicated their program. In an impressive display of regulatory intelligence, the province then asked our group to prospectively evaluate its future drug cost-containment initiatives, and even agreed to let us help design some new experimental policies and test their outcomes in a randomized trial.

GRAPPLING WITH DRUG PRICES

In a more information-rich environment, manufacturers of absurdly expensive products that offer little advantage over existing medicines would have to reduce what they charge in order to retain any market share at all. But stronger medicine will be needed to address the fact that Americans still pay up to twice what citizens of other nations do for the same drugs, made by the same multinational companies. Because of those companies' lobbying clout, U.S. price controls don't seem likely in the near future. But other regulatory solutions are much more feasible.

PATENT LAW: BACK TO FIRST PRINCIPLES

When the founding fathers decided to reward inventors by giving them a period of exclusive ownership of their discoveries, the goal was to encourage innovation, not to stifle competition indefinitely. Critics have complained that the large pharmaceutical firms have lost their capacity to innovate. I disagree; their lawyers have been remarkably creative in developing hitherto undreamed-of ways to stretch patent protection for years beyond any plausible duration. Legislators, the courts, and the marketplace have rewarded the companies so handsomely for this kind of innovation that for many it has become as lucrative to play the patent extension game as it is to invest in the demanding and costly task of discovering important new treatments. Enforcing the patent laws' original goals could have two very useful outcomes. First, it would allow generic drugs to enter the marketplace in a timely way as originally intended, making a big dent in drug costs. Second, it would create a healthier scientific and economic climate in which companies will prosper only when they invest in genuinely innovative drug research.

GLOBALIZATION TO THE RESCUE

Protection of intellectual property isn't the only industry petard on which drug companies might find themselves hoisted in the coming years. The same may prove true of the right to move easily across national borders, wherever business opportunity beckons. Consumers can play the globalization game as well, and that may prove to be one of the most potent forces eroding the high price of drugs in the United States. In a worldwide economy, how long will it be possible for the same company to sell the same drug for $4 a pill in the United States, $2 in Canada, and 40 cents in Mexico? Transnational trade in medications is bound to grow, and has already spawned booming businesses of its own—exactly as proponents of globalization would have predicted and advocated. Prohibiting this is as irrational as it is xenophobic; in a truly global economy, such bans cannot last long. Either drug prices will shoot up around the world or they will fall in the United States. Don't bet on the former.

The flap over demon drugs imported from Canada will soon sound like the pathetic whinings of temperance zealots at the end of Prohibition. It is becoming nearly impossible to stop Americans from buying high-quality medications at half price from non-U.S. sources, with or without a prescription. If some manufacturers react by refusing to ship their products to participating pharmacies in those countries, this will just open the door to generic manufacturers in other nations that don't share our views about patent laws. Some of those products will be well made, as potent and pure as those from the American innovator companies. But others will not be; beyond the reach of the FDA, some offshore vendors could indeed sell products that are diluted, counterfeit, or even contaminated. Ironically, this would be made more likely by American manufacturers' denial of product to legitimate clients in Canada and other developed countries. The companies could yet play the pivotal role in bringing about the toxic fantasies they themselves invented.

One solution to that problem would be to create a central authority that could certify the safety and purity of such drugs, backed by the force of law. Such a governmental agency could evaluate the adequacy of a particular vendor's manufacturing processes, and also require a minimum set of credentials in medicine for prescribers, and in pharmacy for dispensers. Some very useful papers, books, and laws were written on these subjects during the period 1900–1910. The ideas they embodied were roundly criticized at the time by conservatives, some manufacturers, and a host of freelance healers, all of whom argued that the government had no right to restrain their lucrative trade. Despite this opposition the Progressive movement prevailed, and set the stage for the flowering of modern prescription drug manufacture and use. Perhaps it's time to reinvent that movement, just in time for its centennial.

PUTTING BUSINESS INTO PERSPECTIVE

Implementing the tough love changes outlined here and in the preceding chapters would impose more marketplace discipline on an increasingly pudgy pharmaceutical industry. It would help to contain the cost of existing drugs and postpone the imposition of price controls. At the same time, it would help redirect manufacturers' R&D efforts toward discovering truly useful new products, the only real way to maintain our balance-of-trade advantage in this sector of the economy. The resulting situation won't be as exorbitantly lucrative as the one the industry enjoyed in the 1980s and 1990s, but those days will soon have gone the way of other implausible economic arrangements like NASDAQ 5,000 and the dot-com bubble.

Despite dire predictions to the contrary, innovative drug discovery will continue, and will probably become better focused. It will still be fueled by NIH-supported research; those who worry about the supply of new medicines would do well to strengthen that key component of the pipeline. The industry's R&D tax credit will help protect its own cutting-edge work, and could even be enhanced to make up for declining revenues from bloated sales of overpriced products. The changes outlined above could trim billions of dollars from the growth path of ballooning governmentally supported drug budgets; those large sums could be recycled into publicly funded biomedical research, where so many important discoveries begin.

Despite short-term dislocations in the prices of drug stocks, all this would have a beneficial effect on businesses in the other 98.5 percent of the economy. U.S. industry is uniquely burdened with the responsibility of paying for the world's most costly drugs and most overpriced medical care for its workers and retirees. Our inefficient and expensive health care system imposes a hefty virtual tax on U.S. corporations—a real disadvantage vis-à-vis competitors in countries with health care systems that are more efficient and/or governmentally subsidized. If the rate of increase in prescription expenditures were slowed, American manufacturers would see moderation in the galloping growth of their outlays for health coverage, and thus in their overall cost of doing business. It would also help take pressure off the increasingly contentious labor disputes over medical benefits that have become so disruptive for both workers and corporations in all sectors of the economy.

THE ULTIMATE FREE MARKET

Like the sorcerer's apprentice, we may find that the accelerating forces in medication use may not stop just where we want them to. Three trends may take us considerably further, eroding the traditional definitions of doctor, patient, pharmacist, and drug maker. We've considered these forces before: the internet, globalization, and free markets. Working in new and inadvertent synergy, their impact may soon resemble that of the universal solvent—that mythical chemical we heard about in high school that could dissolve any material it touched. The joke was that no one could devise a container to put it in.

Taken to its logical extreme, the "killer app" for medicine may be that one day patients will directly access decision-support software on the world wide web to decide which drugs they need, and then use the internet to purchase those drugs directly. Patients have to go to surgeons for their technical capacities and their dexterity, skills we haven't yet succeeded in replicating with circuitry. But why do they come to internists like me? For my fund of medical knowledge, my information-processing and decision-making skills, the fact that I can provide legal access to prescription drugs, and a continuing personal relationship—not necessarily in that order. The last of these, like the surgeon's dexterity, is still a human monopoly. The third is an administrative convention; it is there primarily because of the first two. But if the prescribing decision could draw on the entire universe of medical knowledge as well as all available facts about a given patient, might it be made as well by a computer as a physician? If so, why couldn't the patient just access the computer directly?

The internet is getting smart enough that if provided with the right data inputs, it will soon be able to make many prescribing decisions at least as well as most flesh-and-blood doctors. A well-written program would have all the probabilities and recommendations of medical science at its instantaneous command, something I can't pull off even on a good day. Already dealt multiple blows by the commodification of medicine, our current concept of the personal physician could be in grave danger. The term of art for this is "disintermediation," the high-tech version of what we used to call getting rid of the middleman.

Many pages ago, I cited the old saw about the progress of medicine that held that it wasn't until some time in the early 1900s that the average patient seeing the average doctor had more than a fifty-fifty chance of benefiting from the encounter. In the next decade or two, apart from the enormously important human element, for many common conditions the average patient accessing a computer-assisted diagnosis-and-prescription program could have a fifty-fifty chance of ending up with a more appropriate treatment plan than if he or she had seen the average doctor. With the continuing dehumanization of the medical visit brought on by ever fewer minutes and ever greater frustration by both doctor and patient, it's not clear how much longer we living healers will have the edge on the caring front either. The more the efficiency demands of commercial medicine make doctors act like automatons, the easier it will be to replace many of us with a suite of differential equations.

Although most patients still have to get a prescription from a physician in order to buy a drug from a licensed pharmacist, it's useful to recall that this was not the way things worked before the twentieth century, and it's not clear that it is the only way things will work after the twentieth century. Required prescriptions? A doctor's permission? Fixed prices? Ha! Just as pornography was the leading edge of internet adoption for many Americans, so Viagra was the edge of the wedge in eliminating the need for an in-person doctor or local pharmacist to obtain a prescription drug. Log on to any search engine, type in those six letters, and you'll be flooded with websites—many of them offshore—that will ask you a few questions, take your credit card number, and FedEx you a handsome supply of little blue pills overnight. Viagra has quickly been followed by blood pressure pills, arthritis pills, insulin, and nearly everything else—the sites are cropping up like mushrooms. The process raises important problems of product authenticity and quality control that are real, but not insurmountable.

In controlled doses, the automation of prescribing could even have some good outcomes. Consider sore throats, urinary tract infections, or hypertension, some of the most common problems in primary care. What would the drug regimens for each look like if devised by an expert-built decision tree using information provided by the patient, aided by a technician to take the throat or urine culture or measure the blood pressure? The prescriptions would be based on the best current information, and would surely result in far less improper antibiotic use for the first two conditions, and less reliance on overpriced drugs-of-the-moment for the last. Such consultations would be available instantaneously at any hour of the day or night, and their unit cost would be minuscule. At the end of the encounter the recommended drug (if any) and dose would appear on the screen; a few clicks later the patient could log on to his or her favorite website to buy the medicine.

This vision wouldn't mean the end of doctoring, but it would sure change the power relationships in the clinical encounter. If patients can subscribe to clinical decision-making software and patronize freestanding technicians to take their blood pressure or listen to their lungs or draw their blood, and if they don't need my legal imprimatur to buy their algorithm-recommended medicines on the web, what am I still good for? I had better offer something valuable in the human domain, or I'm professional road-kill littering the information highway.

There is one aspect of medicine that will surely survive our universal sol-vent: the need for a compassionate, competent person to help another con-front the suffering of illness. It is the oldest aspect of medicine, it has been the most fragile in our recent upheavals, but it may prove to be the most durable in the face of the changes that are coming.

Prescribing could thus join the long list of occupations that had to adapt to new technology; John Henry faced a similar problem. So did artists, with the advent of photography in the mid-nineteenth century. Painters who continued in the realist mode eventually became passé. But the change also led eventually to van Gogh, Monet, and Picasso, who each offered some-thing a mere camera could not. It will be interesting to see what parallel developments await medicine as technology continues to transform the present realities of drug use.

SO HERE IS WHERE we've ended up. We can take concrete steps to assemble the evidence about the comparative effectiveness and safety of similar drugs; to stack up those attributes against the drugs' costs; and to disseminate that information to doctors and patients to improve their medication choices. We can do those things, and we must. It will help blunt the unsustainable rise in the nation's drug costs, and will improve clinical outcomes for patients who have access to care. But it won't be enough to address one problem we have not yet considered: many Americans cannot get the medi-cines they need because they have no health insurance. Curing that aspect of our drug-use problem will take more than just palliation; it will require us to think outside the medicine box and deal with some thorny underlying policy issues. Some aspects of prescription drug use can be healed only by changing the larger context of the health care system as a whole.

CONFRONTING THE BIG PICTURE

The vision of medicine as just another business has made it difficult for the United States to provide the universal drug coverage that virtually every other advanced industrial nation offers. This problem will be exacerbated by the cost-increasing structure of the new Medicare drug benefit. With so many doctors functioning as small entrepreneurs or working on a piece-work basis for large insurers, and with few means in place to constrain the drug-use preferences of most patients and physicians, simply increasing drug coverage is likely to lead to even heavier promotion and use of the most expensive products. Patients will demand them, as the direct-to-consumer ads prompt them to do. Most physicians, primed by "market conditioning" and other promotion aimed at them, will have little incentive to resist. The drain on the federal Treasury will grow to a torrent.

The problem that will haunt the new Medicare drug program is the same one that has stymied implementation of a universal drug entitlement for all patients. We cannot afford to further expand (or even to maintain) a medical care system driven by the premise that all participants—insurance companies, specialists, primary-care physicians, HMOs, patients, hospitals, drug makers, device makers—are expected to "work the system" for their own benefit, and if necessary at the expense of the other participants.

Most proposed policy solutions for health care in general and drug coverage in particular, including the new Medicare drug benefit, originate from stale perspectives. Traditionally, conservatives have resisted generous public funding, even where health is concerned. Instead, they have pushed for the transfer of medical care payment and delivery into private hands, with consequent reduction in the resources available to the public sector. Liberals have called for increasing governmental support of entitlements within our existing bizarre bazaar of commercial medicine, hoping that throwing even more money at the problem will fix it. Others on the left have concluded that simply having the government run most of health care would be the best possible answer. Such proposals may well flow from a love of humanity, but it is useful here to recall the definition of love as the triumph of imagination over intelligence.

When it comes to medications and other aspects of health policy, workable solutions to our problems of access, affordability, and appropriate use will require us to move beyond conventional perspectives of conservative and liberal, and instead to build on what works best in the vision of each—a policy style that's been called ideologically androgynous. Conservatives will need to take a hard look at the waste and inequities that the commercialization of health care has created. For their part, liberals will need to keep an open mind about the efficiencies and responsiveness that a pluralistic system could offer, if properly tamed and closely regulated. The left will also have to consider whether a decentralized system of care, coupled with gentle economic incentives for doctors and patients to use resources wisely, might promote rather than threaten our goal of universal access, affordability, and accountability.

The idea would be to take advantage of the pluralism that has enabled America to become innovative and successful in other aspects of the economy. But how can we move in this direction without hurtling into the all-against-all game-the-system vision that has worked out so badly in medicine? From the left we would take the bedrock assumption that every American should have a right to affordable, quality health care. Supporting that access is the responsibility of all, mediated the same way we pay for other social goods—through taxation. From the right would come the insight that giving people choices can help maximize quality and value. But we would not jump to the foolish premise that medical goods and services can simply be treated as if they were part of a well-functioning free market, which health care never was and probably never can be.

A COMPREHENSIVE VISION

One good way to give medical "power to the people" would be for the government to ensure that every American has coverage enough to buy a respectable basic health insurance package of his or her choice—and to be respectable, it would have to provide a good drug benefit. Medical services would be delivered through a pluralistic collection of heavily regulated comprehensive health care organizations, among which consumers could choose. Each would be required by law to provide a defined set of core benefits. Ideally, I would prefer such organizations to be run on a not-for-profit basis, to prevent the abuses that have been so common in for-profit health care insurance companies. However, because so much American medicine has been privatized in the last two decades, and because these interests are so powerful politically, it will be hard to reach this goal in the near future. Failing that, all such organizations would be rigorously supervised by an active and aggressive regulatory body. Legislation would forbid the practices that have given many managed care companies such a bad name, including the reluctance to enroll sick people, and unwillingness to pay for expensive needed drugs and services. Whatever its corporate structure, no health care organization would be permitted to collect a large excess of premiums over amounts spent on direct patient care. Requiring and enforcing a basic benefit package would make it impossible to compete or profit on the basis of reduced provision of services.

In this vision, every American would have a tax-funded voucher that would be used to enroll in the system of his or her choice, but for nothing else. People could pay more out of pocket if they wanted to purchase amenities like unlimited specialist visits or diagnostic imaging tests, house calls, private hospital rooms, cosmetic surgery, or nonformulary drugs. Government would monitor and regulate these organizations very closely, but otherwise would get out of the way. Employers could escape their increasingly onerous role of health care broker. Most would be pleased to be rid of this middleman function as long as the transition were revenue-neutral. This would give consumers more choices of plans to join, and make it easier to leave one care system and enroll in another with considerable freedom. But no one could opt out of securing basic coverage, just as no car owner can opt out of auto liability insurance in most states.

These plans would compete on the basis of quality, not through a "race to the bottom" in charging the lowest premiums. Consumer choice would be exercised by deciding which regulated health care system to invest one's voucher in, and which physicians to consult within that system. This is where choosing would make the most sense, rather than at the level of particular clinical decisions like which heart medicine to buy. The organization one signed up with in any given year would be an integrated system that provides (and doesn't simply pay for) primary care, medications, specialist consultations, hospitalization, and all diagnostic tests. For drugs, this would overcome the current dysfunctional separation between prescriber, pharmacist, patient, and payer, each in a separate—often competing—economic sphere. Instead, they could all work together as part of the same health care organization and share a common computer-based information system. Doctors would be more accessible and accountable for participation in educational and quality-improvement programs, since these would be provided by the organization that employs them. The pharmacist who dispenses a prescription would be a member of the same team as the physician who wrote it. Patients would not have to worry that their doctor was denying them a needed medication because of some ulterior financial motive on his part or that of the health care system, as such profit-based incentives would be forbidden by law.

Even if it were not possible to redefine all HMOs and other insurers as nonprofits, some of their worst excesses could be contained by aggressive legislation. Every organization would be required to offer a comprehensive formulary of medications in all categories, but would not be required to pay for every prescription drug on the market. Instead, each could choose which products in a class it offered, and would be able to negotiate with manufacturers to get the best prices in exchange for inclusion on the covered drug list. That vital flexibility would be nearly impossible to achieve in a single government-run system.

THE POWER OF DATA

To remain eligible to accept patients' health care vouchers, each organization would have to participate in an intense program of data-driven accountability. Every year, each would be required to report information on a wide variety of utilization patterns, expenditures, and outcomes to answer questions like these:

- What fraction of voucher-derived revenues was spent on direct medical care, and how much for administration or other purposes?
- How was the organization ranked by its enrollees in a standardized national survey of patient satisfaction?
- What is the ratio of practicing full-time clinicians to patients?
- What is the median length of an office visit?
- How many physicians have recently passed board certification renewal or other competency testing?
- What is the annual rate of disenrollment, broken down by age group and gender?

There would also be a host of condition-specific questions that could be readily answered from the system's information systems. A few examples of some drug-related measures:

- What proportion of hypertensive patients have their blood pressure in good control?
- What is the rate of noncompliance in patients taking specific medications chronically, and what programs are in place to address it?
- Is the rate of diagnosis and treatment of depression above or below the expected rate predicted by the system's demographics?
- Of patients on anticoagulants, what proportion have had the laboratory tests required for safe use, and how many are in the proper therapeutic range?
- Are tests to evaluate cholesterol levels, bone density, or glaucoma being done at the appropriate frequency, and are patients with abnormal tests being treated properly?

The data needed to respond to most of these questions can be gathered if an organization's computer systems are adequate—this would be a necessity in any case. The results would guide regulators in their oversight responsibilities and consumers in their choices. Outcomes of annual audits would be made widely available, something like the *U.S. News and World Report* rankings of hospitals and colleges that so fascinate consumers. A recurring pattern of poor performance on quality measures, high disenrollment rates, or other signs of problems would lead to increased regulatory scrutiny and then to stiff economic sanctions. Such data would also provide health services researchers and epidemiologists with nearly limitless opportunities for useful studies that could inform ongoing quality improvement programs.

With such scrutiny and tight controls in place, over time the hot money of investors eager for quick profits would flee for-profit HMOs and insurers as the industry came to look more like a well-regulated public utility (remember them?). That would leave the sector a bit leaner fiscally, but dominated by those whose main interest is in providing appropriate medical care and being paid fairly to do so.

An overview of this vision was necessary to convey some understanding of how much easier it would be to choose, pay for, and assess drugs in a saner system of comprehensive health care delivery. The benefits would extend far beyond covering the uninsured. For all patients, there would be far less wasteful working at cross-purposes. Each system would have the scale and the wherewithal to run programs to keep physicians educated about rational and cost-effective drug choices, to communicate with patients about their medicines in a non-product-driven way, and to monitor the effectiveness of those interventions. Bringing together primary care, specialist consultations, hospitalizations, laboratory testing, and prescriptions in the same organizational structure would marshal powerful information to manage the quality of medication use and its outcomes.

Far from being implausible, nearly all aspects of this approach to organizing and funding health care are already in place and working rather well in various combinations throughout the industrialized world, and in some of this nation's more advanced health care systems. The current U.S. mode of piecework health care delivery, with its all-against-all assumptions, its perverse incentives, its absurdly high costs, its embarrassingly large numbers of uninsureds, its tattered patchwork of uncoordinated services, and its frequent denial of care—*that* is the system that's implausible.

There is much that we can do now to improve medication use even within the framework of our current dysfunctional nonsystem; we can't afford to wait for fundamental change before we take some of the more modest steps that lie before us. But in the end, the most powerful medicine for curing our shared drug problem will be reorganizing the way we deliver and pay for all of medical care in a more sensible, efficient, and humane way.

EPILOGUE:
THE TRIPLE-EDGED SWORD

In shaping the nation's approach to medications, it would be helpful for all stakeholders—patients, doctors, policy makers, manufacturers—to ask themselves some old questions posed by Rabbi Hillel around 20 B.C. in a very different context:

> If I am not for myself, who will be for me?
> And if I am for myself only, what am I?
> And if not now, when?

We've gotten pretty good at asking the first question. Maybe it's time we all moved on to the next two.

It has been said that the mark of a good scientist is the ability to keep two contradictory ideas in mind at the same time. The same skill is needed to get a thoughtful grip on how we can make the best use of prescription drugs. The answers are within reach, but we won't find them if we settle for simplistic one-sided solutions. There are many paradoxes to confront, but we can take comfort in realizing that in a paradox, the contradictions may be more apparent than real.

THE RANDOMIZED CONTROLLED TRIAL is the best way ever invented to determine whether a drug works or is better than another; not only is it an unparalleled scientific tool, it is also a social tool for informing policy. But it leaves us far short of all the answers we need about how to deploy treatments in the real world of complex patients seen by typical doctors in everyday settings.

By contrast, observational studies can lead us in horribly wrong directions if they are done imperfectly, or if their results are overinterpreted. Yet they remain our best hope for answering hundreds of pressing drug questions for which randomized trials simply can't or won't be done.

Comparing a drug's cost to its impact on disability and death can help us understand which treatments provide the best value per dollar for a given condition, and can help us solve our growing problem of drug affordability. But pushed too far, such analyses can reach beyond their quantitative and ethical limits and risk becoming both silly and immoral.

Despite the obvious triumph of free markets over state-run economies, a laissez-faire approach is unlikely to provide the solutions we need in caring for the sick or disabled. Relying on commerce alone to allocate drugs and other medical resources properly can cause exorbitant waste as well as unconscionable pain to those who lack the knowledge or the capital to play the game. Yet patients will do best if they are given some individual choice about the health care systems in which they participate.

Many pharmaceutical company researchers perform vital work developing useful new medicines, and the industry can be one important source of drug discoveries as well as an innovation engine for the economy as a whole. Yet few benefit when the creative potential of that industry is diverted into promotion-driven distractions that produce overpriced products of little value, or into corporate efforts to protect dangerous drugs rather than the patients who take them.

We waste billions of dollars a year on prescription drugs that are excessively priced, poorly prescribed, or improperly taken. Yet for a sum no greater than our current drug budget, medications could provide every American with the most productive and cost-effective interventions in all of health care.

WE LIVE AT the dawn of an amazing new era. Decades of brilliant progress in physiology, pharmacology, biochemistry, and now genetics have given us a capacity to prevent and treat disease that would have seemed impossible to our ancestors, or even our grandparents. Small miracles occur millions of times every day thanks to these accomplishments. But every day people also become ill or die when they don't get the drugs they need, either because their doctors didn't prescribe them or because they couldn't afford to pay for them or because they failed to take them. And the triumph of modern pharmacology continues to be marred by lethal adverse effects that could have been averted.

The work of generations of researchers and physicians has produced a triple-edged medication sword with awesome powers to help or harm in the domains of benefits, risks, and cost. That sword must be wielded carefully by all of us—patients, doctors, pharmacists, nurses, policy makers, drug companies, regulators, and all the organizations that pay the bills in our balkanized medical care system. In our own ways, each of us can use that sword to fight the illnesses that plague our species. Or we can swing it recklessly and inflict needless wounds on ourselves and on each other. With the stakes on all fronts higher than ever in human history, the choices we make will determine how well we use this powerful gift.

NOTES

These notes are intended both for the general reader who wants to learn more about a particular topic and for medical professionals and researchers who want to investigate an area in greater depth. Abstracts to articles in the medical literature can be accessed at no cost by anyone with internet access via www.nlm.nih.gov. This is the PubMed site of the National Library of Medicine, which provides access to over 12 million medical citations from some 4,600 journals going back to the mid-1960s. These generally include the abstract for a given paper; full text is increasingly available online as well, and is sometimes free. References are also listed below for subject-specific websites through which a reader can follow up on particular topics of interest. The frequency of citations to the work of our group merely reflects the book's focus on that research; many other important citations from other centers could have been listed if space had permitted. These notes are not intended to be exhaustive, but to present a limited number of representative articles and links. Additional material, updates, links to references, and corrections will be periodically added at the book's website, www.powerfulmedicines.org.

PROLOGUE: DIFFERENT STROKES

4 Stroke prevention in atrial fibrillation: Evidence had accumulated by the early 1990s that drugs like warfarin could reduce the risk of stroke by two thirds in such patients. See, for example, a review by the Atrial Fibrillation Investigators, "Risk Factors for Stroke and Efficacy of Antithrombotic Therapy in Atrial Fibrillation," *Archives of Internal Medicine* 154 (1994): 1449–1457.

6 PPA and stroke: W. N. Kernan et al., "Phenylpropanolamine and the Risk of Hemorrhagic Stroke," *New England Journal of Medicine* 343 (2000): 1826–1832.

8 Underuse of drugs in patients who can't afford them: M. A. Steinman, L. P. Sands, and K. E. Covinsky, "Self-Restriction of Medications Due to Costs in Seniors Without Prescription Coverage," *Journal of General Internal Medicine* 16 (2001): 793–799.

9 Drugs vs. angioplasty in heart attack: T. Aversano et al., "Thrombolytic Therapy vs. Primary Percutaneous Coronary Intervention for Myocardial Infarction," *Journal of the American Medical Association* 287 (2002): 1943–1951.

10 Comparison of commonly used medications for high blood pressure: ALLHAT Officers, "The Antihypertensive and Lipid-Lowering Treatment to Prevent Heart Attack Trial (ALLHAT)," *Journal of the American Medical Association* 288 (2002): 2981–2997. Numerous follow-up papers appeared after the publication of ALLHAT, including new clinical trial data; several came to different conclusions. These can be found via the "Related Articles" link in PubMed.

14 Deaths from Posicor: A former FDA official commented on this in a letter to the *British Medical Journal*. See L. Landow, "FDA Approves Drugs Even When Experts on Its Advisory Panels Raise Safety Questions," *British Medical Journal* 318 (1999): 944. See also L. W. Po and W. Y. Zhang, "What Lessons Can Be Learnt from Withdrawal of Mibefradil from the Market?" *Lancet* 351 (1998): 1829.

16 Medications as a cause of reduced death from cardiovascular disease: See M. J. Wald and M. R. Law, "A Strategy to Reduce Cardiovascular Disease by More Than 80%," *British Medical Journal* 326 (2003):1419–1420.

1: THE PREGNANT MARE'S LESSON

27 Problematic evidence that estrogens prevent heart disease: For example, see F. Grodstein et al., "A Prospective, Observational Study of Postmenopausal Hormone Therapy and Primary Prevention of Cardiovascular Disease," *Annals of Internal Medicine* 133 (2000): 933–941.

28 Early pro-estrogen literature directed at patients: R. A. Wilson, *Feminine Forever* (New York: Evans and Lippincott, 1966).

31 Adverse effects of hormone replacement therapy: The first large randomized controlled trial to test long-term estrogen replacement therapy in women was the HERS study: S. Hulley et al., "Randomized Trial of Estrogen Plus Progestin for Secondary Prevention of Coronary Heart Disease in Postmenopausal Women," *Journal of the American Medical Association* 280 (1998): 605–613. The main results of the Women's Health Initiative study were published as J. E. Roussouw et al., "Risks and Benefits of Estrogen Plus Progestin in Healthy Post-Menopausal Women," *Journal of the American Medical Association* 288 (2002): 321–333. On the doubling of risk of developing symptoms of Alzheimer's-like senility with estrogen use: S. A. Shumaker et al., "Estrogen Plus Progestin and the Incidence of Dementia and Mild Cognitive Impairment in Post-Menopausal Women," *Journal of the American Medical Association* 289 (2003): 2651–2662.

32 The Tuskegee experiment: See James H. Jones, *Bad Blood: The Tuskegee Syphilis Experiment* (New York: Free Press, 1993).

2: LEAVING THE DARK AGES BEHIND, MOSTLY

39 The plague: Barbara Tuchman, *A Distant Mirror: The Calamitous Fourteenth Century* (New York: Knopf, 1978).

40 Holmes on drugs: "Lecture at Harvard Medical School," cited in John Bartlett, *Bartlett's Familiar Quotations,* 10th ed. (Boston: Little, Brown, 1919).

43 Evolution of drug studies: See Harry Marks, *The Progress of Experiment: Science and Therapeutic Reform in the United States, 1900–1990* (Cambridge: Cambridge University Press, 1997).

43 History of the FDA and the evolution of drug regulatory policy: See Philip J. Hilts, *Protecting America's Health: The FDA, Business, and One Hundred Years of Regulation* (New York: Knopf, 2003).

47 Placebo effect: L. Lasagna et al., "A Study of the Placebo Response," *American Journal of Medicine* 16 (1954): 770–779. See also H. L. Fields and D. D. Price, "Toward a Neurobiology of Placebo Analgesia," in A. Harrington, ed., *The Placebo Effect: An Interdisciplinary Exploration* (Cambridge, Mass.: Harvard University Press, 1997).

48 The first clinical trial: Daniel 1.

50 Scurvy: James Lind, *A Treatise on the Scurvy* (Edinburgh: A. Kincaid and A. Donaldson, 1753). Excerpts from the book and much related material on the evolution and logic of clinical trials can be found on a website created by the Royal College of Physicians of Edinburgh to commemorate the 250th anniversary of the publication of Lind's work: www.jameslindlibrary.org.

54 Karl Popper: His most important work in this connection is *Logik der Forschung* (*The Logic of Scientific Discovery*) (Vienna: Julius Springer Verlag, 1935). He wrote on the implications of his work for social policy in *The Open Society and Its Enemies* (London: Routledge, 1945). A website devoted to his work can be found at www.eeng.dcu.ie/~tkpw/.

57 Statistical significance: An interactive way to experience the logic of the cointoss experiment is at www.probability.ca/jeff/java/utday/. A good discussion of the perils of simpleminded reliance on arbitrary definitions of statistical significance can be found in Kenneth J. Rothman, *Epidemiology: An Introduction* (New York: Oxford University Press, 2002), Ch. 6.

60 Sodom and Gomorrah: Genesis 18–19.

63 Existentialism and medical practice: Albert Camus, *The Plague,* trans. Stuart Gilbert (New York: Vintage, 1991; orig. ed., 1948).

64 Supplements: The Dietary Supplement Health and Education Act of 1994 is Public Law No. 103-417. See also P. B. Fontanarossa, D. Rennie, and C. D. DeAngelis, "The Need for Regulation of Dietary Supplements—Lessons from Ephedra," *Journal of the American Medical Association* 289 (2003): 1568–1570; C. Morris and J. Avorn, "Internet Marketing of Herbal Products," *Journal of the American Medical Association* 290 (2003): 1505–1509.

67 Postmodernism: An important but painfully obscure work applying a kind of postmodernist analysis to medicine is Michel Foucault, *The Birth of the Clinic: An Archaeology of Medical Perception* (New York: Vintage, 1994; orig. ed., 1963).

3: THE FAT IS IN THE FIRE

72 Paracelsus: The National Library of Medicine established a Paracelsus home page to commemorate the 500th anniversary of his birth. It contains an excellent overview of his work and of the world of alchemy in which it occurred: www.nlm.nih.gov/exhibition/paracelsus/paracelsus_1.html.

73 Wyeth: This company is not likely to win an award from the National Organization for Women; its corporate umbrella also came to include the manufacturer of the Dalkon Shield, an intrauterine contraceptive device that produced sterility and serious infections, and Norplant, a sustained-release birth-control delivery system that led to frequent side effects, widespread litigation, and concerns over its effectiveness; it has now been taken off the U.S. market.

74 The fen-phen story is told in great detail in Alicia Mundy, *Dispensing with the Truth* (New York: St. Martin's, 2001). The pivotal French study was L. Abenheim et al., "Appetite Suppressant Drugs and the Risk of Primary Pulmonary Hypertension," *New England Journal of Medicine* 335 (1996): 609–616.

79 Brigham letter to the editor: K. Dillon, K. Putnam, and J. Avorn, "Death from Irreversible Pulmonary Hypertension Associated with Short-Term Use of Fenfluramine and Phentermine," *Journal of the American Medical Association* 278 (1997): 1320. The same case was described in E. J. Mark et al., "Fatal Pulmonary Hypertension Associated with Short-Term Use of Fenfluramine and Phentermine," *New England Journal of Medicine* 337 (1997): 602–606.

82 Heart valve damage: H. M. Connolly et al., "Valvular Heart Disease Associated with Fenfluramine-Phentermine," *New England Journal of Medicine* 337 (1997): 581–588.

84 FDA's required drug surveillance studies don't get done: Food and Drug Administration, "Report on the Performance of Drugs and Biologics Firms in Conducting Postmarketing Commitment Studies," *Federal Register,* May 21, 2003, pp. 27822–27823. Described at www.fda.gov/bbs/topics/answers/2003/ans.01223. html.

4: TOO SWEET TO BE TRUE

87 *Los Angeles Times* reporting on Rezulin: Much information on the story behind Rezulin's approval was reported by David Willman of the *Los Angeles Times* and published in a series of investigative articles beginning in late 2000.

90 Conflict of interest at NIH: D. Willman, "Drug Maker Hired NIH Researcher," *Los Angeles Times,* December 7, 1998. See also M. Cimons, "NIH Opens Conflict-of-Interest Investigation," *Nature Medicine* 5 (1999): 129–130.

91 The underuse of liver function monitoring in Rezulin patients: D. J. Graham et al., "Liver Enzyme Monitoring in Patients Treated with Troglitazone," *Journal of the American Medical Association* 286 (2001): 831–833.

94 British view of Rezulin debacle: E. A. M. Gale, "Lessons from the Glitazones: A Story of Drug Development," *Lancet* 357 (2001): 1870–1875.

5: COLD COMFORT

100 Yale study: W. N. Kernan et al., "Phenylpropanolamine and the Risk of Hemorrhagic Stroke," *New England Journal of Medicine* 343 (2000): 1826–1832.

6: GETTING RISKS RIGHT

105 John Snow: The most recent and comprehensive retelling of his story is in Peter Vinten et al., *Cholera, Chloroform and the Science of Medicine: A Life of John Snow* (Oxford: Oxford University Press, 2003). A fine website describing Snow's work is maintained by the UCLA Department of Epidemiology: www.ph.ucla.edu/epi/snow.html.

106 Bob Dylan: "Subterranean Homesick Blues" is from his 1965 album *Bringing It All Back Home,* an appropriate title in this context.

112 Russian trio: The programming for all of the epidemiological studies from our group was conducted by Igor Choodnovskiy, Helen Mogun, and Raisa Levin, to whom I am deeply indebted.

114 Pharmacoepidemiology in general: A good introduction to this field is Brian Strom, *Pharmacoepidemiology* (New York: Wiley, 2000). In addition to the Rothman book cited in the notes to Chapter 2, a more advanced text is his *Modern Epidemiology* (Philadelphia: Lippincott, Williams & Wilkins, 1998).

116 Calcium-channel blockers and heart attacks: B. M. Psaty et al., "The Risk of Myocardial Infarction Associated with Antihypertensive Drug Therapies," *Journal of the American Medical Association* 274 (1995): 620–625.

117 Glaucoma medications and lung disease: J. Avorn et al., "Adverse Pulmonary Effects of Topical Beta-Blockers Used in the Treatment of Glaucoma," *Journal of Glaucoma* 2 (1993): 158–165.

118 Prozac and suicidal tendencies: M. H. Teicher, C. Glod, and J. O. Cole, "Emergence of Intense Suicidal Preoccupation During Fluoxitene Treatment," *American Journal of Psychiatry* 147 (1990): 207–210.

120 Bendectin: A comprehensive evaluation of the published research concluded that it was definitely not a teratogen (cause of birth defects), but that its notorious history of litigation made it "the most prevalent *tortogen*": R. L. Brent, "Bendectin: Review of the Medical Literature of a Comprehensively Studied Human Non-Teratogen," *Reproductive Toxicology* 9 (1995): 337–349.

121 Use of cholesterol drugs and "immortality": R. J. Glynn et al., "Paradoxical Relations of Drug Treatment with Mortality in Older Persons," *Epidemiology* 12 (2001): 682–689.

123 Berton Roueche, *Eleven Blue Men and Other Narratives of Medical Detection* (Boston: Little, Brown, 1953).

130 Aging and medical care: See J. Avorn, "Medicine, Health, and the Geriatric Transformation," *Daedalus* 115 (1986): 211–225. This paper was reprinted in A. Pifer and L. Bronte, eds., *Our Aging Society: Paradox and Promise* (New York: Norton, 1986). The book is a good overview of the effects of a growing elderly population on many aspects of American life.

132 For a fuller discussion of medication effects in the elderly, see J. Avorn, J. H. Gurwitz, and P. Rochon, "Principles of Pharmacology," in C. Cassel et al., eds., *Geriatric Medicine,* 4th ed. (New York: Springer, 2003). This text is one of the best books on geriatrics overall. Also see J. Avorn and P. S. Wang, "Prescribing Psychotropic Drugs for the Elderly: Epidemiologic and Policy Considerations," in C. Salzman, ed., *Clinical Geriatric Psychopharmacology,* 4th ed. (New York: McGraw-Hill, 2004).

133 Underrepresentation of elderly in drug studies: J. H. Gurwitz, N. Col, and J. Avorn, "Exclusion of Elderly and Women from Clinical Trials in Acute Myocardial Infarction," *Journal of the American Medical Association* 268 (1992): 1417–1422. An update of these findings, with distressingly similar results, appeared nine years later in *Journal of the American Medical Association* 286 (2001): 708–713.

135 Medication-induced symptoms mistaken for new Parkinson's disease: J. Avorn et al., "Neuroleptic Drug Exposure and Treatment of Parkinsonism in the Elderly: A Case-Control Study," *American Journal of Medicine* 99 (1995): 48–54. See also J. Avorn et al., "Increased Incidence of L-dopa Therapy Following Metoclopramide Use," *Journal of the American Medical Association* 274 (1995): 1780–1782; J. Avorn et al., "Clinical Assessment of Extra-Pyramidal Signs in Nursing Home Patients Given Antipsychotic Medication," *Archives of Internal Medicine* 154 (1994): 1113–1117; S. C. Kalish et al., "Antipsychotic Prescribing Patterns and the Treatment of Extra-Pyramidal Symptoms in Older People," *Journal of the American Geriatrics Society* 43 (1995): 967–973. Much of this work was funded by the National Institute on Aging of the NIH.

142 Faustus: An appealing little website prepared by Professor D. L. Ashliman pulls together several Faust legends and links to a variety of literary and musical variations on this theme: www.pitt.edu/~dash/faust.html.

144 Making structured decisions in the face of uncertainty: The classic work here is Howard Raiffa, *Decision Analysis* (New York: McGraw-Hill, 1997; orig. ed., 1968).

145 Clinical uses of decision analysis: The standard reference work is Marthe Gold, Siegel Gold, and Milton Weinstein, *Cost-Effectiveness in Health and Medicine* (New York: Oxford University Press, 1996).

146 Anticoagulation to prevent stroke: See Atrial Fibrillation Investigators, "Risk Factors for Stroke and Efficacy of Antithrombotic Therapy in Atrial Fibrillation," *Archives of Internal Medicine* 154 (1994): 1449–1457.

9: IMPERFECT MEASURES

152 An earlier version of some of the arguments presented here first appeared in J. Avorn, "Benefit and Cost Analysis in Geriatric Care: Turning Age Discrimination into Health Policy," *New England Journal of Medicine* 310 (1984): 1294–1301.

153 Quantifying the quality-of-life contribution of Viagra: K. J. Smith and M. S. Roberts, "The Cost-Effectiveness of Sildenafil," *Annals of Internal Medicine* 132 (2000): 933–937.

154 Framing and decision making: A comprehensive collection of the work of the two cognitive psychologists who founded this area of inquiry: Daniel Kahneman and Amos Tversky, eds., *Choices, Values, and Frames* (Cambridge: Cambridge University Press, 2000). An early seminal paper was A. Tversky and D. Kahneman, "The Framing of Decisions and the Psychology of Choice," *Science* 211 (1981): 453–458.

154 Bernoulli's paradox: The original paper, first published in 1738, was reprinted 216 years later as D. Bernoulli, "Exposition of a New Theory on the Measurement of Risk," *Econometrica* 22 (1954): 23–36.

157 NICE is discussed further in Chapter 20.

158 Improving patient decision making: A brief recent overview is A. M. O'Connor et al., "Standard Consultations Are Not Enough to Ensure Decision Quality Regarding Preference-Sensitive Options," *Journal of the National Cancer Institute* 95 (2003): 570–571.

10: WHOSE RISK IS IT, ANYWAY?

164 *PDR: Physicians' Desk Reference,* 57th ed. (Montvale, N.J.: Thomson Publishing, 2003).

166 Communicating about risk: D. Powell and W. Leiss, *Mad Cows and Mother's Milk: The Perils of Poor Risk Communication* (Montreal: McGill-Queen's University Press, 1997).

169 Viagra risk: R. A. Kloner, "Sex and the Patient with Cardiovascular Risk Factors," *American Journal of Medicine* 109, supp. A (2000): 13S–21S.

11: A BALANCING ACT

174 Treatment of septic shock with Activated Protein C: The pivotal study was first published as G. R. Bernard et al., "Efficacy and Safety of Recombinant Human Activated Protein C for Severe Sepsis," *New England Journal of Medicine* 344 (2001): 699–709. For follow-up studies and debate, see also *New England Journal of Medicine* 347 (2002): 993–1000 and 1027–1034.

175 FDA advisory committee reports: The FDA website (www.fda.gov) has a search function that makes it possible to find all mentions of any drug throughout the agency's site. Adding "Advisory Committee" to the search term will access the public transcripts of a panel's deliberations.

180 Thalidomide and risk management: G. J. Annas and S. Elias, "Thalidomide and the *Titanic:* Reconstructing the Technology Tragedies of the 20th Century," *American Journal of Public Health* 89 (1999): 98–101.

180 Accutane and pregnancy: A. A. Mitchell et al., "A Pregnancy-Prevention Program in Women of Childbearing Age Receiving Isotretinoin," *New England Journal of Medicine* 333 (1995): 124–125.

184 Drug-induced illness in long-term-care facilities: J. H. Gurwitz et al., "Incidence and Preventability of Adverse Drug Events in Nursing Homes," *American Journal of Medicine* 109 (2000): 87–94.

12: LIVE CHEAP OR DIE

194 Reductions in essential drug use after New Hampshire "cap" policy: S. B. Soumerai, J. Avorn, S. Gortmaker, et al., "Payment Restrictions for Prescription Drugs in Medicaid: Effects on Therapy, Cost, and Equity," *New England Journal of Medicine* 317 (1987): 550–556. Its effects on clinical outcomes: S. B. Soumerai, D. Ross-Degnan, J. Avorn, et al., "Effects of Medicaid Drug-Payment Limits on Admission to Hospitals and Nursing Homes," *New England Journal of Medicine* 325 (1991): 1072–1077.

196 Current state policies to limit drug expenses under Medicaid, as well as many other developments related to prescription drug coverage, are tracked well on the website of the Henry J. Kaiser Family Foundation: www.kff.org.

13: FILLING THE PIPELINE

199 OTA report on R&D and pharmaceutical companies: Office of Technology Assessment, *Pharmaceutical R&D: Costs, Risks, and Returns* (Washington, D.C.: Government Printing Office, 1993).

199 Public research funding and drug development: See M. Gluck, *Federal Policies Affecting the Cost and Availability of New Pharmaceuticals* (Washington, D.C.: Georgetown University Institute for Health Care Research, 2002). This work was commissioned by the Henry J. Kaiser Family Foundation and is available on their website: www.kff.org/content/2002/3254/GluckFinalReportweb3254.pdf.

201 Coxib discovery: U.S. Patent No. 6,048,850 (issued April 11, 2000): "Method of Inhibiting Prostaglandin Synthesis in a Human Host." Judge Larimer's decision: *University of Rochester v. G. D. Searle,* 249 F. Supp. 2d 216 (Western Dist. New York 2003).

202 Vioxx side effects: D. H. Solomon et al., "Relationship Between Selective Cyclooxygenase-2 Inhibitors and Acute Myocardial Infarction in Older Adults," *Circulation* 109 (2004): 2068–2073.

203 Report on public funding and Taxol, requested by Senator Wyden: General Accounting Office, *NIH–Private Sector Partnership in the Development of Taxol* (Washington, D.C.: General Accounting Office, 2003). Available at www.gao.gov/cgi-bin/getrpt?GAO-03-829.

204 Innovation and large pharmaceutical companies: National Institute for Health Care Management, *Changing Patterns of Pharmaceutical Innovation* (Washington, D.C.: NIHCM Foundation, 2002). Available at www.nihcm.org/innovations/pdf. A wide-ranging critique of the industry's approach to research

and to business can be found in M. Angell and A. Relman, "America's Other Drug Problem," *The New Republic,* December 16, 2002.

205 Economic analysis of the drug industry: *Health Care Industry Market Update: Pharmaceuticals,* the federal government's calculations about the industry's expenditures, prepared by the Department of Health and Human Services, can be found at www.cms.hhs.gov/reports/hcimu.

206 The Securities and Exchange Commission site containing required corporate filings is www.sec.gov/edgar.shtml.

206 These data are from the report by Families USA, *Profiting from Pain: Where Prescription Drug Dollars Go* (Washington, D.C.: Families USA, 2002). Available at www.familiesusa.org. A few caveats are in order. The subparts of the "sales, general, and administrative" category are generally not broken down in the reports that companies make to the SEC, so we cannot know how much of that lump sum is spent on marketing and advertising on the one hand versus general administration on the other. Most estimates put the industry's direct promotion to prescribers at about $20 billion annually, with another $2 billion spent each year on company-sponsored educational events designed to promote product sales. An additional $3 billion is devoted to direct-to-consumer advertising. Adding in a modest expenditure for the administration of these programs, the total for promotion-related activities comes to nearly $30 billion a year of the $200 billion the nation spends on prescription drugs, or about one out of every seven dollars.

207 The story of Gleevec's discovery: J. Waalen, "Gleevec's Glory Days," *Howard Hughes Medical Institute Bulletin,* December 2001 (www.hhmi.org/bulletin/dec2001/gleevec). For the perspective from the Dana-Farber Cancer Institute, see "Gleevec: The Dana-Farber Connection," *Paths of Progress,* fall/winter 2001 (www.dfci.harvard.edu/res/research/gleevec.asp). The manufacturer's website is www.gleevec.com.

209 Medicare overpayments to oncologists for chemotherapy: Government Accounting Office, *Medicare: Payments for Covered Out-Patient Drugs Exceed Providers' Cost* (Washington, D.C.: GAO, 2001), Report GAO-01-1118, available at www.gao.gov.

213 The growing influence of business in academia: Derek Bok, *Universities in the Marketplace: The Commercialization of Higher Education* (Princeton, N.J.: Princeton University Press, 2003).

14: WHAT THE TRAFFIC WILL BEAR

217 Cost of prescription drugs: The Department of Health and Human Services estimated that the nation would spend $204.7 billion on prescription drugs in 2004. This does not include medications used in hospitals and nursing homes. The figure represents 11.5 percent of total estimated national health expenditures of $1.78 trillion. See *National Health Care Expenditures Projections* at www.cms.hhs.gov/statistics/nhe/projections-2002/.

218 Underuse of drugs by elderly: M. A. Steinman, L. P. Sands, and K. E. Covinsky, "Self-Restriction of Medication Use Due to Cost in Seniors Without Prescription Coverage," *Journal of General Internal Medicine* 16 (2001): 793–799.

220 Cross-national comparison of expenditures on drugs and other health care: Organisation for Economic Co-operation and Development, *Health at a Glance* (Paris: OECD, 2001). Available through www.oecd.org.

220 Five-country survey: This is an ongoing study conducted by researchers at the Harvard School of Public Health, supported by the Commonwealth Fund. Two recent reports are R. J. Blendon et al., "Common Concerns amid Diverse Systems: Health Care Experience in Five Countries," *Health Affairs* 22 (2003):106–121; and R. J. Blendon et al., "Inequities in Health Care: A Five-Country Survey," *Health Affairs* 21 (2002): 182–191. More information on the studies is available at the Commonwealth Fund's website: www.cmwf.org.

225 Statements by the Federal Trade Commission chairman: F. M. Muris, "Competition in the Pharmaceutical Industry," testimony before the U.S. Senate Committee on Commerce, Science, and Transportation, April 23, 2002, and testimony before the U.S. House of Representatives Subcommittee on Health, October 9, 2002. Available at www.ftc.gov.

227 Drug industry profitability: *Fortune,* April 14, 2003.

15: NAVIGATING THE THIRD DIMENSION

240 The economic discussion here also draws on my essay "Benefit and Cost Analysis in Geriatric Care," *New England Journal of Medicine* 310 (1984): 1294–1301.

242 More recent human-capital approaches: C. J. L. Murray and A. D. Lopez, eds., *The Global Burden of Disease* (Cambridge, Mass.: Harvard University Press, 1996). For a skeptical view, see S. Anand and K. Hanson, "Disability-Adjusted Life-Years: A Critical Review," *Journal of Health Economics* 16 (1997): 685–702.

242 Willingness to pay: For two reviews of this and related approaches, see F. D. Johnson, E. E. Fries, and H. S. Banzhaf, "Valuing Morbidity: An Integration of the Willingness-to-Pay and Health-Status Index Literatures," *Journal of Health Economics* 16 (1997): 641–665; and K. Blumenschein and M. Johannesson, "Incorporating Quality of Life Changes into Economic Evaluations of Health Care: An Overview," *Health Policy* 37 (1996): 199–204.

246 Expected utility approach: J. von Neumann and O. Morgenstern, *Theory of Games and Economic Behavior* (Princeton, N.J.: Princeton University Press, 1944).

247 Futilon: These numbers are not so unrealistic; lifelong use of many drugs to manage risk states like high blood pressure or cholesterol yield only about a month of added life, on average, in many subgroups of patients.

250 The GUSTO study: Some controversy continues about the validity of the GUSTO findings, but our discussion gets complicated enough without considering this. For simplicity, we'll ignore those arguments and treat the trial data as if they are the last word on the subject, even though some doubt whether that's true. Our economic analysis was published as S. Kalish, J. H. Gurwitz, H. Krumholz, et al.,

"A Cost-Effectiveness Model of Thrombolytic Therapy for Acute Myocardial Infarction," *Journal of General Internal Medicine* 10 (1995): 321–330. A similar study by investigators at Duke University independently came up with a strikingly similar number in their analysis of the cost-effectiveness of the two drugs.

256 The cost of a quality-adjusted life-year: W. C. Winkelmayer et al., "Health Economic Evaluations: The Special Case of End-Stage Renal Disease Treatment," *Medical Decision Making* 22 (2002): 417–430.

257 The cost of a good erection: K. J. Smith and M. S. Roberts, "The Cost-Effectiveness of Sildenafil," *Annals of Internal Medicine* 132 (2000): 933–937.

259 Utilitarianism: J. Bentham, *An Introduction to the Principles of Morals and Legislation* (Oxford: Blackwell, 1948; orig. ed., 1789).

262 Underuse of statins in Europe: A. K. Mantel et al., "Undertreatment of Hypercholesterolaemia: A Population-Based Study," *British Journal of Clinical Pharmacology* 55 (2003): 389–397.

263 Treating very costly hemophilia patients: A. B. Colowick, R. L. Bohn, J. Avorn, et al., "Immune Tolerance Induction in Hemophilia Patients with Inhibitors: Costly Can Be Cheaper," *Blood* 96 (2000): 1698–1702.

265 The policy aspects of these questions are taken up in Part Five.

16: SIGNALS, NOISE, AND THE BIG VOID

269 Signal transduction: For a good review, see J. D. Scott and T. Pawson, "Cell Communication: The Inside Story," *Scientific American* 282 (2000): 72–79.

273 The ALLHAT study: See ALLHAT Officers, "The Antihypertensive and Lipid-Lowering Treatment to Prevent Heart Attack Trial (ALLHAT)," *Journal of the American Medical Association* 288 (2002): 2981–2997.

275 High-dose chemotherapy with bone marrow transplantation for the treatment of cancer: E. A. Stadtmauer et al., "Conventional-Dose Chemotherapy Compared with High-Dose Chemotherapy Plus Autologous Hematopoietic Stem-Cell Transplantation for Metastatic Breast Cancer," *New England Journal of Medicine* 342 (2000): 1069–1076. For a good overview of the policy aspects of this treatment, see M. M. Mello and T. A. Brennan, "The Controversy over High-Dose Chemotherapy with Autologous Bone Marrow Transplant for Breast Cancer," *Health Affairs* 20 (2001): 101–117.

278 The website for the federal CERTs program is www.certs.hhs.gov.

285 Noncompliance: see M. Monane et al., "Compliance with Antihypertensive Therapy: The Role of Age, Gender, and Race," *American Journal of Public Health* 86 (1996): 1805–1808; J. Avorn et al., "Persistence of Use of Lipid-Lowering Medications: A Cross-National Study," *Journal of the American Medical Association* 279 (1998): 1458–1462; J. S. Benner et al., "Long-Term Deterioration in Persistence with Statin Therapy," *Journal of the American Medical Association* 288 (2002): 455–461.

286 FDA history: The story of the agency's thwarted attempts to require that accurate and impartial patient information be included with prescriptions is well

detailed in a presentation to the agency by consumer advocates: L. D. Sasich and S. M. Wolfe, "Public Citizen's Health Research Group's Comments on the Status of Useful Written Prescription Drug Information for Patients," FDA Docket No. 00N-0352, March 1, 2000; available at www.fda.gov/ohrms/dockets/dailys/00/mar00/032200/co1.pdf. The results of the analysis the FDA commissioned to study the problem can be found in B. L. Svarstad and J. K. Mount, "Evaluation of Written Prescription Information Provided in Community Pharmacies, 2001"; available at www.fda.gov/cder/reports/prescriptionInfo/default/htm.

288 Direct-to-consumer drug advertising: This section is based in part on J. Avorn, "Advertising and Prescription Drugs: Promotion, Education, and the Public's Health," *Health Affairs,* 2003; available at www.healthaffairs.org/webexclusives/Avorn_web_excl_022603.htm.

17: INFORMATIONAL KUDZU

293 Kudzu: Weird pictures of cars and houses overtaken by kudzu overgrowth can be found at www.jjanthony.com/kudzu/.

294 Early study of the effect of advertising versus data on doctors' drug knowledge: J. Avorn, M. Chen, and R. Hartley. "Scientific vs. Commercial Sources of Influence on Physician Prescribing Behavior," *American Journal of Medicine* 73 (1982): 4–8.

298 Promotion-driven patterns of prescribing for high blood pressure: M. Monane et al., "Trends in Medication Choices for Hypertension in the Elderly: The Decline of the Thiazides," *Hypertension* 125 (1995): 1045–1051. See also E. L. Knight et al., "Failure of Evidence-Based Medicine in the Treatment of Hypertension in Older Patients," *Journal of General Internal Medicine* 133 (2000): 128–135.

303 How-to manual for drug detailers: D. Currier and J. Frost, *Be Brief, Be Bright, Be Gone: Career Essentials for Pharmaceutical Representatives* (San Jose, Calif.: Writers Club Press, 2001).

305 Drug industry's data: *Industry Profile, 2002* (Washington, D.C.: Pharmaceutical Research and Manufacturers of America, 2002). Available at www.phrma.org.

305 Drug promotion: The major publication for this aspect of the industry is *Medical Marketing and Media.* Much candid and interesting content from its issues can be accessed through www.cpsnet.com. The broad menu of promotional services offered by the Grey Healthcare Group can be viewed at www.ghgroup.com.

306 *British Medical Journal* issue on drug promotion, May 31, 2003: Its contents are available free online at www.bmj.com. Of particular interest are the editorial and the paper by Lexchin analyzing the relationship between pharmaceutical company sponsorship of studies and the results they report.

306 The "No Free Lunch" site (www.nofreelunch.org) contains a comprehensive list of readings on the relationship between the drug industry and the medical profession, as well as a ready-to-use slide-lecture presentation on this topic. It also offers a "pen amnesty" program in which a free No Free Lunch ballpoint is offered to any health care worker in exchange for a pen or other bauble received from a drug manufacturer.

309 Some of the websites mentioned: www.WebMD.com; www.medicalletter. com; www.UpToDate.com; www.ePocrates.com. Information is also available at www.medlineplus.gov and www.micromedex.com.

310 Paradoxical counterproductivity: I. Illich, *Medical Nemesis* (New York: Random House, 1976).

310 Chronic stunning in heart failure: E. B. Braunwald and R. A. Kloner, "The Stunned Myocardium," *Circulation* 66 (1982): 1146–1149.

18: DEVISING AN ANTIDOTE

315 The government's agricultural extension service is still at work; its current activities are described at www.reeusda.gov.

318 The cocaine paper was published as J. Avorn, "The Role of Cocaine in Treating Intractable Pain in Terminal Disease," in R. Jeri, ed., *Cocaine: Proceedings of the Interamerican Seminar of Medical and Sociological Aspects of Coca and Cocaine* (Lima, Peru: Pan-American Health Organization, 1979), pp. 227–235.

325 Academic detailing: The first paper published on this topic was J. Avorn and S. B. Soumerai, "Improving Drug-Therapy Decisions Through Educational Outreach: A Randomized Controlled Trial of Academically Based 'Detailing,'" *New England Journal of Medicine* 308 (1983): 1457–1463. A follow-up paper defined the financial aspects of the process: S. B. Soumerai and J. Avorn, "Economic and Policy Analysis of University-Based Drug 'Detailing,'" *Medical Care* 24 (1986): 313–331. The work done by the team at Vanderbilt University can be found in W. Schaffner et al., "Improving Antibiotic Prescribing in Office Practice," *Journal of the American Medical Association* 250 (1983): 1728–1732. See also J. Avorn and S. B. Soumerai, "A New Approach to Reducing Sub-Optimal Drug Use" (editorial), *Journal of the American Medical Association* 250 (1983): 1752–1753. By 1990 there was so much interest in the practical aspects of how to run these programs that we published an expanded version of the original grant proposal I had written in 1979, laying out the rationale and methods of academic detailing. This appeared as S. B. Soumerai and J. Avorn, "Principles of Educational Outreach ('Academic Detailing') to Improve Clinical Decisionmaking," *Journal of the American Medical Association* 263 (1990): 549–556. The literature on academic detailing has now become large enough that the Cochrane Collaborative has established a systematic ongoing review of papers published on this topic: M. A. Thomson O'Brien et al., "Educational Outreach Visits: Effects on Professional Practice and Health Care Outcomes," in *Cochrane Library,* issue 3 (Oxford: Update Software, 2003). See www.cochrane.org/cochrane/revabstr/AB000409.htm. For a review of similar studies, see J. G. Cauffman et al., "Randomized Controlled Trials of Continuing Medical Education," *Journal of Continuing Education in the Health Professions* 22 (2002): 214–221.

328 Problematic drug use in nursing homes: M. Beers, J. Avorn, S. B. Soumerai, et al., "Psychoactive Medication Use in Intermediate-Care Facility Residents," *Journal of the American Medical Association* 260 (1988): 3016–3020.

329 Misuse of drugs in board-and-care facilities: J. Avorn, P. Dreyer, K. Connelly, et al., "Use of Psychoactive Medication and the Quality of Care in Rest Homes: Findings and Policy Implications of a State-Wide Study," *New England Journal of Medicine* 320 (1989): 227–232.

332 Outcomes of the "academic detailing" geriatrics project: J. Avorn et al., "A Randomized Trial of a Program to Reduce the Use of Psychoactive Drugs in Nursing Homes," *New England Journal of Medicine* 327 (1992): 168–173. See also D. E. Everitt, D. Fields, J. Avorn, et al., "Resident Behavior and Staff Distress in the Nursing Home," *Journal of the American Geriatrics Society* 39 (1991): 792–798. This work was supported by the John A. Hartford Foundation.

334 The Brigham division: Its website is www.drugepi.org. Some of the division's work is described in J. Avorn, "Balancing the Cost and Value of Medicines: The Dilemma Facing Clinicians," *Pharmacoeconomics* 20, supp. 3 (2002): 67–72.

337 Reducing excessive antibiotic use: see D. H. Solomon et al., "Academic Detailing to Improve Use of Broad-Spectrum Antibiotics at an Academic Medical Center," *Archives of Internal Medicine* 161 (2001): 1897–1902.

338 Dutch study of academic detailing: M. E. Van Eijk, J. Avorn, A. J. Porsius, et al., "Reducing Prescribing of Highly Anticholinergic Antidepressants for Elderly People: A Randomised Trial of Group Versus Individual Academic Detailing," *British Medical Journal* 322 (2001): 654–657.

338 Karl Popper: See the references to his work in the notes to Chapter 2.

19: THE EMPEROR'S FASHION CRITICS

343 I. Semmelweis, *The Cause, Concept, and Prophylaxis of Childbed Fever* (Madison: University of Wisconsin Press, 1893; orig. ed., 1861); K. S. Carter, S. Abbot, and J. L. Siebach, "Five Documents Relating to the Final Illness and Death of Ignatz Semmelweis," *Bulletin of the History of Medicine* 69 (1955): 255–270. The newest biography describes Semmelweis' downfall in engaging detail: S. B. Nuland, *The Doctor's Plague: Germs, Childbed Fever, and the Strange Story of Ignac Semmelweis* (New York: Norton, 2003).

344 The Boston contribution: O. W. Holmes, *The Contagiousness of Puerperal Fever*, Harvard Classics, vol. 38, part 5 (New York: Collier, 1910).

20: SAME LANGUAGE, DIFFERENT ACCENTS

349 Australia's cost-effectiveness requirement: Difficulties in the early stages of this program are described in S. R. Hill et al., "Problems with the Interpretation of Pharmacoeconomic Analyses," *Journal of the American Medical Association* 283 (2000): 2116–2121.

351 The website for the Australian National Prescribing Service contains a good description of the program as well as many useful educational materials about drugs: www.nps.org.au.

353 The British National Institute for Clinical Excellence (NICE) is at www. nice.org.uk. The decision-support software developed by the National Health

Service for that nation's practitioners can be accessed by anyone at www.prodigy. nhs.uk. It also contains useful material for patients about specific drugs and diseases. Two helpful sources of information about prescription and over-the-counter medications are also based in the United Kingdom but are available globally: the British National Formulary (www.bnf.org) and the Electronic Medicines Compendium, distributed through the Virtual Health Network (www.emc.vhn.net).

355 Canadian evaluations of drugs and other medical interventions can be found at the site maintained by the Canadian Coordinating Office for Health Technology Assessment: www.ccohta.ca. The University of British Columbia has been particularly active in this area. Its Centre for Health Services and Policy Research tracks work done in these fields across the entire country (www.chspr.ubc.ca), and its Therapeutics Initiative produces excellent materials on optimal drug use, as well as providing links to related sites: www.ti.ubc.ca. The province of Saskatchewan has a comprehensive provincewide academic detailing program that regularly disseminates and updates comparative information on drugs. The impressive materials it uses in its physician education programs are available free at www.rxfiles.ca. In Alberta, the Canadian Centre for Health Evidence publishes an internet-based *User's Guide to Evidence-Based Practice* for patients, practitioners, and policy makers at www.cche.net.

21: PULLING THE FACTS TOGETHER

360 E. O. Wilson, *Consilience: The Unity of Knowledge* (New York: Knopf, 1998).

366 The work of the Cochrane Collaborative can be found at www.cochrane.org and www.cochranelibrary.com.

366 Other programs that perform health care technology assessment: Some of these consider medications only peripherally, but their methods and output on other technologies provide a model of what this approach can accomplish. See, for example, www.ecri.org; www.icsi.org; www.bcbs.com/tec/; www.metawork.com; www.ahcpr.gov/clinic/epcix.htm; www.hayesinc.com.

366 Consumer Reports site: Go to www.crbestbuydrugs.org. The Oregon drug assessment initiative: Go to www.ohsu.edu/drugeffectiveness/.

370 R. Kuttner, *Everything for Sale: The Virtues and Limits of Markets* (New York: Knopf, 1998).

372 The work of Dr. Sidney Wolfe and colleagues at the Public Citizen Health Research Group can be found at www.citizen.org/hrg/.

381 A better way to assess new drugs: W. Ray, M. Griffin, and J. Avorn, "Evaluating Drugs After Approval for Clinical Use," *New England Journal of Medicine* 329 (1993): 2029–2032. See also A. J. Wood, C. M. Stein, and R. Woosley, "Making Medicines Safer—the Need for an Independent Drug Safety Board," *New England Journal of Medicine* 339 (1998): 1851–1854.

387 Efficacy of Lipitor: C. P. Cannon et al., "Intensive Versus Moderate Lipid Lowering with Statins After Acute Coronary Syndrome," *New England Journal of Medicine* 350 (2004): 1495–1504.

22: TURNING KNOWLEDGE INTO ACTION

393 Savings from more appropriate treatment of blood pressure: M. A. Fischer and J. Avorn, "Economic Implications of Evidence-Based Prescribing for Hypertension," *Journal of the American Medical Association* 291 (2004): 1850–1856.

397 Medical informatics as seen from the 1970s: J. Avorn, "The Future of Doctoring: Information Technology and Health Care Delivery," *Atlantic Monthly* 234 (1974): 71–79. For a more recent perspective, see D. W. Bates and A. A. Gawande, "Improving Drug Safety with Information Technology," *New England Journal of Medicine* 348 (2003): 2526–2534.

23: MARKETS AND MEDICINES

403 Standards for optimal medication use in older patients: E. L. Knight and J. Avorn, "Quality Indicators for Appropriate Medication Use in the Care of the Vulnerable Elderly," *Annals of Internal Medicine* 135 (2001): 703–710. This was one of several papers from the ACOVE project that were published in the October 16, 2001, issue of the *Annals.* Further information is at www.acponline.org/sci-policy/acove/. The project was supported by Pfizer, which provided unrestricted funding for the work but exercised no control over its content.

405 British Columbia policy reduces drug costs without clinical harm: S. Schneeweiss et al., "Outcomes of Reference Pricing for ACE Inhibitors," *New England Journal of Medicine* 346 (2002): 822–829. That study was funded by the U.S. Agency for Healthcare Research and Quality; Dr. Schneeweiss' ongoing policy research in British Columbia is also funded by the National Institute on Aging of NIH.

411 "Ideologically androgynous policy": The term is from Matthew Miller, *The Two Percent Solution: Fixing America's Problems in Ways Liberals and Conservatives Can Love* (New York: Public Affairs, 2003).

INDEX

Abenheim, Lucien, 78
academic detailing, 314–38, 349–52, 356, 390, 394
Accutane, 180
ACE-inhibitors, 41, 165, 236, 299
acetaminophen, 147, 295
acetylcholine, 127
acne, 150, 180, 238
Activated Protein C (APC), 173–5
adherence, poor, 284–5
adult learning theory, 320
advertising, drug, 282–3, 353; antidote to, 322–4, 330–1; direct-to-consumer, xvii, 288–91; in medical journals, 293; *see also* marketing, pharmaceutical
Advil, xvii, 127
ageism, 130–1
Agency for Health Care Policy and Research (AHCPAR), 277–8, 373
AIDS, 80, 180, 235, 264, 359, 382; in Africa, 241–2, 389; side effects of drugs for, 149
alcohol, 161
alendronate, 281
Aleve, xiv
alglucerase, 199
allergy medications, 116
ALLHAT randomized trial, 116, 264, 273
alternative medicine, 64–8

Alzheimer's disease, 91, 104, 121, 131; estrogen replacement and, 23, 27, 31, 33, 34; prevention of, 359; sedation of patients with, 127–8, 328, 332
American Association of Retired Persons (AARP), 287
American Heart Association, 33, 195
Aminorex, 73
amphetamine, 5, 96, 98
angina, 12, 47, 116, 150, 168, 169, 190, 335
angioplasty, 9, 10, 140, 143
Annals of Internal Medicine, 153–4, 271, 403
antianxiety drugs, 226
antibiotics, 62, 104, 173, 183; broad- versus narrow-spectrum, 336–7; drug interactions with, 116, 147; overprescription of, 44, 281, 319, 321–2, 345, 350, 397; *see also specific drugs*
anticholinergics, 129, 134–5
anticoagulants, 4, 41, 145–8, 182–3, 264, 281, 335, 414
antidepressants, ix–xiii, 42, 118–19, 136, 240, 282; *see also specific drugs*
antipsychotics, 41, 127–9, 135–7, 179, 183; overprescription to elderly of, 327, 328, 330

anxiety, 47
Archimedes, 36
Aristotle, 388
Arrowsmith (Lewis), 339
arthritis, 109, 122, 127, 140, 210, 236, 409; Cox-2 drugs for, 282; interactions of medications for, 147; placebo effect in, 47; in quality-adjusted life-year analysis, 152, 154; *see also* rheumatoid arthritis
Ashcroft, John, 93
aspirin, xvi, xvii, 40, 58, 64; drug interactions with, 147; effectiveness of Darvon compared with, 295, 297, 318, 319, 324; for heart attack prevention, 15, 41, 142, 282
Assessing Care of Vulnerable Elders (ACOVE), 403
asthma, 44, 47, 58, 62, 104, 181–2, 184, 195, 238
AstraZeneca, 278
atherosclerosis, 296
atorvastatin, 387
atrial fibrillation (AF), 4, 15–16, 41, 145–8, 183, 281, 335, 421n
Australia, 338, 348–52, 356; National Prescribing Service (NPS), 349, 351
Aventis, 278
average wholesale price (AWP), 209
Ayds, 96
Ayerst, 25, 28
AZT, 195

back pain, chronic, 277
bacteria, antibiotic-resistant, 44, 320, 336, 337, 345, 350
barbiturates, 44
Bates, David, 182, 398
Bathish, Joe, 77
BCR-ABL, 207, 208
Beaver Dam Outcomes Study, 153–4, 257
Beecher, Henry, 47
Beers, Mark, 328
behavioral economics, 156
Bellergal, 44

Bendectin, 120–2, 180, 425n
Benner, Josh, 285
Bentham, Jeremy, 259
Bernoulli, Daniel, 154
Berra, Yogi, 132
beta-blockers, 13, 41, 112, 116, 236, 298–9
Beth Israel Hospital (Boston), 90, 318
Bextra, xiv, xvi, xvii, xviii
Bible, 48–9, 60–1
birth control pills, 144–5, 156, 167
birth defects, 44, 102, 120–1, 180, 425n
Black Death, 51, 220
blood clots, 171, 335; birth control pills and, 144, 167; estrogen replacement and, 31, 34, 38, 167, 168, 273, 309
Blue Cross/Blue Shield, 204
Bohn, Rhonda, 115
Bok, Derek, 213
bone density tests, 414
bone marrow transplantation, 274–5
Boston Lying-In Hospital, 346–7
Braunwald, Eugene, 310–11
breast cancer, 28, 34, 38, 141, 157, 166–8, 273–5, 309
Brigham and Women's Hospital, 9, 79, 173, 175, 253, 263, 282, 347, 398; Division of Pharmacoepidemiology and Pharmacoeconomics, 333–7; Pharmacy and Therapeutics Committee, 92, 335–6
Bristol-Myers Squibb (BMS), 203, 226, 278
Britain, 348, 349, 356, 402; General Practitioner Research Database, 284; Medicines Control Agency, 92; National Formulary, 354; National Health Service (NHS), 157, 338, 352–4, 366; National Institute for Clinical Excellence (NICE), 353–5, 370, 434n
British Columbia, 405
British Medical Journal, 306, 366, 432n
bronchodilators, 44, 62, 190
Bush, George W., xix, xx, 244, 305, 380, 381

BuSpar, 226
Butler, Robert, 130, 131

caffeine, 98, 162
calcium-channel blockers (CCBs), 7,
116, 302, 382, 387; marketing of, 281,
289, 298; thiazide diuretics versus,
298–9, 393, 398
California, University of, at Los
Angeles, 395
Camus, Albert, 99, 323n
Canada, xix, xxi, 348, 354–6, 364, 375,
405; Centre for Health Evidence,
435n; Coordinating Office for
Health Technology Assessment
(CCOHTA), 355–6; reimportation of drugs from, 222–4, 291,
406
cancer, 46, 139, 140, 160, 167, 171,
263, 264, 311, 359; drugs for
treatment of, 80, 149, 203, 207–12,
226, 230, 235–7, 383; in elderly,
133; estrogen replacement and, 23,
27–9, 34, 157; evaluation of dietary
supplements for prevention of,
64; fatigue and weakness due to,
290; see also specific types of
cancer
cannabis, 161
Cannuscio, Carolyn, xv
cardiovascular disease, 139, 165–6,
190, 195; cholesterol-lowering
drugs and, 236, 237, 387; estrogen
replacement and, 23, 26–31, 33, 34,
36–8, 107, 167, 273, 309, 380;
obesity and, 74, 75, 81; phenylpropanolamine and, 97; testosterone and, 161, 171; see also
congestive heart failure; heart
attacks
case-control studies, 78, 100, 114
cataracts, 277, 278
Celebrex, xiv, xvi, xvii, xviii, 127, 201,
202, 282
Center for Science in the Public
Interest, 97

Centers for Disease Control and
Prevention (CDC), 373, 384
Centers for Education and Research in
Therapeutics (CERTs), 278–9
cephalexin, 318
Ceredase, 199
channeling, 117–19
chemotherapy: high dose, 274–5;
see also cancer, drugs for treatment of
childbed fever, 341–6
children, drug testing in, 133
Chiron, xix
chlorpromazine, 127
cholera, 105–6, 341
cholesterol, 104, 414; drugs for
lowering, 121–2, 157, 256, 262, 264,
236, 237, 288, 302, 382, 384, 387, 402;
elevated, 15, 62, 109, 311; estrogen
and, 26, 380; noncompliance and, 285
chronic myelogenous leukemia (CML),
207–8
chronobiology, 329–30
Churchill, Winston, 270
churn rate, 262
Ciba-Geigy, see Novartis
ciglitazone, 86
Clarinex, 225, 310
Claritin, 225
Clark, Roberta, 321
Clinical Evidence, 366
clinical trials, 376–80; funding of, 378;
mandate for, 377–8; methodology
for, 376–7; see also randomized
controlled trials
Clinton, Bill, 32, 223
Clinton, Hillary, 133, 380
clot-dissolving drugs, 9–10, 140, 143,
248–50, 263
clozapine, 179–80, 183
cocaine, 98
Cochrane Collaboration, 338, 366
Col, Nananda, 133
cold remedies, 5–6, 45, 96–101
colon: cancer of, 34, 167; ischemia of,
177, 179

Colowick, Alan, 263
Comtrex, 5
confounding by indication, 116–17
congestive heart failure, 15, 41, 58, 62, 150, 310–11, 398
Congress, U.S., 93, 214, 283, 361, 380, 381, 396; consumer information bill passed by, 286; extension of drug patents by, 133, 225; Office of Technology Assessment (OTA), 199, 276–7, 287; pharmaceutical industry and, 43–4, 200, 202; and reimportation of drugs from Canada, 223; supplement industry lobby and, 65
Connolly, Heidi, 82
Constitution, U.S., 55
Contac, 5, 96
contract research organizations, 384
control group, 54
copayments, 404–5
Coricidin, 5, 96
coronary artery disease, 116, 161, 335
coronary thrombosis, see heart attack
corporate welfare, 202–4
Corporation for Public Broadcasting, 367
cost-benefit analysis, 237–44; human-capital approach to, 239–42; willingness-to-pay approach to, 242–4
cost-effectiveness assessment, 150, 244–64, 274–6, 335, 380, 384–5, 389, 418; opposition to, 276–9
Coumadin, see warfarin
Cox-2 (coxibs), xiv–xviii, 201–2, 282
cross-sectional studies, 135
curare, 58, 64
Customs Service, U.S., 223
Cycloplasmol, 296, 323

Dalkon Shield, 424n
Dang Shen, 65
Dartmouth Medical School, 158
Darvon, 295, 297, 318, 319, 324
dead bowel syndrome, 8
decision analysis, 139–48; qualitative issues in, 149–60

decision-support software, 354
deep-vein thrombophlebitis, 144
Defense Department, U.S., 273
depression, 46, 118–19, 121, 235, 236, 321, 403, 414; in elderly, 319, 332; estrogen replacement and, 23, 27, 31, 33; herbal treatments for, 64; placebo effect in, 47; quality-adjusted life years and, 150; underdiagnosis and undertreatment of, 288, 311
Descartes, René, 123
detailers, 300–4
Dexatrim, 96
dexfenfluramine, 75–6, 80, 82
diabetes, 85, 98, 109, 147, 190, 195, 263, 264, 288; in elderly, 104; gender-based symptoms in, 168–9; hypertension and, 299; kidney failure in, 41; obesity and, 74, 75, 81, 82; in quality-adjusted life-year analysis, 154; Rezulin for, 86–95, 141, 164
dialysis, 8, 152
Dietary Supplement and Health Education Act (1994), 65, 66
Dietch, Marc, 83
diet drugs, 71–84, 164, 311; over-the-counter, 96, 99, 101
digitalis, 40
digoxin, 62, 64, 112, 190
Dimetapp, 5
discount rates, 157, 258
disintermediation, 408–9
Distant Mirror, A (Tuchman), 39
diuretics, 62, 193; see also thiazides
DNA, 202
Doctor's Dilemma, The (Shaw), 339
Dole, Bob, 288
dopamine, 127–9
double-blind studies, 54
Drazen, Jeff, xiv
dropsy, 58
drotrecogin alfa activated, see Activated Protein C
drug assessment: funding of, 374–5; information synthesis for, 363–6; mandate for, 372–4;

marketplace approach to, 368–70; methodology for, 375–6; organizational structures for, 366–8; risk data in, 370–2; *see also* cost-effectiveness assessment

Drug Enforcement Agency (DEA), 223, 279

drug interactions: with antibiotics, 117, 147; with supplements and herbal remedies, 66; with Viagra, 169–70

Druker, Brian, 208

Dylan, Bob, 106

dyspepsia, 47

Dzau, Victor, 334

Eastman, Richard, 90

echinacea, 65–6

educational outreach, 390–6; to patients, 396–7; *see also* academic detailing

educational theory, 316, 320

Einstein, Albert, 264

Eisenhower, Dwight, 215–16

elderly, 104, 126–38, 311, 398; guidelines for drug use in, 403; national health insurance for, *see* Medicare; oversedation of, 326–33; prescription of useless drugs to, 295–6, 319, 323

Electronic Data Gathering, Analysis and Retrieval (EDGAR), 206

Eleven Blue Men (Roueche), 123

Elizabeth I, Queen of England, 313

emphysema, 152, 190

end-stage disease, 122

endometrial cancer, 27

endorphins, 47

Enemy of the People, An (Ibsen), 340–1

Enlightenment, 50

Environmental Protection Agency (EPA), 244

ephedrine, 58, 98

ePocrates, 310

erectile dysfunction, 86, 153–4, 159, 202, 257, 288; diabetes and, 169–70

erysipelas, 345

estrogen replacement, 23–40, 68, 111, 125, 128, 170–1, 387; blood clots and, 31, 34, 38, 167, 168, 273, 309; cancer and, 23, 27–9, 34, 157; cardiovascular disease and, 23, 26–31, 33, 34, 36–8, 107, 166–8, 273, 309, 380; combined with tranquilizers, 44; HERS study of, 31–5; internet sources on, 308–9, 354; stroke and, 23, 26, 33, 38, 167, 168, 273, 309

Everything for Sale (Kuttner), 370

evidence-based medicine, 316

exercise, prescribing, 323–4

existentialism, 63, 99, 333

expected utility theory, 246

Families USA, 206

Farmer, Richard, 156

Faust, 142, 157

Federal Aviation Agency (FAA), 373

Federal Trade Commission (FTC), 225–6

Fein, Rashi, 241

Feldene, 127

Feminine Forever (Wilson), 25–6

fenfluramine, 73–6, 78–84, 164; *see also* fen-phen

fen-phen, 74–6, 77–80, 99

fetal abnormalities, *see* birth defects

Fischer, Michael, 173, 393

Fleming, Alexander, 339

flu shot, xix

Food and Drug Administration (FDA), 6, 14, 17, 49, 71–3, 162, 353, 355, 371–6, 406; adverse drug event surveillance by, 104–5, 110–11, 371–3, 374–5; Advisory Committee on Endocrinologic and Metabolic Drugs, 92; Advisory Committee on Gastrointestinal Drugs, 177–9; age guidelines for clinical test subjects of, 133–4; alternative approval approach for, 380–86; and cancer-drug research, 203, 207, 211; decision analysis in, 140, 142; drug advertising standards of, 26, 282–3, 288; Drug Efficacy Study Implementation

Food and Drug Administration (FDA)
(*continued*)
(DESI), 45, 96–7, 296, 386;
effectiveness requirement of, 52,
59–61, 63, 108–9, 236, 249, 273, 279,
299, 314; and estrogen replacement,
28–31, 34–5, 309; Kefauver Act
changes in, 44; labeling requirements
of, 164, 165, 286–7; medical device
industry and, 42; underestimation of
risks by drug companies to, 73–8,
82–5, 87–9, 92–4; new drug applications (NDAs) submitted to, 204, 205;
reimportation of drugs from Canada
opposed by, 223–4, 291; risk management approach of, 172–6, 179–81,
373; and safety of grandfathered
over-the-counter drugs, 96–101, 120;
supplements excluded from regulatory control of, 64–6, 68, 265–6;
tobacco and, 160, 162, 171
Fortune 500 companies, 227
Fortune magazine, 297
Fosamax, 281
Frist, Bill, 381
Fuchs, Victor, 236

Gale, Edwin, 94–5
Galen, 26, 42, 52, 56, 65, 317
gallbladder disease, 31, 34
game theory, 141
Gaucher's disease, 199, 260
Genentech, 248–52
General Accounting Office (GAO),
203, 209
General Electric, 221
General Motors, 221
generic drugs, 7, 290, 299
germ theory of disease, 341–2, 343–4
ginseng, 65, 66
glaucoma, 62, 109, 117–18, 262, 414
GlaxoSmithKline, xii, 278, 302
Glaxo-Wellcome, 88–90, 178, 179, 180
Gleevec, 207–9
Gluck, Michael, 200
Glynn, Robert, 121

Goethe, Johann Wolfgang von, 142, 265
Gold, Arnold, xxi
Gold, Sandra, xxi
Gottlieb, Gary, 334
Gounod, Charles, 142
graft-versus-host disease, 275
Graham, David, xviii, 91
Great Depression, 129
Greeks, ancient, 124
Gresham's law, 313–14, 319
Grey Healthcare Group, 305
Griffin, Marie, 381
Gurwitz, Jerry, 133, 182
GUSTO study, 250–6, 430*n*

Haldol (haloperidol), 126, 127, 129,
136, 137, 327, 331
Hartford, John A., Foundation, 330
Harvard University, 194, 213, 360, 364;
Business School, 321; Dana-Farber
Cancer Institute, 208; Medical
School, 18, 40, 47, 79, 118, 123, 126,
158, 191, 272, 280, 294, 316, 318,
346, 347, 360 (*see also* Brigham and
Women's Hospital); School of Public
Health, 318, 430*n*
Harvey, Ken, 349–50
Hassan, Fred, 77
Hatch, Orrin, 64–5
headaches, 47; migraine, 104
Health and Human Services (HHS),
U.S. Department of, 90, 205, 206,
221, 223–4, 287, 373, 429*n*
Health Care Financing Administration,
195
Health Research Group, 207, 287, 372
Heart and Estrogen-progestin
Replacement Study (HERS), 31–5
heart attacks, 8, 62, 108, 116, 146, 157,
166, 202, 218, 242, 298–9, 345;
aspirin for prevention, 15, 41, 142,
282; clot-busting drugs for, 9–10, 143;
cholesterol and, 62, 236, 281;
diabetes and, 168–70; estrogen
replacement and, 166–8; in elderly,
133; GUSTO study of drugs for,

251–4; smoking and, 241; *see also* cardiovascular disease
heart valve abnormalities, 82, 111
hemophilia, 262–3
heparin, 335
hepatitis, 104, 109, 113
herbal supplements, 64–7, 366
high blood pressure, *see* hypertension
Hillel, Rabbi, 417
hip fractures, 167, 218, 262; oversedation and, 329
histamine blockers, 236
Holmes, Oliver Wendell, Sr., 40, 344–7
hormone replacement therapy (HRT), *see* estrogen replacement
Horwitz, Ralph, 100
Houghton, Amo, 277
House of Representatives, U.S., 6, 200, 225
Hughes, Howard, Medical Institute, 195, 207–8
human-capital approach, 239–42
Human Genome Project, 230
hypertension, 6–9, 11–15, 109, 116, 183, 273, 321, 382, 387, 398, 409, 414; congestive heart failure and, 310–11; cost-effectiveness assessment of drugs for, 256, 260, 262; as drug side effect, 97, 202; in elderly, 62, 190; labeling requirements for drugs for, 165–6; marketing of drugs for, 7, 11–13, 281, 298–9, 302, 304, 393; mild to moderate, 235, 236; noncompliance and, 285; obesity and, 74, 81, 82; patient education on, 397; in quality-adjusted life-year analysis, 154; pulmonary, 74–9, 81–8; stroke and, 8–9; undertreatment of, 288, 289, 311
hypogonadism, 171
hysterectomy, 27–8

Ibsen, Henrik, 340–1
ibuprofen, xvi, xvii, 127, 200, 201, 282, 295
idiopathic diseases, 128

Illich, Ivan, 310
immunosuppressive drugs, 262
impersistence, 284–5
impotence, *see* erectile dysfunction
IMS America, 294
incontinence, 27, 33, 131, 159, 288
incrementally modified drugs (IMDs), 204
inflammatory bowel disease, 359
information: existing, pulling together, 363–6; failure to apply, 281–2; for patients, 285–8; inadequacy of, 273–4; internet sources of, 308–10; promotional, *see* advertising; marketing; systems for transfer of, 389–400
informed consent, 162–3
insomnia, 47
insulin, 86–7, 92, 190, 195, 241, 409
International Society for Pharmaco-Epidemiology, 103
Introduction to the Principles of Morals and Legislation (Bentham), 259
irritable bowel syndrome (IBS), 176–80
isotretinoin, 180

Janssen, 278
Joint Commission on Accreditation of Healthcare Organizations, 395
Journal of the American Medical Association (JAMA), 12, 31, 65, 79, 116, 270–1, 308, 309, 328

Kabi, 250
Kahneman, Daniel, 154, 155
Kalish, Susan, 250
Kaufman, Ewing Marion, 297
kava kava, 66
Kefauver, Estes, 43–5
Keflex, 318–20, 322, 324
Kelsey, Frances, 43–4
Kessler, David, 64, 162
kidney disease, 8, 152, 299
Knight, Eric, 285, 298, 403
Kuttner, Robert, 370

labeling, 164–5
Lancet, xiii, 47, 94, 97, 271, 387
Larimer, David, 201
last case bias, 145
L-dopa, 129, 137
learning theory, 320
Lederle, 278
LeLorier, Jacques, 72, 285
leprosy, 180
leukemia, 104, 207–8
Leukemia and Lymphoma Society of America, 208
leukotriene inhibitors, 184
Levine sign, 9
Lewis, Richard, 80, 83
Lewis, Sinclair, 339
Lilly, 173
Lind, James, 50–1
Linnen, Mary, 78–9
Lipitor, 289, 387
Lister, Joseph, 50
Los Angeles Times, 77, 90
Lotronex, 176–80, 184
lung cancer, 150, 241
Lutwak, Leo, 77
lymphoma, 104, 184

Maclure, Malcolm, 364
malaria, 51
Marax, 44
Marion Laboratories, 296–7
marketing, 281, 292–312, 393; antidote to, 314–38; of expensive drugs, 298–9; by medical communications companies, 307–8; public relations and, 305–6; by sales representatives, 300–4; of unsafe drugs, 87–8; of useless drugs, 294–7; *see also* advertising
Massachusetts: Board of Registration in Medicine, 280–1; Department of Public Health, 330
Massachusetts Institute of Technology (MIT), 75
Massengill Massacre, 43
May, Frank, 350
Mayo Clinic, 82, 83

Medicaid, 6, 203, 273, 320, 391, 403; as data source, 111, 112, 189, 298, 325, 375, 385, 386; nursing homes and, 327; passage of, 231; prescription drug coverage under, 7, 8, 189–97, 217–18, 222, 232, 285, 316
medical communications companies, 307–8
medical education, 134, 271–2, 389–91; *see also* academic detailing
Medical Letter, 309–10
Medical Nemesis (Illich), 310
Medicare, xx, 130, 132, 192, 193, 262, 273; cutbacks in, 79, 212; chemotherapy reimbursements by, 203, 209, 211; as data source, 111, 112, 385, 386; fixed payments to hospitals under, 249; passage of, 231, 235; prescription drug coverage under, 218–19, 245, 380, 410–11
Medicine Equity and Drug Safety Act (2000), 223
Medline, 270
Mellaril, 127
Mencken, H. L., 339, 401
menopause, 150; treatment of, *see* estrogen replacement
menstrual symptoms, 47
Merck, xiv, xv–xviii, 201, 202, 278, 302, 328
miasma, 105, 341, 342
migraine, 104
minoxidil, 86
Misbin, Robert, 92–3
Monane, Mark, 285, 298
Monistat-7, 292
monoclonal antibodies, 184
Moody's, 368–9
Morgenstern, Oskar, 246
morphine, 40, 44, 47–8, 58, 64, 240, 259, 295
Morris, Charles, 65
Mosholder, Andy, xii
Motrin, xvi, xvii, 200, 282, 295, 324
Mulley, Al, 158
multiple sclerosis, 104
Muris, Timothy, 225–6

Nader, Ralph, 213, 372
naloxone, 47
National Academy of Sciences, 386;
    Institute of Medicine of, 374
National Cancer Institute, 133, 208
National Center for Health Care
    Technology Assessment, 276
National Center for Health Services
    Research, 194, 316
National Committee on Quality
    Assessment, 395
National Endowment for the Arts, 367
National Institute for Health Care
    Management (NIHCM), 204
National Institutes of Health (NIH), 10,
    30–1, 34, 52, 198, 202, 212, 215, 277,
    318, 373, 384; Division of Diabetes,
    Endocrine, and Metabolic Diseases,
    90–1; National Eye Institute, 54;
    National Institute on Aging, 130;
    pharmaceutical companies and,
    199–200, 203, 226, 407; "Science of
    Placebo" interdisciplinary grant
    program of, 48; Women's Health
    Initiative (WHI), 31–4, 273, 309
National Library of Medicine, 270
National Pharmaceutical Council,
    194–5
National Transportation Safety Board,
    373
Nature, 90
Netherlands, 338
neuroleptics, 127
neurotransmitters, 58, 118, 127–9
new drug applications (NDAs), 204
New England Journal of Medicine, 6,
    12, 56, 78, 83, 100, 174, 194, 195,
    249, 270, 325, 333, 381, 405
new molecular entities (NMEs),
    204
Newton, Isaac, 53, 57–8
New Yorker, The, 123
New York magazine, 240
Nexium, 225, 310, 353
nicotine, 162
nitrates, 190
nitroglycerine, 169–70

nocebo response, 53
noncompliance, 284–5, 414
Norplant, 424*n*
Norvasc, 387
Novartis, 207, 208
null hypothesis, 55
nursing home residents, 104;
    overprescription of sedatives to,
    326–33
nutritional deficiencies, 50–1

Oakar, Mary, 99
obesity, 74, 75, 81–3
observational studies, 102–25, 417–18;
    bias and erroneous conclusions in,
    111–22; computer models for,
    111–14; experimental research
    versus, 106–11
Office of Management and Budget
    (OMB), 244
Office of Technology Assessment
    (OTA), 276–7
olanzapine, 127, 209, 281
oncology, medical, *see* cancer, drugs for
    treatment of
opiates, 47, 62; *see also* morphine
oral contraceptives, *see* birth control
    pills
order-entry system, computer-based,
    334–5, 398–9
Oregon, drug assessment program in,
    364
Organization for Economic Co-
    operation and Development
    (OECD), 220
osteoporosis, 28, 41, 62, 262, 281;
    patient education on, 397; *see also*
    hip fractures
over-the-counter drugs, 96, 99, 101,
    209; *see also specific drugs*
OxyContin, 295

package inserts, 164–5
pain medications, 200–1, 236; *see also*
    opiates; *specific drugs*
Pan American Health Organization
    (PAHO), 318

Paracelsus, 72, 230, 401
Parke-Davis, 87–93
parkinsonism, 126, 128–9, 135–7, 330
Pasteur, Louis, 132, 339
Pasteurella pestis, 51, 52
Patent and Trademark Office, 226
patents, 201–2, 224–6, 299, 405–6
patients' rights, 162
Pavabid, 44
Paxil, ix, xii, xiii
penicillin, 32, 46, 318, 368
Pfizer, 169, 202, 278, 302, 387
Pharmacia, 201, 202, 278
pharmacogenetics, 183–4
phentermine, 74, 80; *see also* fen-phen
phenylpropanolamine (PPA), 5–6, 45,
    96–101, 114, 119–20, 141
Physicians' Desk Reference (PDR),
    163–4, 170, 363
Pinel, Philippe, 329
placebo effect, 47–8, 53
plague, 39, 51–2, 54, 56–7, 59, 220
Platinol, 226
pneumonia, 46, 263
Pondimin, 73–6, 80, 81, 83, 85
Popper, Karl, 54, 338, 340, 347
Posicor, 11–14
pragmatic clinical trials, 377
pregnancy, 144–5; drugs taken during,
    43–4, 102, 120–1, 180
Premarin, 23–6, 30, 73
Prempro, 23, 28, 168
prescription benefit management
    companies (PBMs), 392–3, 395
prescription drug prices, 217–34; future
    of, 231–3; globalization and, 406–7;
    information on, 396; in other
    countries, 220–2; patents and, 224–6,
    299, 405–6; patient awareness of,
    403–5; reimportation and, 222–4,
    291; as social and political construct,
    226–7
Prescription Drug User Fee Act
    (PDUFA), 93, 374
Prilosec, xvii, 209, 225, 236, 281, 353
Procrit, 290

progestin, 27, 28
Progressive movement, 43, 374, 407
promotional information, 282–3
propoxyphene, *see* Darvon
prostaglandins, 200–1
prostate disease, 64, 159, 277; cancer, 161
proton pump inhibitors (PPIs), 236,
    353–4
protopathic bias, 119–20
PROWESS (PROtein C Worldwide
    Evaluation in Severe Sepsis), 173–5
Prozac, ix, xiii, 118–19, 236, 289, 311
pseudoephedrine, 6, 99, 101
psychology of risk assessment, 141
public relations, 305–6
puerperal fever, 341–6
pulmonary embolus, 144
pulmonary hypertension, 74–9, 81–4
Pure Food and Drug Act (1906), 43, 231
p-value, 59

quality-adjusted life-year (QALY)
    analysis, 150–5, 247, 255–7, 260
quantum mechanics, 57
quinine, 51, 64

Raiffa, Howard, 144
RAND Corporation, 403
randomized controlled trials (RCTs),
    53–7, 120, 376, 417; of anticoagu-
    lants, 146; of antihypertensive drugs,
    116; of birth control pills, 144; of
    cholesterol-lowering drugs, 122, 387;
    of de-marketing, 316–25; observa-
    tional studies and, 107–9, 115, 122–3
Ray, Wayne, 381
Reagan, Ronald, 191, 287
recall bias, 120–21
Redux, 75–8, 80, 81, 83–5, 101, 111,
    141, 164
regulations, inadequacy of, 279–81
reimportation of drugs, 222–4, 291
renal failure, 150, 152
Republican Party, 277
research and development (R&D),
    funding of, 198–216, 310, 407

retinopathy, diabetic, 168
Rezulin, 86–95, 99, 101, 141, 164, 165, 179, 180, 368
rheumatoid arthritis, 104, 181–2, 184, 359
risk-benefit decisions, *see* decision analysis
risk management, 175–81, 370–3; new technologies and, 183–5; over time, 181–2; systems approach to, 182–83
risks, communication of, 162–71; information sources and, 163–4; informed consent and, 162–3; language barriers in, 164–7
risk stratification, 174–5
Risperdal, 127
risperidone, 127
Ritalin, 162
Roche, 180, 278
Rochester, University of, 200–1
Rogaine, 86
Romans, ancient, 124
Roueche, Berton, 123
Royal College of Physicians, Edinburgh, 50–1

Saint-John's-wort, 64
sales representatives, drug-company, 300–4, 320, 324–6
Salk, Jonas, 339
sawgrass palmetto, 64
schizophrenia, 41, 127–8, 136, 139–40, 145, 150, 179, 359
Schneeweiss, Sebastian, 405
Science, 47
scurvy, 50–1
Securities and Exchange Commission (SEC), 206, 429*n*
selective serotonin reuptake inhibitors (SSRIs), 118–19, 236
selenium, 64
Semmelweis, Ignaz, 341–4, 346, 347
Senate, U.S., 6, 200, 219, 225
septic shock, 173–5, 333, 343
Shalala, Donna, 223
Shaw, George Bernard, 248, 339

signal transduction, 269–70, 275, 310
Silagy, Chris, 350
sleeping pills, 311, 327–30
smallpox vaccine, 140
Smith, Adam, 156
Snow, John, 105–6, 341
Social Security, 212
Solomon, Dan, xiv, xv, 281–2, 337
Sorcerer's Apprentice, The, 271
sore throats, 409; antibiotics prescribed for, 44
Soumerai, Steve, 189, 192–4, 318, 324, 325
Spitzer, Eliot, xii
Standard & Poor's, 368–9
steroids: inhaled, 104, 184, 190, 195; oral, 181–2
stimulants, 162
streptokinase, 248–53, 255, 256
streptomycin, 44
stroke, 3–16, 150, 161, 218, 311, 345; anticoagulants to prevent, 4, 41, 146–8, 421*n*; cholesterol and, 62, 281; clot-dissolving drugs and, 9–10, 143, 252, 254; in elderly, 133; estrogen replacement and, 23, 26, 33, 38, 167, 168, 273, 309; hypertension and, 6–9, 298–9, 398; phenylpropanolamine and, 5–6, 45, 97–101, 114, 119–20, 141
Sudafed, 6, 99
sulfanilamide, 43
Sullivan, Louis, 214
supplements, 64–7, 283, 366
surgery, informed consent for, 163
syphilis, 32, 162

tachyphylaxis, 98
tacrine, 91
tamoxifen, 141–2
Taxol, 64, 203, 226
testosterone, 125, 160–1, 171
thalidomide, 43–4, 180
Theory of Games and Economic Behavior (von Neumann and Morgenstern), 246

thiazides, 7, 13, 264, 273, 289, 298–9, 393, 398
Thinz, 96
thioridazine, 127
Thompson, Tommy, xxi, 224
Thorazine, 127
thrombolytic drugs, *see* clot-dissolving drugs
thrombophlebitis, 144
thyroid disease, 319
TNF inhibitors, 184
tobacco, 161, 162, 171, 241
tPA, 248–56
tranquilizers, 44, 136, 226, 238, 311; major, *see* antipsychotics; over-prescription to elderly of, 326–33
Triaminic, 96
troglitazone, *see* Rezulin
tuberculosis, 119
Tuchman, Barbara, 39, 51, 220
Tuskegee experiment, 32–4, 162
Tversky, Amos, 154, 155
Tylenol, 147, 295, 318, 319

ulcers, 200, 236
United Health Group, 366
United Kingdom, *see* Britain
United Nations Global Burden of Disease program, 242
UpToDate, 310
urinary tract infection, 321, 409
uterus, cancer of, 141–2
utilitarianism, 259–60

vaccines, 140, 141, 224, 237, 264
vaginitis, 292, 305
vasodilators, cerebral and peripheral, 295–7, 318, 319, 322, 323
Veterans Administration (VA), 30, 375, 385, 390, 392, 399, 402
Veterans Affairs, U.S. Department of, 273
Viagra, 86, 140, 169–71, 202, 257, 288, 409
Victoria, University of, 364

Vioxx, xiv–xviii, 201, 202, 281
Virchow, Rudolf, xx
vitamin B_{12} deficiency, 319
vitamins, 50–1, 64
Voltaire, 41
von Neumann, John, 246

Wang, Phil, 282
warfarin, 145–8, 182–3, 281, 421*n*
watchful waiting, 159
watershed infarct, 14
Waxman, Henry, 93
WebMD, 309, 354
weight loss, 71–84
Weil, Andrew, 318
Wennberg, Jack, 158
willingness to pay, 242–4
Willman, David, 90
Wilson, E. O., 360
Wilson, Fred, 74–5
Wilson, Robert, 25–6
Winkelmayer, Wolfgang, 256
Wisconsin Alumni Research Foundation, 182
Withering, William, 3
Witte, Owen, 207–8
Wolfe, Sidney, 287, 372
Wood, Alistair, 381
World War II, 47, 129, 276
Worst Pills, Best Pills (Wolfe), 372
Wyden, Ron, 9, 203
Wyeth, 25, 26, 28, 34–5, 73, 75–7, 83–4, 278, 320, 424*n*

Xigris, *see* Activated Protein C

Yale Medical School, 6, 100, 114
Yeats, William Butler, 314
yin and yang, 106–7, 124–5
Young, Donald, 200

Zantac, xvii, 236
Zerhouni, Elias, 203
Zoloft, ix, xii, xiii, 288
Zyprexa, 127

EATING IN THE DARK
America's Experiment with Genetically Engineered Food
by Kathleen Hart

Most Americans eat genetically modified food on a daily basis, but few are aware of it. Kathleen Hart explores biotechnology's real potential to enhance nutrition and cut farming expenses. She also reveals how American government agencies decided not to label genetically modified food and not to require biotech companies to perform even basic safety tests on their products.

Science/Current Affairs/0-375-72498-2

PLAGUE TIME
The New Germ Theory of Disease
by Paul W. Ewald

Conventional wisdom claims that genes and lifestyles are the most important causes of the deadly ailments of our time, but in this controversial book, the eminent biologist Paul W. Ewald offers some revolutionary arguments. Germs appear to be at the root of heart disease, Alzheimer's, schizophrenia, and many forms of cancer, but the medical establishment has so far ignored the evidence that implicates these germs—to the detriment of our public health.

Health/Medicine/0-385-72184-6

WHY WE GET SICK
The New Science of Darwinian Medicine
by Randolph M. Nesse, M.D. and George C. Williams, Ph.D.

In this groundbreaking book, two pioneers of the emerging science of Darwinian medicine argue that illness as well as factors that predispose us to it are subject to the laws of natural selection. Deftly summarizing the latest research on maladies ranging from cancer to Huntington's chorea, *Why We Get Sick* fundamentally alters our attitudes toward illness and will intrigue laypersons and medical practitioners alike.

Science/Medicine/0-679-74674-9

VINTAGE AND ANCHOR BOOKS
Available from your local bookstore, or call toll-free to order:
1-800-793-2665 (credit cards only).